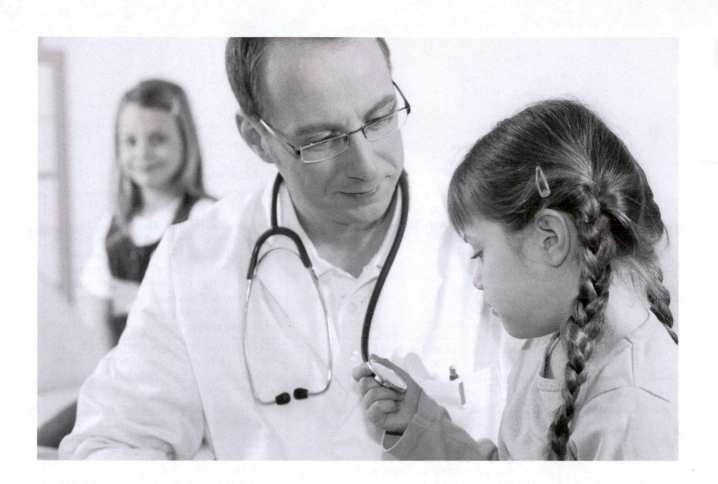

BMJ Clinical Review:

Paediatrics

Edited by
Babita Jyoti & Rebecca Saunders

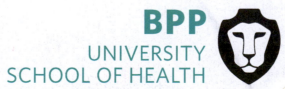

BPP
UNIVERSITY
SCHOOL OF HEALTH

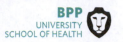

First edition July 2015

ISBN 9781 4727 3934 6
eISBN 9781 4727 4403 6
eISBN 9781 4727 4411 1

British Library Cataloguing-in-Publication Data
A catalogue record for this book is available
from the British Library

Published by
BPP Learning Media Ltd
BPP House, Aldine Place
London W12 8AA

www.bpp.com/health

Printed in the United Kingdom by
CPI Antony Rowe

Bumper's Farm
Chippenham
Wiltshire
SN14 6LH

Your learning materials, published by BPP Learning
Media Ltd, are printed on paper sourced from
sustainable, managed forests.

The content of this publication contains articles from The
BMJ which have been selected, collated and published
by BPP Learning Media under a licence.

The contents of this book are intended as a guide
and not professional advice. Although every effort
has been made to ensure that the contents of this
book are correct at the time of going to press, BPP
Learning Media, the Editor and the Author make no
warranty that the information in this book is accurate
or complete and accept no liability for any loss or
damage suffered by any person acting or refraining
from acting as a result of the material in this book.

Every effort has been made to contact the copyright
holders of any material reproduced within this
publication. If any have been inadvertently overlooked,
BPP Learning Media will be pleased to make the
appropriate credits in any subsequent reprints or
editions.

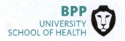

About the publisher

BPP Learning Media is dedicated to supporting aspiring professionals with top quality learning material. BPP Learning Media's commitment to success is shown by our record of quality, innovation and market leadership in paper-based and e-learning materials. BPP Learning Media's study materials are written by professionally-qualified specialists who know from personal experience the importance of top quality materials for success.

About The BMJ

The BMJ (formerly the British Medical Journal) in print has a long history and has been published without interruption since 1840. The BMJ's vision is to be the world's most influential and widely read medical journal. Our mission is to lead the debate on health and to engage, inform, and stimulate doctors, researchers, and other health professionals in ways that will improve outcomes for patients. We aim to help doctors to make better decisions. BMJ, the company, advances healthcare worldwide by sharing knowledge and expertise to improve experiences, outcomes and value.

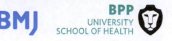

Contents

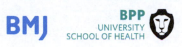

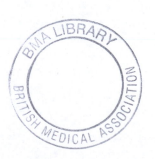

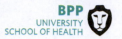

About the editors

Dr Babita Jyoti is a Radiation Oncologist with a special interest in Paediatric Proton Therapy. She graduated in Medicine in India followed by training in UK and obtained MRCP (UK) & FRCR (UK). She trained as a Clinical Oncologist at Clatterbridge Cancer Centre. She is currently working at the University of Florida Health Proton Therapy Institute in Paediatric Proton Therapy. She has been a PBL tutor and an OSCE examiner at Manchester Medical School.

Miss Rebecca Saunders is a Specialty Trainee in General Surgery working in the Mersey deanery. She graduated from the University of Manchester in 2009 and after foundation years started her surgical training. She became a Member of the Royal College of Surgeons of Edinburgh in 2012.

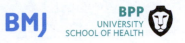

Introduction to Paediatrics

BMJ Clinical Review: Paediatrics is an up to date collection of review articles first published in the BMJ. It has been compiled as a helpful, concise review of topics frequently encountered by GPs, Paediatricians and Emergency physicians around the world.

BMJ Clinical Review articles are written by experienced clinicians and aimed at non-specialist hospital doctors, trainees and candidates preparing for post-graduate examinations. Each article offers a broad update of developments and expected applications in primary and secondary care. By reviewing recent good quality evidence the articles give an evidence-based understanding of the area. Suggestions are made for further reading and highlight important articles in that field. The authors give advice for non-specialists, including when to refer the patient to secondary care and details of the treatment they would expect to receive.

An emphasis on patient partnership has lead to many articles including a section *How patients were involved in the creation of this article as well* as information on how the condition affects quality of life and what information and resources are useful for patients and families.

We have carefully selected and collated the most relevant reviews on frequently encountered and important topics that will help clinicians in their everyday practice.

Articles included cover a wide range of subjects; from nutrition, common developmental, gastroenterology and respiratory problems to oncological and mental health conditions. This book will give readers a comprehensive and up to date overview of common Paediatric conditions.

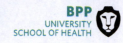

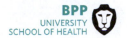

The extremely premature neonate: anticipating and managing care

Natalie K Yeaney consultant in neonatology[1], Edile M Murdoch consultant in neonatology[1], Christoph C Lees consultant in obstetrics and fetal-maternal medicine[2]

[1]Department of Neonatology, Addenbrooke's Hospital, Cambridge University Hospitals NHS Foundation Trust, Cambridge CB2 2QQ

[2]Department of Fetal-Maternal Medicine, Addenbrooke's Hospital

Correspondence to: C Lees christoph. lees@addenbrookes.nhs.uk

Cite this as: *BMJ* 2009;338:b2325

‹DOI› 10.1136/bmj.b2325
http://www.bmj.com/content/338/bmj.b2325

Preterm deliveries are increasing in absolute numbers and as a proportion of all births. According to NHS data for England in 2006, 2000 births—0.3% of all births—were extremely preterm (23-25+6 weeks' gestation).[1] Similar numbers are reported by other western European countries. Preterm births have increased by 20% over the past two decades in the United States, mainly because of the 42% increase in twin births.[2] Advances in neonatal intensive care for babies born at the margins of viability have improved survival, but these infants are more likely to have long term morbidities and to use healthcare resources extensively in the first 2 years of life. Data from the Neonatal Research Network show that babies born before 26 weeks' gestation spend at least 111 days in hospital during infancy and incur intensive care costs of more than £100 000 (€114 000; $160 000).[3] An emotional and financial burden is often placed on families and community support systems. One or more family member may leave paid work to care for the baby, or skilled day care providers may help care for a child with serious ongoing medical conditions.[4]

Disability is highest in extremely preterm infants, but the numbers of children with disability and the implications for public health and social care are greatest in children born moderately prematurely.[5] Although extremely premature infants are cared for perinatally as inpatients, any clinician who deals with pregnant women could benefit from an awareness of advances in care and the evidence that underpins best practices to advise, refer, and support women who are at risk of or have had an extremely preterm delivery.

Why are babies born extremely preterm?

This may occur because of spontaneous preterm vaginal delivery, when planned delivery before 26 completed weeks is the safest option for delivering the baby alive (almost never carried out before 24 weeks), or when planned early delivery is necessary because of maternal illness. Complications that can cause spontaneous preterm delivery include rupture of membranes, chorioamnionitis, placental abruption, polyhydramnios, and multiple pregnancy. Reasons for an intended delivery include fetal distress, severe pre-eclampsia, acute or chronic maternal conditions such as renal disease, decompensation of congenital heart disease, or connective tissue disorders. Severe early onset fetal growth restriction at 24-26 weeks does not normally lead to intended delivery because the outcome of growth restricted premature babies less than 450 g is poor.[6] The box lists antenatal interventions that might reduce premature birth (box).

Why has survival improved for these infants?

The administration of maternal antenatal corticosteroids has become standard practice—a systematic review and large cohort study have shown that this is associated with increased survival in moderately preterm and extremely preterm infants.[7] Improvements within organised neonatal and perinatal networks for predelivery (in utero) transfer enable the fetus to be delivered at a specialist centre with appropriate resources and staffing and thereby avoid the complications that attend transfer of a preterm neonate.[8]

Events in the first hours after birth affect neonatal mortality and morbidity. Many units give surfactant routinely to extremely preterm infants in the first moments of life. Maintaining normothermia, controlling acid-base status, and rapidly obtaining intravenous access to prevent hypoglycaemia by infusing glucose are also important. Neonatal care has become less invasive for the baby and aims to limit central blood pressure monitoring. Ventilator strategies have changed, with increased use of non-invasive continuous positive airway pressure and the acceptance of relatively higher concentrations of carbon dioxide (hypercapnia), in an effort to reduce barotrauma. High oxygen saturation (hyperoxia) is avoided in an effort to reduce lung inflammation from oxygen toxicity. Other contributions include improved neonatal nutritional practices and curtailment of the use of corticosteroids postnatally. A randomised trial has shown that caffeine improves the outcome of preterm neonates because of its neuroprotective effect.[9] A focus on the developmental environment of the neonate in intensive care has resulted in minimal handling and a reduction in noise levels.[10]

SOURCES AND SELECTION CRITERIA

We used our knowledge of the current literature, guidance statements from national organisations, and searches of the PubMed database. We carried out literature searches for data on survival, morbidity, and acute and long term clinical outcomes. We focused on national studies rather than local unit studies.

POTENTIAL ANTENATAL INTERVENTIONS TO REDUCE PREMATURITY

- Legislation to reduce the number of embryos transferred into the uterus during in vitro fertilisation (already present in the UK)
- Measurement of fetal fibronectin and assessment of cervical length by transvaginal ultrasound may help define which women admitted to the delivery unit require transfer to a specialist unit. Their role in this context has not yet been defined
- Cervical cerclage or progesterone prophylaxis may benefit women at risk of preterm delivery

---

SUMMARY POINTS

- Improvements in neonatal care mean that many extremely preterm infants now survive, but neurodevelopmental and other morbidities are common
- The incidence of extremely preterm birth is increasing
- Survival rates improve greatly with each week of gestation
- The use of antenatal corticosteroids and the baby's sex, birth weight, and condition at delivery affect survival and should inform decisions about resuscitation
- Guidelines can aid the clinician at delivery, but detailed discussions with parents, obstetricians, and neonatologists should be undertaken, ideally before delivery
- Sustained support of families is essential
- Prevention is the best way to limit the mortality and morbidity associated with extreme prematurity

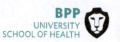

What is the chance of survival for these infants?

The lowest gestation at which survival is possible is currently 22 weeks. However, it is rare for a baby born this early to survive without serious morbidity in the neonatal period and long term disability.

Survival data are available from the United Kingdom, France, northern Europe, and the US for extremely preterm births from the mid-1990s to 2003 (table). Most neonates born at 22 weeks' gestation were not resuscitated; survival varied from 0% to 5%. Survival increased greatly with each successive week of gestation: at 23 weeks' gestation, 11-43% survived until discharge from hospital; this improved to 26-61% at 24 weeks' gestation and 44-77% at 25 weeks.[3] [11] [12] [13] [14] [15]

Information about numbers of extremely preterm infants surviving to hospital discharge in a particular neonatal database should be qualified, because data can be reported as the proportion of all births, all live births, or all babies admitted to neonatal intensive care that survive. When using survival statistics in counselling or decision making, clinicians should consider which cohort is most applicable to the clinical situation. For example, it would be most relevant to consider the proportion of all neonates who survive when engaging in a prenatal discussion on the delivery unit with parents.

What is the long term outcome for these infants?

Many infants have serious disabilities that affect quality of life. Magnetic resonance imaging of the central nervous system shows that up to 80% of premature infants have diffuse white matter injury.[16] Outcome studies use varied definitions of impairment, including any abnormal neurological finding, changes in coordination, cerebral palsy, blindness, deafness, or cognitive deficits. The data all reflect practice at least five, and in many cases, more than 10 years ago. The further into childhood the neurological evaluation is performed, the more predictive it will be of adult function. Statistics on neurodevelopmental impairment can be difficult to put into context; for example, a Finnish multicentre trial found that 43% of children had any neurological abnormality, but only 14% had function limiting cerebral palsy at 2 years.[13] If profound impairment includes an IQ more than two standard deviations below the mean, uncorrectable blindness or deafness, or cerebral palsy that precludes ambulation, then about a third of those born at 23-24+6 weeks, and a half of those born at 25-26+6 weeks, survive without profound impairment.[8]

Two recent national cohort studies from the UK and France provide data on survival and long term neurodevelopmental outcome. Epicure is the first UK national study of long term outcome for babies born at 25 weeks' gestation or less.[11] Disability was common, and follow-up at 8 years has given insight into school performance. The children who were extremely preterm scored an average of 24 points lower on cognitive testing than their age matched school peers (IQ 82 v 106). The Epipage study group studied a similar cohort of preterm infants and reported that the incidence of cognitive and neurological impairment at 5 years increased with decreasing gestational age.[5]

Preterm infants are at risk of other long term morbidities; very low birthweight babies (<1500 g) are more likely to develop insulin resistance, glucose intolerance, and hypertension in early adult life.[17] Respiratory problems such as asthma can persist throughout childhood, and growth usually remains below average.[18] Immediate neonatal morbidities such as chronic lung disease, necrotising enterocolitis, patent ductus arteriosus, retinopathy of prematurity, and late onset sepsis have not changed substantially in incidence.[19]

Obstetric decision making when extreme preterm delivery is likely

Difficult management decisions around the time of delivery need a multidisciplinary approach involving the parents, midwives, obstetric staff, and paediatric staff. This must include a plan for delivery (mode of delivery and fetal monitoring) and for managing the baby afterwards, either by active intervention or palliative care.[20] An accurate gestational age, ideally from a 10-14 week ultrasound, should be ascertained. A recent scan describing the estimated fetal weight, presentation, amniotic fluid, and—in fetal growth restriction—Doppler arterial and venous blood flow indices is invaluable for tailoring management to individual circumstances. Corticosteroids should be given to the mother if delivery is expected within 48 hours. Tocolytics are sometimes given to delay early spontaneous preterm labour—to allow time for transfer to a specialist neonatal care unit or for steroids to take effect—although no benefit on perinatal mortality has been shown.[21] [22]

Evidence on which to base a decision on vaginal delivery or caesarean section at 24-26 weeks is scant. No adequate randomised studies exist because of recruitment difficulties.[23] Some trials have indicated that caesarean section confers a survival advantage, whereas others have found no difference.[24] [25] If spontaneous vaginal delivery is anticipated, the indications for an operative delivery should be discussed with the parents. If the parents do not want operative intervention, the fetal heart rate should probably not be monitored. When delivery is planned, a caesarean section is usually performed rather than induction of labour so that the baby is born under optimal condition. In tertiary obstetric practice, operative intervention may be considered after 25+0 weeks' gestation. Before 26 weeks, however, a classic caesarean is often performed, in which a vertical incision is made in the uterus because the lower uterine segment is poorly developed. This increases the risk of uterine rupture in a subsequent pregnancy and mandates future delivery by caesarean.

Proportion of live births surviving to hospital discharge						
	Data source (time period)					
Gestational age (weeks)	US NICHD (1998-2003)	Finland (1996-7)[13]	Sweden (1992-8)[12]	Norway (1999-2000)[14]	UK Epicure study (1995)	France Epipage study (1997)
22	5	5	—	0	1	0
23	26	11	43	16	11	0
24	56	41	61	44	26	31
25	75	63	77	66	44	50

NICHD=National Institute of Child Health and Human Development.

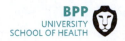
What guidance can be given about active resuscitation versus palliative care?

The decision not to begin intensive care for an extremely preterm infant is an important and difficult judgment. Staff must tell the parents if a baby is unlikely to survive or will have a high risk of severe disability and discuss the purpose of resuscitation with them. The Nuffield Council on Bioethics and the British Association of Perinatal Medicine have issued recent resuscitation guidelines.[26] [27] Resuscitation is not recommended at 22 weeks' gestation, whereas 23-24 weeks is a "grey area" in which the decision relies heavily on parental wishes and the clinical condition of the baby. Doctors should remember that parents are more likely than professionals to favour intervention.[28]

What other factors influence survival?

Factors other than gestational age at birth influence survival. The US Neonatal Research Network study published in 2008 confirmed the findings from large international databases. A birth weight more than 100 g above the average for gestation, female sex, and adequate administration of antenatal steroids all improved the chances of survival.[11] Delivery by caesarean was also associated with increased survival, although this may be influenced by surgery being performed in more favourable circumstances or an association between chorioamnionitis and vaginal birth.[11]

Multiple birth and birth outside a specialist centre reduced survival, but race and ethnicity did not.[11]

Ongoing support for families

The decision of whether to resuscitate, the effect of long term morbidities, and the loss of a baby can place serious psychological pressures on parents. The average length of hospital stay is 111 days at 25 weeks' gestation, and this rises to 222 days at 22 weeks' gestation.[3] Parents often rely on neonatal nurses to help them cope with their baby's illness and establish their role as caregivers.[29] Parent support groups are a useful resource for both parents and staff. Developmental care programmes help support parents during hospital stay and after discharge.[30] Irrespective of the outcome, it is usual practice to provide follow-up obstetric debriefing and discussion of risks for future pregnancies. If the child has died, bereavement support can be offered both in hospital and in community settings.

Ongoing community and paediatric support must be available for these babies as they grow, to identify developmental delays and to intervene when, for example, learning difficulties and speech problems occur. It should not be forgotten, however, that many extremely preterm babies who survive the neonatal period will live healthy and fulfilling lives.

Karen Faminial (about her son Elijah), Bottisham, Cambridge

Contributors: NKY and EMM searched the literature. All authors wrote parts of the review and jointly edited and revised the article. CCL is guarantor.

TIPS FOR NON-SPECIALISTS

- Ascertain the levels of care and predelivery (in utero) transfer policies in your local maternity and neonatal network units
- Be aware of both national and local outcome statistics
- Aim for multidisciplinary communication with parents before delivery
- Competent initial resuscitation, thermoregulatory care, and respiratory care in the first hour after delivery decreases the risk of morbidity
- Parents may have powerful trauma and grief reactions, which can persist
- Fathers' reactions are sometimes forgotten when a preterm baby is born
- Resources such as preterm support groups should be offered to parents
- Psychological support from staff can help families struggling to cope with a baby's critical illness, both in hospital and in the community

---

ADDITIONAL EDUCATIONAL RESOURCES

Information resources for health professionals

- British Association of Perinatal Medicine (www.bapm.org)—Information on neonatal networks and the management of in utero transfers
- Nuffield Council on Bioethics (www.nuffieldbioethics.org/go/ourwork/neonatal/introduction)—Considers the ethical problems raised by critical care decisions in fetal and neonatal medicine

Information resources for parents

- BLISS (www.bliss.org.uk)—Special care baby charity that provides free information and advice to families
- SANDS (www.uk-sands.org)—Charity that supports parents whose baby has died during pregnancy or after birth

---

A PATIENT'S PERSPECTIVE

I began bleeding at home on the evening that I gave birth to Elijah. I was just starting to enjoy the pregnancy and then the baby was already out. I hadn't heard of anybody giving birth at less than seven months, but Elijah was born at 23 weeks and 6 days' gestation, weighing just 680 g. I was in shock when the doctors tried to discuss whether to resuscitate my baby, but I think the right decision was made. I come in each day happy to see him. If we get good news I go home happy. If the news is bad, such as when he recently needed surgery for patent ductus arteriosus ligation, I go home upset. During the pregnancy, I had dreams of how wonderful it would be to experience the birth of my baby and to take him home with me. Now, I feel I have to let go of those dreams and start another chapter of my life. It took 10 days before my husband began taking pictures of Elijah. We were both so afraid to become attached. Elijah is now 30 days old and we take a photo every day .

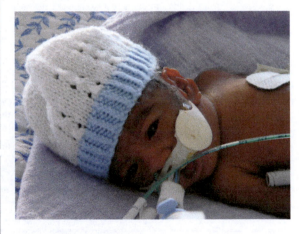

Competing interests: None declared.

Provenance and peer review: Commissioned; externally peer reviewed.

Patient consent obtained.

1. NHS. *NHS maternity statistics UK 2005-2006.* 2007. www.ic.nhs.uk/statistics-and-data-collections/hospital-care/maternity/nhs-maternity-statistics-2005-06.
2. Martin J, Kung HC, Mathews TJ, Hoyert DL, Strobino DM, Guyer B, et al. Annual review of vital statistics:2006. *Pediatrics* 2008;121:788-801.
3. Tyson J, Prarikh N, Langer J, Green C, Higgins R. Intensive care for extreme prematurity—moving beyond gestational age. *N Engl J Med* 2008;358:1672-81.
4. Gilbert WM, Nesbitt TS, Danielsen B. The cost of prematurity: quantification by gestational age and birthweight. *Obstet Gynecol* 2003;102:488-92.
5. Larroque B, Ancel PY, Marret S, Marchand L, André M, Arnaud C, et al. Neurodevelopmental disabilities and special care of 5 year old children born before 33 weeks of gestation (the EPIPAGE study): a longitudinal cohort study. *Lancet* 2008;371:813-20.
6. Kamoji VM, Dorling JS, Manktelow BN, Draper ES, Field DJ. Extremely growth-retarded infants: is there a viability centile? *Pediatrics* 2006;118:758-63.
7. The EPIPAGE study group. Impact of the use of antenatal corticosteroids on mortality, cerebral lesions and 5 yr developmental outcomes of very preterm infants: the EPIPAGE cohort study. *BJOG* 2008;115:275-82.

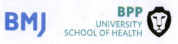

8   Fenton AC, Leslie A, Skeoch CH. Optimising neonatal transfer. *Arch Dis Child Fetal Neonatal Ed*2004;89:F215-9.

9   Schmidt B, Roberts RS, Davis P, Doyle LW, Barrington KJ, Ohlsson A, et al. Long-term effects of caffeine therapy for apnea of prematurity. *N Engl J Med*2007;357:1893-902.

10 Brandon DH, Ryan DJ, Barnes AH. Effect of environmental changes on noise in the NICU. *Neonatal Netw*2007;26:213-8.

11 Marlow N, Wolke D, Bracewell M, Samara M. Neurologic and developmental disability at six years of age after extremely preterm birth. *N Engl J Med*2005;352:9-19.

12 Serenius F, Ewald U, Farooqi A, Holmgren PA, Håkansson S, Sedin G. Short-term outcome after active perinatal management at 23-25 weeks of gestation. A study from two Swedish tertiary care centres. Part 2: infant survival. *Acta Paediatr*2004;93:1081-9.

13 Mikkola K; for the Finnish ELBW Cohort Study Group. Neurodevelopmental outcome at 5 years of age of a national cohort of extremely low birth weight infants who were born in 1996-1997. *Pediatrics*2005;116:1391-9.

14 Markestad T; on behalf of the Norwegian Extreme Prematurity Study Group. Early death, morbidity, and need of treatment among extremely premature infants. *Pediatrics*2005;115:1289-98.

15 Larroque B, Bréart G, Kaminski M, Dehan M, André M; for the Epipage Study Group. Survival of very preterm infants: Epipage, a population based cohort study. *Arch Dis Child Fetal Neonatal Ed*2004;89:F139-44.

16 Volpe JJ. Brain injury in preterm infants: a complex amalgam of destructive and developmental disturbances. *Lancet Neurol*2009;8:110-24.

17 Hovi P, Andersson S, Eriksson J, Jarvenpaa A, Strang-Karlsson S, Makitie O, et al. Glucose regulation in young adults with very low birth weight. *N Engl J Med*2007;356:2053-63.

18 Bracewell MA, Hennessy EM, Wolke D, Marlow N. The EPICure study: growth and blood pressure at 6 years of age following extremely preterm birth. *Arch Dis Child Fetal Neonatal Ed*2008;93:F108-14.

19 Fanaroff AA, Hack M, Walsh MC. The NICHD neonatal research network: changes in practice and outcomes during the first 15 years. *Semin Perinatol*2003;27:281-7.

20 Ahluwalia J, Lees C, Paris JJ. Decisions for life made in the perinatal period; who decides and on which standards? *Arch Dis Child Fetal Neonatal Ed*2008;93:F332-3.

21 Gabriel R, Grolier F, Graesslin O. Can obstetric care provide further improvement in the outcome of preterm infants? *Eur J Obstet Gynecol Reprod Biol*2004;15:S25-8.

22 King JF. Tocolysis and preterm labour. *Curr Opin Obstet Gynecol*2004;16:459-63.

23 Grant A, Penn ZJ, Steer PJ. Elective or selective caesarian section of the small baby? A systematic review of the controlled trials. *BJOG*1996;103:1197-2000.

24 Naylor CS, Vanderhal A, Hoble C, Forbis S, Sola A. Cesarean delivery for extremely low birth weight infants 500 to 750 grams in breech presentation. What are the benefits? *Am J Obstet Gynecol*2001;184:S194.

25 Riskin A, Riskin-Mashiah S, Lusky A, Reichman B; Israel Neonatal Network. The relationship between delivery mode and mortality in very low birthweight singleton vertex-presenting infants. *BJOG*2004;111:1365-71.

26 Nuffield Council on Bioethics. Critical care decisions in fetal and neonatal medicine: ethical issues. 2006. www.nuffieldbioethics.org/go/ourwork/neonatal/publication_406.html.

27 Wilkinson AR, Ahluwalia J, Cole A, Crawford D, Fyle J, Gordon A, et al. Management of babies born extremely preterm at less than 26 weeks gestation: a framework for clinical practice at the time of birth. *Arch Dis Child Fetal Neonatal Ed*2009;94:F2-5.

28 Streiner DL, Saigal S, Burrows E, Stoskopf B, Rosenbaum P. Attitudes of parents and health care professionals toward active treatment of extremely premature infants. *Pediatrics*2001;108:152-7.

29 Miles MS, Carlson J, Funk SG. Sources of support reported by mothers and fathers of infants hospitalized in a neonatal intensive care unit. *Neonatal Netw*1996;15:45-52.

30 Saigal S. An overview of mortality and sequelae of preterm birth from infancy to adulthood. *Lancet*2008;608:261S-9S.

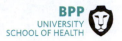

Managing common breastfeeding problems in the community

Lisa H Amir principal research fellow[1] medical officer[2]

[1]Judith Lumley Centre, La Trobe University, Melbourne, VIC 3000, Australia

[2]Breastfeeding Service, Royal Women's Hospital, Parkville, VIC 3052, Australia

Correspondence to: L H Amir l.amir@latrobe.edu.au

Cite this as: BMJ 2014;348:g2954

‹DOI› 10.1136/bmj.g2954
http://www.bmj.com/content/348/bmj.g2954

Breast feeding is universally acknowledged as the first step in the promotion of health and wellbeing of children and their families. The World Health Organization recommends breast feeding for two years or beyond,[1] with solids introduced around 6 months of age. Since WHO and Unicef established the baby friendly hospital initiative in 1991, maternity services around the world have been improving support within hospitals for breastfeeding initiation. Support for breast feeding in the community has not received the same attention, however, and women often cease breast feeding in the early weeks when they encounter or perceive problems. Medical practitioners may not receive education in managing breastfeeding problems and at times may provide advice that is inappropriate or unhelpful.

The two most common problems faced by breastfeeding women are nipple and breast pain and low (or perceived low) milk supply. About 30% of women experience at least one breastfeeding problem at two weeks post partum,[2] and many will seek help from their general practitioner or other health professional. This article provides medical practitioners with up to date evidence on how to manage common problems associated with breast feeding.

What are the common causes of breast and nipple pain?

Mastitis

Mastitis means inflammation of the breast. Although the term has been used by some authors for painful breast conditions, it should be reserved for conditions that involve breast inflammation as well as systemic symptoms.[3] It is generally agreed that a continuum exists from a blocked duct or engorgement to mastitis to breast abscess.[4] In mastitis an area of the breast, typically a wedge-shaped section, becomes red, firm, and tender. In addition, affected women have systemic symptoms such as fever, rigors, lethargy, muscle aching, depression, nausea, or headache.[5] In the past, mastitis was referred to as "milk fever," which captures the notion that the symptoms are not confined to the breast. Milk or products in the milk get into the

SOURCES AND SELECTION CRITERIA

I searched the Cochrane database of systematic reviews, guidelines of the UK National Institute for Health and Care Excellence and US Academy of Breastfeeding Medicine, and my own EndNote library. I also searched PubMed using the terms "breastfeeding management", "mastitis", "abscess", "nipple pain", "sore nipples", "low milk supply", and "insufficient milk".

bloodstream, leading to symptoms similar to those of an incompatible blood transfusion.[4] [6]

Mastitis can be infectious or non-infectious. There is no easy way to determine whether an infection is present, but it is more likely to occur in the early weeks post partum in the presence of obvious nipple damage, which allows entry of bacteria into the breast. Mastitis occurring in the absence of nipple damage and secondary to poor drainage of the breast is likely to be non-infectious; common examples are external pressure on the breast from clothing or car seat belts, or extended periods between feeds when a child first sleeps through the night. Although textbooks have stated that each breast contains 15-20 ducts, recent ultrasound studies indicate that the average number may be around 10 (range 4-18).[7] Thus one blocked duct can affect 25% of the breast.

Management of mastitis

The WHO review of mastitis recommends first line treatments for 24 hours before antibiotics are started.[3] Research evidence on the management of mastitis, including the use of antibiotics,[8] is lacking; the management strategies described here are based on expert opinion.[9]

First line management involves improved drainage of the breast. This might be achieved by increasing frequency of feeds, improving the attachment of infants to the breast, and positioning infants at the breast with their chin pointed towards the blockage, as the tongue applies a wave-like movement to the underside of the breast. Heat is often applied before the feed (shower, warm face cloth, or heat pack) to improve the mother's relaxation and milk flow.

If infants are not feeding effectively, expressing milk by hand or pump, focusing on the affected area, can help. Breast massage should not be rough; oil on the fingers avoids breast skin becoming grazed. Physiotherapists use therapeutic ultrasound as another modality to apply heat to the affected area; anecdotally this can be useful but has not been confirmed by randomised trials.[10]

Antibiotics and mastitis

A Cochrane review on antibiotics for mastitis in breastfeeding women concluded that there is little evidence for the effectiveness of antibiotics and that high quality randomised controlled trials are urgently needed to establish the role of antibiotics in mastitis.[8] The review included one small trial (25 participants) comparing amoxicillin with cephradine. The study found no difference between the antibiotics,

SUMMARY POINTS

- Breastfeeding rates are lowest in groups most at risk of ill health: preterm infants, low socioeconomic status, and mothers who are young, overweight, or obese

- General practitioners play a key role in managing breastfeeding problems in the community

- Women experiencing nipple pain should be referred to a local infant feeding expert to ensure optimal attachment of the infant to the breast

- In addition to nipple pain and damage from poor attachment, pain may be caused by anatomical problems, such as infant tongue-tie, maternal infection (bacterial, thrush, herpes), dermatitis, or nipple vasospasm

- There is a continuum from engorgement or blocked duct (swollen area of breast with redness or systemic symptoms) to mastitis (red, painful, firm area of breast with fever or systemic symptoms) to breast abscess

- Ongoing maternal milk supply is under local (autocrine) control: removal of milk stimulates the breast to produce more milk

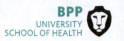

and an older study comparing breast emptying alone as "supportive therapy," antibiotic therapy plus supportive therapy, and no therapy, which suggested faster clearance of symptoms for women who used antibiotics. Given the paucity of data, the Academy of Breastfeeding Medicine has based recommendations on expert opinion[9] and has not changed the WHO recommendations of attempting first line measures for 24 hours before starting antibiotics. However, antibiotics are recommended immediately for women who are acutely ill, or in the early postpartum period when nipple damage is present.[9]

Staphylococcus aureus is the most common pathogen in the milk of women with mastitis.[11] The table summarises antibiotic treatments, which are based on the antibiotic guidelines prepared in Australia by an expert writing group, representing independent consensus opinion, based on the best evidence available at the time of publication.[15] Usual treatment is with a penicillinase resistant antibiotic, such as flucloxacillin; initially 500 mg four times a day for five days, continuing for another five days if inflammation is not resolved, with cephalexin or clindamycin used for women who are allergic to penicillin.[15] Local guidelines may vary.

Milk samples are not collected routinely, but WHO guidelines recommend that a clean catch specimen should be sent for culture if the mastitis does not resolve within 48 hours or appears to be severe or unusual.[3] If the affected area of the breast remains firm after feeds, a diagnostic ultrasound may be necessary to exclude a deep abscess.[9]

Postpartum women and infants are at increased risk of community acquired meticillin resistant *S aureus* (CA-MRSA).[16] In recent years, MRSA has been isolated from the milk of women with mastitis and from aspirates of breast abscesses.[17] Clinicians should be aware of the likelihood of CA-MRSA in their area and increase microbiological testing of milk if the risk of MRSA is high. If CA-MRSA is suspected or isolated, local protocols or advice should be sought from local infectious disease experts.

Non-mastitis causes of nipple and breast pain

Nipple pain is common in the early weeks post partum: over half (56%, 183/326) of the first time mothers in our recent cohort study reported nipple pain at three weeks post partum.[18] New mothers should be encouraged to seek help to resolve breastfeeding associated pain.

Feeding problems

Poor infant attachment is the most common cause of nipple pain and damage. Health professionals can help new mothers optimise attachment of the infant to the breast (figs 1 and 2 and box 1). Maternal and infant anatomy can negatively affect attachment—for example, if the nipples are inverted or hard to grasp, or the infant's jaw is receding or tongue movement is restricted. Figure 1 shows an infant with a poor attachment (the mouth is almost closed and gums will be compressing the nipple rather than the breast) and figure 2 an infant well attached.

Although the importance of infant tongue-tie has been controversial, evidence is mounting from several small trials and several case series that infants who cannot extend their tongue over the lip or successfully cup the breast using wave-like peristalsis may contribute to maternal nipple pain and damage or low milk transfer, or both.[19] [20] Where tongue-tie is evident and breastfeeding difficulties are present, release of the lingual frenulum can be effective. After reviewing the trials and observational studies and consulting with experts, the National Institute for Health and Care Excellence concluded that division of the thin membrane with a small pair of sterile scissors is a safe procedure, causing little distress for the infant.[20]

Nipple damage

When the skin of the nipple is disrupted, the damaged area is usually rapidly colonised with *S aureus*.[21] The nipples should be washed daily[22]; evidence from five randomised controlled trials suggests that application of purified lanolin helps to heal damaged nipples.[23] Although evidence is lacking for the management of nipple damage when skin disruption is major or not resolving, practitioners have found that a topical antibiotic such as mupirocin aids in healing and can be applied after feeds (no need to wash off if used sparingly).[21] [24]

Herpes simplex

Herpes simplex is a rare cause of painful, discrete sores around the nipple or areola (fig 3); if infection with *H simplex* is suspected, newborn infants should not be allowed to breast feed until the sores have resolved, and mothers should express milk and discard to maintain milk supply until lesions have healed.[25]

Drugs used for common breastfeeding problems

Indication*	Drug treatment	Breastfeeding recommendation
Mastitis	Flucloxacillin 500 mg every six hours for 10-14 days; if allergic to penicillin, cephalexin 500 mg four times daily; if highly allergic to penicillin, clindamycin 450 mg three times daily[9]	Small amounts in breast milk not known to be harmful to infants (*British National Formulary* 2014). Compatible with breast feeding[12][13]
Nipple bacterial infection	Mupirocin ointment three times a day after feeds for up to 10 days	Topical treatments should be applied sparingly after breast feeding. Topical preparation is unlikely to cause adverse effects in breastfed infants, as systemic absorption is expected to be minimal[13]
Nipple/breast Candida infection	Mother: miconazole gel or cream for nipples; fluconazole 150 mg every 2nd day × 3, or 100 mg daily × 10 (depending on pain). *British National Formulary* 50 mg daily. Infant: miconazole gel or nystatin oral drops	Compatible with breast feeding.[12][13] Fluconazole is used safely in infants, and amounts present in breast milk are unlikely to be harmful
Nipple vasospasm	Nifedipine 20 mg sustained release daily, increase gradually up to 60 mg daily	Compatible with breast feeding
Nipple/areola dermatitis	Moderately strong steroid (for example, mometasone) ointment once/daily for up to 10 days, after a feed	May be used at recommended dose. Topical application is probably safe but any excess cream or ointment should be wiped from nipple areas before feeding[14]
Low milk supply	Domperidone 10 mg or 20 mg three times daily[12]	Compatible with breast feeding[12][13]

*See Amir et al[14] for guidelines on other commonly used medicines for breastfeeding women.

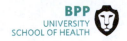

BOX 1 TIPS FOR GOOD ATTACHMENT

Mother
- Body should be supported; leaning back reduces tension in the shoulders and allows the infant's body to be supported by the mother's body
- Mother holds the infant with the arm on the side of breast feeding (cradle hold); the side of the infant's head rests on the forearm and the mother's hand supports the infant's back

Infant position
- Infant's body faces the mother; head, neck, and back in a straight line
- Infant lies diagonally: body under other breast, legs supported on hip
- Chest close against mother's chest
- Nose is in line with mother's nipple
- Chin should be close into the breast (touching)—this stimulates the infant to open his or her mouth wide for latching

Infant latch
- Wait for infant's mouth to be wide open before latching
- The angle of the infant's mouth should be >100° to take the nipple and areola deep into the mouth, allowing the tongue to move in a wave-like manner along the underside of the breast to effectively drain the breast tissue
- Chin should be deep into the breast; nose should be resting on the breast or clear of the breast
- Jaw moves fast initially, but then in a slow, regular motion once the milk has let-down
- Swallowing should be heard
- Cheeks should not be sucked in (indicates "straw sucking movement")

Common pitfalls
- Mother's body leaning over infant
- Infant lying on back (as if bottle feeding)
- Infant's body too far from mother's body, unsupported
- Mother lifting up breast (she can support the breast, but it shouldn't move if she lets go)
- Mother holding the back of the infant's head
- Infant attaching to nipple, rather than to breast

Dermatitis

The nipple and areola can also be affected by skin conditions such as eczema, dermatitis, and psoriasis.[26] Eczema or dermatitis is diagnosed when women describe an itchy, painful condition and erythema is visible, often clearly demarcated, sometimes with flaking or crusting (fig 4). The condition may be atopic in susceptible women, or may be secondary to topical creams or devices such as breast pumps. Psoriasis should be considered when flaking is prominent. Treatment includes application of a moderately strong corticosteroid, such as mometasone, once daily and sparingly after a feed (no need to be washed off) for up to 10 days. When crusting is a feature, the dermatitis is likely to be colonised with S aureus, and mupirocin ointment can be added. Eczema or dermatitis usually responds quickly

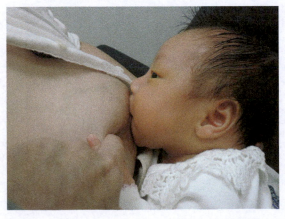

Fig 1 Infant with poor attachment to breast: small mouth, "prissy lips"

to appropriate treatment, so women with a rash on one nipple or areola who do not respond to a moderate steroid should be referred to a surgeon for assessment for the rare condition of Paget's disease.[26]

Fungal infection

"Thrush" or Candida infection of nipple and breast presents as a persistent burning pain in the nipple, with pain occurring during and after feeds. It may also be associated with pain radiating into the breast, particularly after feeds. Infants may have the characteristic white lesions on the buccal mucosas, but signs of thrush in infants are often not present (a coated tongue is non-specific and not diagnostic of oral thrush). Typically, the onset follows antibiotic treatment of the mother or infant. Isolation of Candida from nipple swabs or milk samples has been difficult, leading some authors to conclude that Candida is not associated with radiating breast pain.[27] [28] However, our recently completed cohort study of 346 first time mothers showed that women with burning nipple pain and radiating breast pain were more likely to have Candida isolated from nipple or milk (54%) than women without this pain combination (36%, P=0.014).[29] The proportion of women with a clinical diagnosis of nipple or breast thrush cannot be estimated from this study, but we can confirm that Candida is not just a commensal organism or contaminant.[29] In practice, the diagnosis of Candida infection needs to be made after considering potential differential diagnoses. Treatment includes topical antifungal treatment for the mother's nipples and infant's mouth and oral antifungal treatment for the mother (see table).[30] Topical treatments should always be applied after feeding (or expressing milk); the treatment should be rubbed into the skin of the nipple and areola like hand cream—excess cream, ointment, or gel indicates that too much has been applied. The oral antifungal fluconazole is well absorbed and is compatible with breast feeding.[12] Although not licensed for use in breastfeeding mothers, fluconazole is licensed for use in neonates at higher doses than are likely to be transferred in breast milk.[31]

Nipple vasospasm

Nipple vasospasm (or Raynaud's phenomenon) is the condition where blood flow to the nipples is reduced, abruptly leading to blanching of the nipple (fig 5), and possible nipple colour changes to purple or blue. The only prevalence study is our recent cohort study of 346 primiparous women, which found that about 20% of women noticed these colour changes to the nipple[18] but the pain seemed to be milder than the case studies in the literature.[32] [33] When vasospasm associated pain is problematic it is typically acute and can radiate into the breast and so may be misdiagnosed as Candida infection.[32] [33] Vasospasm tends to occur in thin women with poor circulation,[34] who may have a personal or family history of Raynaud's phenomenon in fingers. Primary nipple vasospasm may be present before breast feeding, but secondary vasospasm is more common, usually developing after nipple pain, damage, or infection.[35] As the pain is worsened by exposure to cold, the most effective first step is avoidance of cold temperatures: nipples should be covered immediately after feeds, heat applied, and warm clothing worn.[36] If these measures are not enough, the calcium channel blocker nifedipine has been used, as this is the most commonly used drug for Raynaud's phenomenon.[37] Nifedipine is compatible with breast feeding, and little of the drug is found in breast

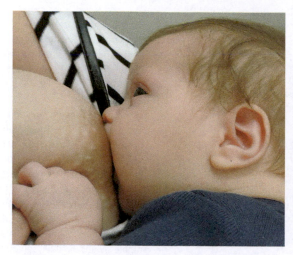

Fig 2 Infant with good attachment to breast: wide mouth, chin touching breast, body close to mother

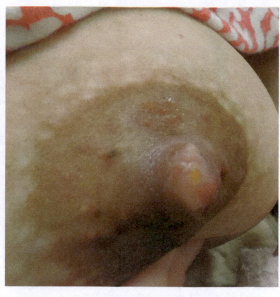

Fig 5 Nipple vasospasm (Raynaud's phenomenon) leading to blanching of nipple

milk.[12] Management of nipple vasospasm has not been the subject of trials, but we generally start nifedipine at a low dose and increase slowly to minimise headache, a common side effect. We recommend starting nifedipine 20 mg slow release once a day and increase as needed by 10 mg a week to a maximum of 60 mg slow release daily. Most women respond to 20 to 30 mg slow release.[24] [38] Treatment can be gradually reduced once the pain has resolved, but personal experience suggests that this may need to be maintained over winter months in cold climates.

Why do women have low milk supply?

An adequate milk supply needs sufficient mammary tissue, normal hormone levels, and regular removal of milk.[39] A small proportion of women have hypoplastic breasts: usually widely spaced breasts with apparently prominent areolas, owing to the lack of glandular tissue. Breast reduction or surgery that interferes with normal nipple sensation can compromise milk supply; other breast surgery is usually not a problem. In pregnancy, high levels of oestrogen and progesterone, along with human placental lactogen and prolactin, stimulate the growth of mammary alveoli and ducts. The delivery of the placenta results in a sudden drop in progesterone, which is the hormonal stimulus for the onset of lactation. Therefore retained placental fragments may interfere with lactogenesis. Normal thyroid function is also required, so women with postpartum thyroiditis or other thyroid conditions may experience difficulties with lactation. Women who experience a large postpartum haemorrhage may have insufficient milk supply, possibly

from a transient lack of blood supply to the pituitary gland affecting prolactin in the important early postpartum period. Ongoing maternal milk supply is under local (autocrine) control: removal of milk stimulates the breast to produce more milk. This is an important concept for clinicians to understand, it means that in certain circumstances women can reduce supply on one side and feed entirely from one breast.

Management of low milk supply

Not producing enough milk is the most common reason women give for ceasing breast feeding. However, it is often the woman's perception that her milk supply is low or a lack of confidence in her ability to produce an adequate milk supply. Many new mothers are not aware that it is normal for their breasts to feel softer and feeds to become shorter as breast feeding becomes established. However, breastfed babies may continue to feed as often as 10 times a day. Monitoring infant weight gain is the best way to assess milk supply. Support for new mothers, from health professionals, family, and peers, is vital.

A systematic review of 30 studies confirmed that early skin-to-skin contact between mother and infant is optimal for establishing milk supply and increasing duration of exclusive breast feeding.[40] If mothers and infants are separated or unwell, early and regular milk expression by hand should be started. Manual compression of the breast while

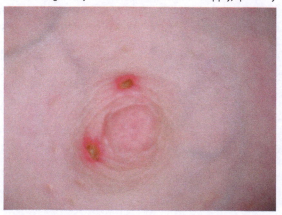

Fig 3 Sores typical of *Herpes simplex* infection of nipple or areola: discrete lesions

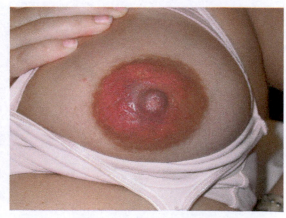

Fig 4 Dermatitis of nipple and areola: well demarcated moist rash

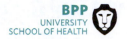

expressing milk maximises milk production.[41] Colostrum is produced for the first two or three days, so infants only require small volumes (7 to 20 mL) initially.

To increase milk supply, better breast drainage is necessary by ensuring effective attachment of the infant at the breast, offering both breasts at each feed or switch feeding (switch sides frequently for sleepy babies), increasing frequency of feeds, or expressing after feeds, as appropriate.

If the above measures are not enough, clinicians may consider prescribing a galactogogue (drug to increase milk supply). In many countries domperidone is used as it increases prolactin levels and is considered compatible with breast feeding.[12] However, a review by the Academy of Breastfeeding Medicine concluded that the evidence for the effectiveness of galactogogues is not strong and further research is needed.[42]

Can women take medicines while breast feeding?

Health professionals and the general public are well aware of the potential risks of using medicines during pregnancy. However, understanding that the risks of medicine use during lactation are significantly reduced compared with pregnancy is poor: the risk of teratogenesis has passed and the breastfed infant receives significantly less drug than the fetus during pregnancy. Few drugs are contraindicated: the latest update from the American Academy of Pediatrics mentions radioactive compounds and anticancer drugs.[13] Most drugs used in children are compatible with breast feeding.[14] Transfer of drugs can be reduced by avoiding systemic medicines where possible: topical applications, sprays, or drops may be available. Clinicians can consult experts or websites, such as LactMed, for evidence based advice. Recommendations are based on knowledge of pharmacokinetics to select drugs with the lowest transfer into milk—for example, high protein binding in maternal plasma means less free drug to transfer; and drugs with short half lives (box 2). In most clinical scenarios involving drug use in breastfeeding women, the benefits for the mother's health outweighs the potential risk for the child.[13]

Competing interests: I have read and understood the BMJ Group policy on declaration of interests and declare the following interests: none.

Provenance and peer review: Commissioned; externally peer reviewed.

Patient consent: Obtained.

1. World Health Organization. Global strategy for infant and young child feeding. WHO, 2003.
2. Binns CW, Scott JA. Breastfeeding: reasons for starting, reasons for stopping and problems along the way. *Breastfeed Rev*2002;10:13-9.
3. World Health Organization. Mastitis: causes and management. WHO/FCH/CAH/00.13. Department of Child and Adolescent Health and Development, WHO, 2000.
4. Inch S, Fisher C. Mastitis: infection or inflammation? *Practitioner*1995;239:472-6.
5. Amir LH, Lumley J. Women's experience of mastitis: 'I have never felt worse.' *Aust Fam Physician*2006;35:745-7.
6. Fetherston CM, Lai CT, Mitoulas LR, Hartmann PE. Excretion of lactose in urine as a measure of increased permeability of the lactating breast during inflammation. *Acta Obstet Gynecol Scand*2006;85:20-5.
7. Ramsay DT, Kent JC, Hartmann PE. Anatomy of the lactating human breast refined with ultrasound imaging. *J Anat*2005;206:525-34.
8. Jahanfar S, Ng CJ, Teng CL. Antibiotics for mastitis in breastfeeding women. *Cochrane Database Syst Rev*2013;2:CD005458.
9. Amir LH, The Academy of Breastfeeding Medicine Protocol Committee. ABM clinical protocol No 4: mastitis, revision, May 2008. *Breastfeed Med*2008;3:177-80.
10. Mangesi L, Dowswell T. Treatments for breast engorgement during lactation (review). *Cochrane Database Syst Rev*2010;9:CD006946.
11. Kvist LJ, Larsson BW, Hall-Lord ML, Steen A, Schalen C. The role of bacteria in lactational mastitis and some considerations of the use of antibiotic treatment. *Int Breastfeed J*2008;3:6.
12. Hale TW. Medications and mothers' milk. 15th edn. Hale Publishing, 2012.
13. Sachs HC, Committee On Drugs. The transfer of drugs and therapeutics into human breast milk: an update on selected topics. *Pediatrics*2013;132:e796-809.

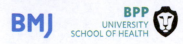

14   Amir LH, Pirotta MV, Raval M. Evidence-based guidelines for use of medicines by breastfeeding women. *Aust Fam Physician*2011;40:684-90.

15   Antibiotic Expert Group. Therapeutic guidelines: antibiotic. Therapeutic Guidelines, 2010.

16   Cataldo MA, Taglietti F, Petrosillo N. Methicillin-resistant Staphylococcus aureus: a community health threat. *Postgrad Med*2010;122:16-23.

17   Reddy P, Qi C, Zembower T, Noskin GA, Bolon M. Postpartum mastitis and community-acquired methicillin-resistant Staphylococcus aureus. *Emerg Infect Dis*2007;13:298-301.

18   Buck ML, Amir LH, Cullinane M, Donath SM, CASTLE study team. Nipple pain, damage and vasospasm in the first eight weeks postpartum. *Breastfeed Med*2014;9:56-62.

19   Kumar M, Kalke E. Tongue-tie, breastfeeding difficulties and the role of frenotomy. *Acta Paediatr* 2012;101:687-9.

20   National Institute for Health and Care Excellence. Division of ankyloglossia (tongue-tie) for breastfeeding. NICE interventional procedure guidance 149, 2005.

21   Livingstone V, Stringer LJ. The treatment of Staphylococcus aureus infected sore nipples: a randomized comparative study. *J Hum Lact*1999;15:241-6.

22   Mass S. Breast pain: engorgement, nipple pain and mastitis. *Clin Obstet Gynecol*2004;47:676-82.

23   Vieira F, Bachion MM, Mota DD, Munari DB. A systematic review of the interventions for nipple trauma in breastfeeding mothers. *J Nurs Scholarsh*2013;45:116-25.

24   University of North Carolina Lactation Program. Breastfeeding-associated pain protocol, 2012. http://mombaby.org/PDF/PainProtocols.v3.pdf.

25   Amir L. Nipple pain in breastfeeding. *Aust Fam Physician*2004;33:44-5.

26   Whitaker-Worth DL, Carlone V, Susser WS, Phelan N, Grant-Kels JM. Dermatologic diseases of the breast and nipple. *J Am Acad Dermatol*2000;43(5 Pt 1):733-51.

27   Hale TW, Bateman TL, Finkelman MA, Berens PD. The absence of Candida albicans in milk samples of women with clinical symptoms of ductal candidiasis. *Breastfeed Med*2009;4:57-61.

28   Carmichael AR, Dixon JM. Is lactation mastitis and shooting breast pain experienced by women during lactation caused by Candida albicans? *Breast*2002;11:88-90.

29   Amir LH, Donath SM, Garland SM, Tabrizi SN, Bennett CM, Cullinane M, et al. Does Candida and/or Staphylococcus play a role in nipple and breast pain in lactation? A cohort study in Melbourne, Australia. *BMJ Open*2013;3:e002351.

30   Royal Women's Hospital. Breast and nipple thrush: clinical practice guideline. 2013. www.thewomens.org.au/uploads/downloads/HealthProfessionals/PGP_PDFs/March_2013/Breast_and_Nipple_Thrush.pdf.

31   Hoddinott P, Tappin D, Wright C. Breast feeding. *BMJ*2008;336:881-7.

32   Page SM, McKenna DS. Vasospasm of the nipple presenting as painful lactation. *Obstet Gynec*2006;108:806-8.

33   Morino C, Winn SM. Raynaud's phenomenon of the nipples: an elusive diagnosis. *J Hum Lact*2007;23:191-3.

34   Flammer F, Pache M, Resink T. Vasospasm, its role in pathogenesis of diseases with particular reference to the eye. *Prog Retin Eye Res*2001;20:319-49.

35   Amir LH. Breast pain in lactating women—mastitis or something else? *Aust Fam Physician*2003;32:141-5.

36   Royal Women's Hospital. Nipple vasospasm: fact sheet. 2013. www.thewomens.org.au/Nipplevasospasm.

37   Goundry B, Bell L, Langtree M, Moorthy A. Diagnosis and management of Raynaud's phenomenon. *BMJ*2012;344:e289.

38   Royal Women's Hospital. Clinical guideline: nipple and breast pain in lactation, 2012. https://thewomens.r.worldssl.net/images/uploads/downloadable-records/clinical-guidelines/nipple-and-breast-pain-in-lactation.pdf.

39   Livingstone VH. Problem-solving formula for failure to thrive in breast-fed infants. *Can Fam Physician*1990;36:1541-5.

40   Moore ER, Anderson GC, Bergman N, Dowswell T. Early skin-to-skin contact for mothers and their healthy newborn infants. *Cochrane Database Syst Rev*2012;5:CD003519.

41   Morton J, Hall JY, Wong RJ, Thairu L, Benitz WE, Rhine WD. Combining hand techniques with electric pumping increases milk production in mothers of preterm infants. *J Perinatol*2009;29:757-64.

42   Powers NG, Montgomery A, Academy of Breastfeeding Medicine Protocol Committee. ABM clinical protocol #9: use of galactogogues in initiating or augmenting the rate of maternal milk secretion (first revision January 2011). *Breastfeed Med*2011;6:41-9.

Related links

bmj.com/archive
previous articles in this series

- Spontaneous pneumothorax (BMJ 2014;348:g2928)
- Management of women at high risk of breast cancer (BMJ 2014;348:g2756)
- Gallstones (BMJ 2014;348: g2669)
- First seizures in adults (BMJ 2014;348:g2470)
- Obsessive-compulsive disorder (BMJ 2014;348:g2183)

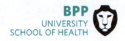

Management of infantile colic

Drug and Therapeutics Bulletin

¹Drug and Therapeutics Bulletin
Editorial Office, London WC1H
9JR, UK

Correspondence to:
dtb@bmjgroup.com

Cite this as: BMJ 2013;346:f4102

‹DOI› 10.1136/bmj.f4102
http://www.bmj.com/content/347/
bmj.f4102

Although infantile colic is considered to be a self limiting and benign condition, it is often a frustrating problem for parents and caregivers. It is a frequent source of consultation with healthcare professionals and is associated with high levels of parental stress and anxiety.[1][2]

Several published reviews of the literature have explored dietary, pharmacological, complementary, and behavioural therapies as options for the management of infantile colic.[1][3] Here, we assess whether these management options are supported by the literature and if there are any novel treatment options.

About infantile colic

Infantile colic has been defined as paroxysmal uncontrollable crying in an otherwise healthy infant less than 3 months of age, with more than three hours of crying per day in more than three days a week and for more than three weeks.[4][5] It is known to have a significant impact on infants and their families, with up to one in six families with children with symptoms of colic consulting healthcare professionals.[6]

Background

Despite the prevalence of the condition, the pathogenesis remains incompletely understood. One hypothesis has suggested that infantile colic is caused by the impact of abnormal gastrointestinal motility and pain signals from sensitised pathways in the gut viscera.[2] Another hypothesis is that inadequate amounts of lactobacilli and increased amounts of coliform bacteria in the intestinal microbiota influences gut motor function and gas production, which subsequently contributes to the condition.[2]

More controversially, behavioural issues such as family tension, parental anxiety, or inadequate parent-infant interaction have also been explored as causative factors for infantile colic.[1] In addition, little is known about concomitant risk factors; however, maternal smoking, increased maternal age, and firstborn status are thought to be associated with the development of infantile colic. No association with feeding method has been noted.[1]

As a consequence of the lack of understanding of the cause of the condition, a wide spectrum of treatment modalities have been suggested, with each one targeted to address a postulated cause.

Diagnosis

Although infantile colic is by definition a benign condition, healthcare professionals should address parental concerns carefully, as the diagnosis is made by exclusion of more sinister causes. Examples of conditions to be excluded are listed in box 1.

A careful generic paediatric history should be taken. In particular this should include the relationship between an infant's behaviour and time of day and duration of crying episodes. Additional red flag features (see box 2) such as apnoeic episodes, cyanosis, respiratory distress, vomiting, or bloody stools should be elicited as these may be suggestive of more uncommon but serious causes, such as intussusception and pyloric stenosis. In addition, other more common conditions such as cow's milk protein allergy or gastro-oesophageal reflux disease, should be considered.

Routine observations such as pulse, respiratory rate and temperature should be performed. The infant's weight should be plotted and compared against previous measurements. In the absence of serial measurements, follow-up weight measurements recorded by a healthcare professional may be necessary to identify infants with faltering growth. A complete physical examination should be undertaken with full exposure to assess the presence of bruises or trauma and identify any visible evidence of non-accidental injuries. If non-accidental injury is suspected, the local clinician responsible for child safeguarding should be contacted immediately.[7] Red flags to be excluded are listed in box 2.[8]

If the history and examination reveal no abnormalities aside from inconsolable crying, there is usually no need for biochemical and radiological examinations.[7]

Management options

There are numerous issues with the methodological rigour of many intervention studies with several systematic reviews on infantile colic describing shortcomings in trial methodology. While some form of randomisation was performed with many of these studies, lack of a clear

---

BOX 1 DIFFERENTIAL DIAGNOSIS OF COLIC SYMPTOMS IN INFANTS

Infection
Meningitis, urinary tract infection, otitis media

Gastrointestinal
Constipation, cow's milk protein allergy, gastro-oesophageal reflux disease, inguinal hernia, intussusception, anal fissure

Metabolic
Hypoglycaemia, inborn errors of metabolism

Neurological
Hydrocephalus

Trauma
Non-accidental injury, accidental trauma

BOX 2 RED FLAGS SIGNS AND SYMPTOMS

Signs
- Irritability, tachycardia, pallor, mottling, poor perfusion
- Petechiae, bruising, tachypnoea, cyanosis, nasal flaring
- Hypotonia, meningism, full fontanelle
- Weight ‹4th centile for age (or decreasing on the centile charts)
- Head circumference ›95th centile (or increasing on the centile charts)

Symptoms
- Bilious or projectile vomiting, bloody stool
- Fever, lethargy, poor feeding
- Perinatal risk factors for sepsis (premature rupture of membranes, maternal fever or infection, group B streptococcus)

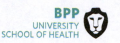

definition for infantile colic, absence of clinically meaningful end points (aside from crying duration), and limited detail on sample size calculations, allocation concealment, and randomisation methods are likely to have affected the validity of the results. It is therefore appropriate to take a cautious approach in translating the outcomes of research to practical recommendations for managing infantile colic.

Diet modification
Based on the theory that infantile colic results from excessive gas production from poor gut digestion of cow's milk proteins, several nutritional interventions have been reviewed.[2]

In practice, any positive impact of diet modification may result from improving symptoms of colic secondary to a previously undiagnosed cow's milk protein allergy in the infant. Therefore, it is important that cow's milk protein allergy is considered during the assessment of an infant with inconsolable crying. There are currently no reported unwanted effects for any of the diet modification studies described below.[9]

Hypoallergenic formula preparations for bottle fed infants
In hydrolysed formulas, whole milk proteins are broken down to prepare them for digestion. These can range from partially hydrolysed to completely hydrolysed formula preparations, with the former often used for lactose intolerance and the latter used in the management of cow's milk protein allergy.[9]

Several systematic reviews have identified studies that demonstrated that completely hydrolysed formulas significantly improved clinical symptoms of infantile colic, such as crying time.[1][9][10] These studies used standard cow's milk formula as the comparator, and improvements were noted from seven days onwards. When carbohydrate and fat content compositions were varied in one study, both proved similarly effective in reducing colic symptoms, suggesting that changes to carbohydrate and fat content had no effect.[9]

In one systematic review, two randomised controlled trials noted that partially hydrolysed formulas reduced colic symptoms after 14 days of feeding. However, the trials did not involve a direct comparison with a regular cow's milk formula but compared partially hydrolysed formulas and soy based formulas.[9]

Where a suspicion of cow's milk protein allergy exists there is some evidence that the use of an empirical time limited trial of a completely hydrolysed formula is a reasonable option.[1][9][10] Correspondingly, while there is some literature advocating the use of partially hydrolysed formula,[9] its use for the dietary management of colic would not be recommended because partially hydrolysed formulas are not hypoallergenic and therefore will not address colic symptoms secondary to a protein allergy.[10]

High fibre formula
High fibre or fibre enriched formulas are those that are fortified, typically with a soy polysaccharide, to increase the dietary fibre concentration. A randomised controlled trial identified by two systematic reviews found no significant difference in symptoms when comparing a high fibre formula with a standard formula.[1][9]

Soy based formula
Two systematic reviews noted several low quality studies that demonstrated a reduction in crying duration when comparing soy based formula with standard cow's milk formula after seven days of feeding.[9][10] However, because of concerns about the levels of phytoestrogens in soy based formula and that soy protein may be an allergen in infancy, its use in infantile colic is not recommended.[10][11]

Hypoallergenic maternal diet for breastfed infants
A hypoallergenic diet for breastfeeding mothers excludes cow's milk products and other possible trigger foods. In comparison to the use of a hypoallergenic infant formula, there is limited evidence supporting the use of hypoallergenic maternal diet, with several studies noting equivocal results.[1][9][10] This has been attributed to the use of an incompletely hydrolysed diet without a thorough exclusion of trigger foods that could have reduced the effect of the intervention.[9]

One systematic review identified a good quality randomised controlled trial in which mothers eliminated dairy foods, eggs, peanuts, tree nuts, wheat, soy, and fish from their diet.[9] The primary end point of the study was a reduction in "cry/fuss" duration of >25% from baseline, with more responders in the low allergen diet group compared with the control group (74% v 37%) and an absolute risk reduction of 37% (95% confidence interval 18% to 56%).[10] Two earlier studies reported similar findings, but neither separated the results for breastfed infants from hypoallergenic formula fed infants.[9]

On balance there is limited evidence to suggest that hypoallergenic diets in mothers may be helpful. If a time limited trial is undertaken, mothers should be advised to exclude trigger foods including cow's milk products from their diet and to ensure that they and their infant receive appropriate nutritional support, including calcium and vitamin D intake. They should also be advised not to discontinue breast feeding while switching to the hypoallergenic maternal diet.[1][9][10]

Lactase therapy
In lactase therapy, galactosidase (lactase) drops are mixed with breast or bottle milk feeds up to 24 hours prior to feeding the infant. A systematic review identified two randomised controlled trials where an improvement in symptoms was noted with the use of lactase therapy. In one randomised controlled trial, a relative decrease in crying time of 22.4% (95% confidence interval 13% to 44%) was noted.[1] This conflicted with several other randomised controlled trials noting no improvement with the use of lactase in either breast or formula milk. In one example, only a 40 minute reduction in crying time was observed compared with placebo.[1]

Pharmacological management
It is hypothesised that the gut's peristaltic cholinergic activity is linked to gastrointestinal discomfort in infantile colic. Consequently, anticholinergics such as dicyclomine hydrochloride and cimetopium bromide, which reduce smooth muscle activity, have been studied. Neither of these drugs are licensed in the UK for use in infants.

In one systematic review, two studies investigating dicyclomine hydrochloride noted improvement in colic symptoms. However, severe adverse effects including respiratory distress and seizures led to its licence

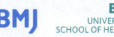

withdrawal in infants less than 6 months of age.[7] One study has reported significant improvements with the use of cimetropium bromide, with only drowsiness noted as a side effect.[1] [3-7]

Simethicone (Infacol), which reduces intraluminal gas and is readily available over the counter, has been studied in two randomised controlled trials. No difference in reducing colic episodes was shown compared with placebo.[1] [7]

Complementary therapies and other interventions

In the absence of safe and effective pharmacological interventions, complementary therapies have taken a more prominent role in the management of infantile colic. These can range from conventional therapies, such as dietary supplements, sugar solutions, herbal extracts, or massage, to controversial options such as chiropractic treatment.

Herbal supplements

A systematic review identified several studies of herbal supplements such as fennel extract and mixed herbal tea that showed a reduction in symptoms of infantile colic.[12] However, the presence of several adverse effects such as vomiting, sleepiness, constipation, and loss of appetite was also noted.[12] Minimal information on extraction and preparation of herbs and lack of standardisation of dosage and formulations have also limited their use.[2]

Sucrose solutions

Two studies compared glucose solutions with placebo and found positive effects in relieving symptoms.[2] However, there are concerns about potential nutritional effects, in particular the content of sugar and alcohol, the lack of formulation standardisation, and the poor quality of the evidence.[2] [12] [13]

Probiotics

Based upon the hypothesis that aberrant intestinal microflora affecting gut function and gas production may contribute to symptoms, the use of probiotics in infantile colic has become more common. Numerous studies have been identified in a systematic review.[12] [14] [15] One randomised double blind placebo controlled trial involving 46 infants used a suspension of freeze dried *Lactobacillus reuteri*. There were significantly more responders (50% reduction in crying time from baseline) in the *L reuteri* group on days 7 (20 v 8, P=0.006), 14 (24 v 13, P=0.007), and 21 (24 v 15, P=0.036). A further randomised controlled trial identified good weight gain and gastrointestinal tolerance.[2]

Massage

One study noted a positive effect in massage using aromatherapy oils, however, the results were not separated between massage and aromatherapy.[16] While several other studies identified in a systematic review[12] [13] showed some improvement on symptoms of colic, overall the quality of these studies is poor.

Swaddling

Swaddling has traditionally been used by some parents to reduce crying in infancy. A systematic review noted that swaddling reduced crying symptoms compared with massage in excessively crying infants with cerebral damage.[17] However, there is a known associated risk of developing hip dysplasia, overheating or sudden infant death syndrome if placed in the prone position. The current evidence base therefore does not support the use of swaddling in the management of infantile colic.

Chiropractic treatment

As a more controversial complementary therapy, chiropractic care is sometimes advocated as a treatment option for infantile colic. Chiropractic care can include, but is not limited to, cranial osteopathy and spinal manipulation therapy. The evaluation of treatment options in this field is challenging because of the absence of good quality randomised controlled trials. Additionally, adverse effects such as vertebral artery dissection have been reported anecdotally.[18] [19]

It is hypothesised that chiropractic care can have a positive effect on symptoms; however, the literature has noted that this may be a consequence of improving parents' coping ability with the condition rather than true effectiveness of chiropractic care.[20]

In several systematic reviews, one good quality single blinded randomised controlled trial was identified noting no differences in outcomes between chiropractic care and placebo, which was infant holding by a nurse.[21] Several other studies were identified noting positive treatment effects, however, these were noted to be of low quality.[12] [18] [19] [21] [22]

Currently, therefore, there is limited evidence from the literature to recommend chiropractic care in infantile colic.

Acupuncture

Several randomised controlled trials evaluating acupuncture were identified, of which two trials noted a shorter duration and intensity of infantile colic symptoms.[23] [24] Another good quality double blinded randomised controlled trial comparing acupuncture with a sham needle insertion noted no major effect on symptoms including feeding, bowel movement frequency, and sleep.[25]

Behaviour modification

Several behavioural interventions were identified that aimed to provide reassurance to parents and offer alternative methods to treat colic.[3]

One systematic review identified two controlled trials where the use of modified parent and infant interaction led to significant reduction in colic symptoms and additional benefits of early gains in development.[1] [26] This has been attributed to increased maternal responsiveness and time spent with infants resulting in increased infant alertness. In another study, entire family involvement using an integrated care model led to the relief of infantile colic symptoms more readily than standard care.[27] The use of "contingent music" was noted to decrease symptoms in another study.[1]

It has been noted that the identification of effective coping strategies and consoling methods to assist parents in managing this stressful condition is imperative.[28] A systematic review identified two studies addressing this; one study used a home based nursing intervention, and another used counselling on specific management techniques and car ride simulation in infants over 6 weeks of age, leading to significant reductions in parental stress and anxiety.[1] [3]

Guidelines

The National Institute for Health and Clinical Excellence guideline on postnatal care advises that holding the baby through the crying episode, and accessing peer support

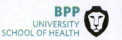

may be helpful; and that the use of hypoallergenic formula in bottle fed babies should be considered for treating colic, but only under medical guidance.[29]

A position statement by the Canadian Paediatric Society on dietary interventions commented that a minority of infants have symptoms of infantile colic secondary to cow's milk protein allergy, and in such cases a maternal hypoallergenic diet for breastfed infants and an extensively hydrolysed formula for bottle fed infants may help.[10] In addition it concluded that there is no proven role for the use of soy based formulas or lactase therapy and insufficient data to make a recommendation on the effect of probiotics.

The Clinical Knowledge Summary noted that "although there are many studies of interventions for infantile colic, most are of poor methodological quality."[30] The guidance suggests that clinicians should "only consider trying medical treatments if parents feel unable to cope despite advice and reassurance." Options listed include a one week trial of simeticone drops (breastfed infants or bottle fed infants); a one week trial of diet modification to exclude cow's milk protein (dairy-free diet for the mother (breastfed infants) or hypoallergenic formula (bottle fed infants)); and a one week trial of lactase drops (breastfed infants or bottle fed infants). However, it should be noted that the Clinical Knowledge Summary guidance was last revised in 2007. A Map of Medicine health guide on infantile colic also cites the Clinical Knowledge Summary guidance.[31]

Other issues

There is evidence of inconsistent advice relating to early infant crying and colic in various media outlets such as parenting magazines.[32] Advice was noted to be "diffuse, varied, and generally unrelated to the current evidence based conceptualization of early infant crying."

Advice for community pharmacists has summarised many of the options available over the counter (including those for which there is little evidence of efficacy, such as gripe water) and highlighted resources and support groups.[33]

Conclusion

Parents with infants with colic commonly consult a healthcare professional. Each case should be thoroughly assessed because of the wide range of other conditions that can present in a similar way. For the majority of cases simple reassurance is all that is required. If the clinician feels intervention is required there are a wide range of options available with a poor evidence base to support any of them.

Currently there are no effective and safe pharmacological management options available over the counter or by prescription. Simeticone, lactase drops, and probiotics are unlikely to be harmful, but there is little evidence to support their use. While complementary treatment options exist, there is currently insufficient evidence to recommend their use. The absence of strong evidence is similarly noted for behavioural modification interventions. Despite this, the absence of side effects makes the argument for a trial of such an intervention more compelling

Where there is a suspicion of cow's milk protein allergy, a short trial of hypoallergenic feeding, through a hypoallergenic formula in bottle fed infants may be considered. The improvement in infants with this approach may in part be as a result of treatment of undiagnosed cow's milk allergy rather than symptomatic improvement of colic. In breastfeeding mothers there is limited evidence

that a fully hypoallergenic exclusion diet may be helpful if undertaken carefully.

Infantile colic, while self limiting and benign, can cause considerable distress to parents, and it is therefore important that parental support is provided. Advice and guidance on where to obtain support outside conventional healthcare sources should be discussed with parents.

This article was originally published with the title *Management of infantile colic* in *Drug and Therapeutics Bulletin* (DTB 2013;51:6-9, doi:10.1136/dtb.2013.1.0153).

DTB is a highly regarded source of unbiased, evidence based information and practical advice for healthcare professionals. It is independent of the pharmaceutical industry, government, and regulatory authorities, and is free of advertising.

DTB is available online at http://dtb.bmj.com.

1. Hall B, Chesters J, Robinson A. Infantile colic: a systematic review of medical and conventional therapies. *J Paediatr Child H* 2012;48:128-37.
2. Savino F, Tarasco V. New treatments for infantile colic. *Curr Opin Pediatr* 2010;22:791-7.
3. Cohen-Silver J, Ratnapalan S. Management of infantile colic: a review. *Clin Pediatr* 2009;48:14-7.
4. Wessel MA, Cobb JC, Jackson EB, Harris GS Jr, Detwiler AC. Paroxysmal fussing in infancy, sometimes called colic. *Pediatrics* 1954;14:421-35.
5. Lucassen PL, Assendelft WJ, Gubbels JW, van Eijk JT, van Geldrop WJ, Neven AK. Effectiveness of treatments for infantile colic: systematic review. *BMJ* 1998;316:1563.
6. Wade S, Kilgour T. Extracts from "clinical evidence": Infantile colic. *BMJ* 2001;323:437.
7. Roberts DM, Ostapchuk M, O'Brien JG. Infantile colic. *Am Fam Physician* 2004;70:735-40.
8. Bolte RG. Intractable crying. In: May HL, et al. *Emergency medicine.* Little, Brown, and Company, 1992: 1810-7.
9. Iacovou M, Ralston RA, Muir J, Walker KZ, Truby H. Dietary management of infantile colic: a systematic review. *Matern Child Health J* 2012;16:1319-31.
10. Canadian Paediatric Society. Infantile colic: is there a role for dietary interventions? *Paediatr Child Health* 2011;16:47-9.
11. Scientific Advice Committee on Nutrition. Subgroup on maternal and child nutrition. *Soya based infant formula.* 2003. www.sacn.gov.uk/pdfs/smcn_03_10.pdf.
12. Perry R, Hunt K, Ernst E. Nutritional supplements and other complementary medicines for infantile colic: a systematic review. *Pediatrics* 2011;127:720-33.
13. Arikan D, Alp H, Gözüm S, Orbak Z, Cifçi EK. Effectiveness of massage, sucrose solution, herbal tea or hydrolysed formula in the treatment of infantile colic. *J Clin Nurs* 2008;17:1754-61.
14. Savino F, Cordisco L, Tarasco V, Palumeri E, Calabrese R, Oggero R, et al. Lactobacillus reuteri DSM 17938 in infantile colic: a randomized, double-blind placebo-controlled trial. *Pediatrics* 2010;126:e526-33.
15. Dupont C, Rivero M, Grillon C, Belaroussi N, Kalindjian A, Marin V. Alpha-lactalbumin-enriched and probiotic-supplemented infant formula in infants with colic: growth and gastrointestinal tolerance. *Eur J Clin Nutr* 2010;64:765-7.
16. Çetinkaya B, Başbakkal Z. The effectiveness of aromatherapy massage using lavender oil as a treatment for infantile colic. *Int J Nurs Prac* 2012;18:164-9.
17. Van Sleuwen B. Swaddling: a systematic review. *Pediatrics* 2007;120:1097-106.
18. Posadzki P, Ernst E. Is spinal manipulation effective for paediatric conditions? An overview of systematic reviews. *FACT* 2012;17:22-6.
19. Posadzki P, Ernst E. Spinal manipulation: an update of a systematic review of systematic reviews. *N Z Med J* 2011;124:55-71.
20. Alcantara J, Alcantara JD, Alcantara J. The chiropractic care of infants with colic: a systematic review of the literature. *J Explore* 2011;7:168-74.
21. Ernst E. Chiropractic spinal manipulation for infant colic: a systematic review of randomised clinical trials. *Int J Clin Prac* 2009;63:1351-3.
22. Ferrance R, Miller J. Chiropractic diagnosis and management of non-musculoskeletal conditions. *Chiropr Osteopathy* 2010;18:14.
23. Landgren K, Kvorning N, Hallström I. Acupuncture reduces crying in infants with infantile colic: a randomised, controlled, blind clinical study. *Acupunct Med* 2010;28:174-9.
24. Reinthal M, Andersson S, Gustafsson M, Plos K, Lund I, Lundeberg T, et al. Effects of minimal acupuncture in children with infantile colic—a prospective, quasi-randomised single blind controlled trial *Acupunct Med* 2008;26:171-82.
25. Landgren K, Kvorning N, Hallström I. Feeding, stooling and sleeping patterns in infants with colic—a randomized controlled trial of minimal acupuncture. *BMC Complement Altern Med* 2011;11:93.
26. Newnham CA, Milgrom J, Skouteris H. Effectiveness of a modified Mother-Infant Transaction Program on outcomes for preterm infants from 3 to 24 months of age. *Infant Behav Dev* 2009;32:17-26.

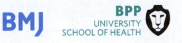

27 Salisbury A, High P, Twomey JE, Dickstein S, Chapman H, Liu J, et al. A randomized control trial of integrated care for families managing infant colic. *Infant Mental Health J* 2012;33:110-22.

28 Kaley F. The psychology of infant colic: a review of current research. *Infant Mental Health J* 2011;32:526-41.

29 National Collaborating Centre for Primary Care. *Postnatal care. Routine postnatal care of women and their babies.* 2006. www.nice. org.uk/nicemedia/pdf/CG037fullguideline.pdf.

30 NHS Evidence Clinical Knowledge Summaries. *Infantile colic.* 2011. www.cks.nhs.uk/colic_infantile.

31 Map of Medicine. *Infantile colic.* 2011. http://healthguides. mapofmedicine.com/choices/map/infantile_colic1.html.

32 Catherine NL, Ko JJ, Barr RG. Getting the word out: advice on crying and colic in popular parenting magazines. *J Dev Behav Pediatr* 2008;29:508-11.

33 Jones W. Colic: how you can help families cope. *Pharm J* 2012;289:128-31.

Related links

bmj.com/archive

Previous articles in this series
- Care of the dying patient in the community (2013;347:f4085)
- Multiple myeloma (2013;346:f3863)
- Diagnosis and management of first trimester miscarriage (2013;346:f3676)
- Glaucoma (2013;346:f3518)
- Managing unscheduled bleeding in non-pregnant premenopausal women (2013;346:f3251)

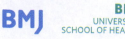

Diagnosis, management, and prevention of rotavirus gastroenteritis in children

Umesh D Parashar lead, viral gastroenteritis epidemiology team[1], E Anthony S Nelson professor of paediatrics[2], Gagandeep Kang professor of microbiology[33] Division of Gastrointestinal Sciences, Christian Medical College, Vellore, India

[1]National Center for Immunizations and Respiratory Diseases, Centers for Disease Control and Prevention, Atlanta, GA 30333, USA

[2]Department of Paediatrics, The Chinese University of Hong Kong, Hong Kong

Correspondence to: U D Parashar
uap2@cdc.gov

Cite this as: BMJ 2013;347:f7204

‹DOI› 10.1136/bmj.f7204
http://www.bmj.com/content/347/
bmj.f7204

Rotavirus is the leading cause of severe childhood gastroenteritis. Each year, rotavirus is responsible for about 25 million clinic visits, two million hospital admissions, and 180 000-450 000 deaths in children under 5 years of age globally.[1] [2] [3] Although rotavirus infection is prevalent worldwide, most deaths from this infection occur in developing countries (fig 1). Gastroenteritis caused by rotavirus cannot be clinically distinguished from that caused by other enteric pathogens; diagnosis requires testing of fecal specimens with commercially available assays. However, rotavirus is not routinely tested for in patients with gastroenteritis because the results do not alter clinical management, which relies mainly on appropriate rehydration therapy. Orally administered live attenuated vaccines that mimic natural infection offer the best protection against rotavirus. Two licensed rotavirus vaccines have been available since 2006 and have been implemented in many countries. We review approaches to diagnosis, management, and prevention of rotavirus gastroenteritis.

How does rotavirus gastroenteritis present clinically?

The clinical spectrum of rotavirus infection ranges from subclinical illness or mild watery diarrhea of limited duration to frequent profuse diarrhea with vomiting and fever that can result in dehydration with shock, electrolyte imbalance, and death. Rotavirus illness usually begins with acute onset of fever and vomiting, followed one or two days later by frequent watery stools. About 30-40% of children may have a moderate fever (temperature >39°C). Vomiting usually lasts for only one or two days and other gastrointestinal symptoms generally resolve in three to seven days.

Although gastroenteritis is the chief manifestation of rotavirus infection, neurologic features—including benign convulsions (usually afebrile but febrile in some cases), encephalitis or encephalopathy, and cerebellitis—have also been described.[4] For example, a multicentre study from Canada reported that 7% of 1359 children admitted to hospital with laboratory confirmed rotavirus had seizures at presentation.[5] A variety of other clinical conditions (such as sudden infant death syndrome, necrotizing enterocolitis, intussusception, Kawasaki's disease, and type 1 diabetes) have been associated with rotavirus gastroenteritis, but a causal association has not been confirmed. A transient rise in serum transaminase concentrations is also often seen in patients with rotavirus gastroenteritis.

Who gets rotavirus disease?

Rotavirus infects nearly all children in developed and developing countries by 3-5 years of age. Neonatal infections occur but are often asymptomatic or mild, possibly because of protection from maternal antibody. The incidence of clinical illness peaks in children aged 4-23 months, who are also at greatest risk of severe disease that requires hospital admission. Although repeat infections are common (three or more rotavirus infections occurred in about 42% of children by 2 years of age in one follow-up study in a cohort of Mexican children), symptoms are milder with each subsequent infection.[6] [7] Therefore, rotavirus infections are usually subclinical or mild in adults, but they can be severe, particularly in immunocompromised and older people.[8] Rotavirus is also an important cause of nosocomial diarrhea.

Case-control studies in industrialized countries have shown that lack of breast feeding, prematurity, and low birth weight are associated with increased risk of hospital admission for rotavirus gastroenteritis.[9] [10] Protracted rotavirus diarrhea with prolonged viral excretion and, in rare instances, systemic dissemination has been described in severely immunodeficient children, particularly those with severe T cell and combined T and B cell deficiencies. People who are immunosuppressed in preparation for bone marrow transplantation are also at risk for severe or even fatal rotavirus disease.

In all regions of the world, rotavirus is the leading cause of hospital admission for gastroenteritis. A systematic review of 131 surveillance studies published from 2001 to 2011 found that rotavirus accounted for 33-49% of hospital admissions for gastroenteritis in countries in different geographic regions and with varying levels of child mortality.[2] However, more than 90% of global deaths from rotavirus occur in low income countries in sub-Saharan Africa and South Asia, mainly because of suboptimal access to healthcare, including basic hydration therapy. In addition, compared with industrialized countries, severe rotavirus gastroenteritis occurs at a younger age in developing countries (up to two thirds of all paediatric

SOURCES AND SELECTION CRITERIA

We looked at recent conference proceedings and searched PubMed, the Cochrane Database of Systematic Reviews, and Clinical Evidence online using the terms "rotavirus", "rotavirus gastroenteritis", and "rotavirus vaccines". We focused on systematic reviews, meta-analyses, and high quality randomized controlled trials published in English within the past 10 years (2004-13).

SUMMARY POINTS

- Rotavirus is the leading cause of severe gastroenteritis in children worldwide, accounting for 35-40% of hospital admissions for gastroenteritis
- Each year, 180 000-450 000 children under 5 years die from rotavirus gastroenteritis, with more than 90% of deaths occurring in developing countries
- Because nearly all children are affected by rotavirus by age 5 years, good sanitation and hygiene alone are inadequate for prevention
- Orally administered live attenuated vaccines offer the best protection against rotavirus; as of December 2013, national immunization programs of 51 countries include rotavirus vaccine
- Such programs have greatly reduced morbidity and mortality from gastroenteritis
- A low risk of intussusception has also been documented post-licensure in some countries, but this risk is greatly exceeded by the health benefits of vaccination

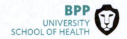

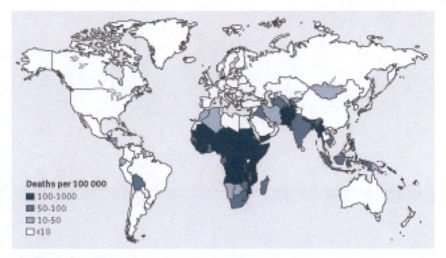

Fig 1 World Health Organization estimates of rotavirus mortality (deaths/100 000 children under 5 years of age) by country in 2008. Reproduced, with permission, from *Lancet Infectious Diseases*[2]

disease occurs in the first year of life) and coinfections with other enteric pathogens are more common.

In temperate climates, rotavirus gastroenteritis shows prominent seasonality, occurring mainly during the fall and winter, with little disease activity during summer months.[11] In tropical countries, rotavirus occurs all year round, although incidence often increases during the cool dry months.

How do rotaviruses cause diarrhea?

Mechanisms of rotavirus pathogenesis have been studied in animal models and humans. The infectious dose of rotavirus is estimated to be 100-1000 viral particles.[12] Transmission of rotavirus occurs mainly through the fecal-oral route, and viral spread can occur through contaminated hands, environmental surfaces and objects, and occasionally food and water. Rotavirus exclusively infects the mature differentiated enterocytes found at the tips of the villi in the small intestine (fig 2). Attachment of rotavirus to its sialoglycoprotein and integrin receptors is mediated mainly by viral protein 4 (VP4), but neutralizing antibodies directed against VP4 or VP7 (or both) can prevent viral binding and penetration. Infection of the enterocyte leads to virus entry, uncoating of the virus, transcription of nucleic acid, translation of viral proteins, formation of viroplasms, and apical release of the virus and viral protein by a non-classic secretory pathway.[13] The progeny virus are produced after 10-12 hours and released in large numbers into the intestinal lumen. Rotavirus can infect neighboring cells, leading to continued replication and shedding, which consists initially of a high viral load. In children, the viral load decreases rapidly as diarrhea resolves, but viral nucleic acid can be detected at low levels for several weeks.[14]

The pathogenesis of rotavirus diarrhea includes effects on absorption and on secretion. Morphologically, rotavirus infection causes enterocyte death and desquamation, leading to the loss of absorptive villous cells and the proliferation of secretory crypt cells.[15] Malabsorption may also result from a virus induced reduction in the expression of absorptive enzymes, as well as paracellular leakage as a consequence of functional changes in tight junctions between enterocytes, which may be mediated by the viral non-structural protein 4 (NSP4). Biopsies show atrophy of the villi and mononuclear cell infiltrates in the lamina propria. Increased chloride secretion and loss of consequent water and electrolyte are mediated by NSP4, which acts as a viral enterotoxin, activating cellular calcium channels and inducing secretory diarrhea. Activation of the enteric nervous system (also thought to be dependent on NSP4) induces secretory diarrhea and increases intestinal motility.[13] Villous brush border enzymes such as sucrase and isomaltase also decrease, resulting in accumulation of undigested sugars in the intestinal lumen. This increases the osmotic gradient, which in turn favours further fluid secretion.

Rotavirus infection was previously thought to be limited to the intestine, but several studies over the past decade have shown that rotavirus causes short term viremia in immunocompetent infants as well as in experimentally infected animals.[16] The clinical relevance of this systemic spread of rotavirus remains unclear, but it may be linked to the extraintestinal clinical manifestations associated with rotavirus infection.

How is rotavirus diagnosed?

Rotavirus can be detected in stool specimens from children with gastroenteritis by several techniques, including electron microscopy, polyacrylamide gel electrophoresis, antigen detection assays, reverse transcription polymerase chain reaction (RT-PCR), and virus isolation. Diagnosis of rotavirus was initially by electron microscopy, with and without agglutination by immune sera. Large numbers of rotavirus particles (up to 10^{11}/g feces) are excreted during the acute phase of infection, and children with severe diarrhea seem to excrete a greater number of viruses.[17] Polyacrylamide gel electrophoresis detects rotavirus RNA extracted directly from stool specimens; the electrophoretic migration pattern of the 11 segments of the double stranded RNA genome permits analysis of the relatedness of circulating strains.[18]

Children with gastroenteritis are not routinely tested for rotavirus because the results do not alter treatment. When testing is performed, antigen detection tests—including commercially available enzyme linked immunosorbent assays (ELISAs) and immunochromatographic assays—are widely used. Most of these tests have high sensitivity and specificity (90-95%).[19] RT-PCR is widely used in research laboratories to detect the viral genome.[20] It provides data on the VP7 and VP4 genotypes that form the basis of binary classification (G and P type, respectively) of rotavirus strains.

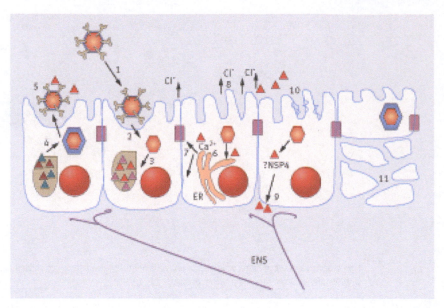

Fig 2 Mechanisms of rotavirus pathogenesis. Most information on rotavirus pathogenesis is derived from small animal models. Infection leads to attachment of the rotavirus to enterocytes (1), uncoating of the virus (2), followed by transcription and translation of viral proteins (3). This leads to the formation of a viroplasm, from which double layered particles assemble (4) and acquire outer coat proteins to form triple layered mature particles, which are shed by a non-classical secretory pathway (5). The viral enterotoxin non-structural protein 4 (NSP4; red triangles) is also released with the mature virions. NSP4 induces the release of intracellular calcium (Ca^{2+}) (6) from the endoplasmic reticulum (ER) and disrupts tight junctions (7), resulting in paracellular leakage of fluid and electrolytes. NSP4 can act on crypt cells to induce chloride ($Cl-$) secretion directly (8) or through the enteric nervous system (ENS) (9), both of which draw water into the lumen. A decrease in brush border enzymes induced by infection (10) results in accumulation of sugars in the lumen and osmotic fluid loss. Destruction of intestinal cells later in infection results in loss of surface area and a malabsorptive diarrhea (11)

How is rotavirus gastroenteritis treated?

The management of acute rotavirus gastroenteritis focuses on the treatment and prevention of dehydration. In most situations the clinician will not be aware at the start of treatment whether the gastroenteritis is caused by rotavirus or another pathogen. Initial assessment therefore focuses on determining the degree of dehydration because this will be used to guide and monitor treatment.

Many evidence based reviews and clinical guidelines are available on various aspects of the assessment and treatment of acute gastroenteritis in young children.[21 22 23 24 25 26 27 28 29 30 31 32 33 34 35 36] However, a recent systematic review of eight guidelines noted considerable variation in their quality, inconsistencies between the recommendations, lack of evidence for many recommendations, and lack of generalisability to general practice.[37] These were suggested as possible reasons why adherence to such guidelines is poor in high income countries. For example, the authors noted that in general practice it was unclear "how" or to "whom" oral rehydration therapy should be given. They concluded that future studies, particularly in general practice, need to determine the value of clinical signs and symptoms in assessing dehydration, the optimal dose of oral rehydration solution for each grade of dehydration, and the validity of reasons why clinicians prescribe other drugs. In contrast, another recent assessment of the quality of clinical practice guidelines for acute gastroenteritis, using the appraisal of guidelines for research and evaluation instrument, concluded that the overall quality of these guidelines was fair.[38]

How should dehydration be assessed?

Several scoring systems have been devised to assess dehydration.[39] The World Health Organization scale is probably most widely used in the developing world (table 1),[40] whereas the modified four point Gorelick score (box) and clinical dehydration scale (table 2) have been used in developed world settings.[32 33 34 39] The clinical dehydration scale has been reported to help predict a longer length of stay and the need for intravenous fluid rehydration.[32] It is generally accepted that conventional clinical signs of dehydration are valid and reliable when used collectively but individually they lack sensitivity and specificity.[41] The Vesikari and Clark scores are used in rotavirus vaccine efficacy trials for assessing the severity of gastroenteritis but are not designed to guide clinical management according to the degree of dehydration.[35]

Oral and intravenous rehydration therapy

Oral and intravenous rehydration is the mainstay of treatment for rotavirus and other causes of acute gastroenteritis. Oral rehydration therapy is the preferred treatment of mild to

---

FOUR POINT MODIFIED GORELICK SCORE[33 34]

1 point for each of the signs listed below:
- Ill general appearance
- Absent tears
- Dry mucous membranes
- Capillary refill >2 s

1 points: maintain hydration (<5% dehydration).

2 points: needs oral rehydration (5-10% dehydration).

3-4 points with normal vital signs: needs intravenous rehydration (>10% dehydration).

Abnormal vital signs (increased heart rate, decreased blood pressure, decreased level of consciousness, increased capillary refill time): needs resuscitation.

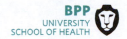

Table 1 World Health Organization guidelines for assessing dehydration in children with acute gastroenteritis[40]

	A	B	C
Condition*			
	Well, alert	Restless, irritable	Lethargic or unconscious
Eyes†			
	Normal	Sunken	Sunken
Thirst			
	Drinks normally, not thirsty	Thirsty, drinks eagerly	Drinks poorly, or not able to drink
Skin pinch‡			
	Skin goes back quickly	Skin goes back slowly	Skin goes back very slowly
Decision			
	No signs of dehydration	Some dehydration if there are .2 signs in B	Severe dehydration if there are .2 signs in C

*Being lethargic and sleepy are not the same. A lethargic child is not simply asleep: the child's mental state is dull and the child cannot be fully awakened; the child may appear to be drifting into unconsciousness.

†In some infants and children the eyes normally appear somewhat sunken. It is helpful to ask the mother if the child's eyes are normal or more sunken than usual.

‡The skin pinch is less useful in infants or children with marasmus or kwashiorkor, and in obese children.

Table 2 Clinical dehydration scale[32]

Characteristic	Score*		
	0	1	2
General appearance	Normal Eyes	Thirsty, restless, or sleepy; irritable when touched	Drowsy, limp, and cold; may be comatose
Eyes	Normal	Slightly sunken	Deeply sunken
Tongue	Moist	Sticky	Dry
Tears	Present	Decreased	Absent

*Total score: 0=no dehydration; 1-4=some dehydration; 5-8=moderate/severe dehydration.

moderate dehydration in children with acute diarrhea.[27] [29] [41] For every 25 children (95% confidence interval 14 to 100) treated one will not respond and will require intravenous rehydration.[27] Expert consensus recommends that children who are very ill, lethargic, drinking poorly, or have shock or near shock are initially treated intravenously. Oral rehydration therapy should not be given to children with intestinal ileus until bowel sounds are audible, or in the presence of glucose malabsorption.[29]

For more than two decades, WHO recommended the standard glucose based oral rehydration solution (90 mmol/L sodium, 111 mmol/L glucose, and a total osmolarity 311 mmol/L).[28] However, subsequent studies have shown that when compared with the standard WHO solution, reduced osmolarity oral rehydration solution is associated with fewer unscheduled intravenous fluid infusions (odds ratio 0.59, 0.45 to 0.79), lower stool volume after randomization, less vomiting, and no increased risk of hyponatremia.[28] In 2002, WHO recommended the routine use of a solution with reduced osmolarity (sodium 75 mmol/L, glucose 75 mmol/L, and total osmolarity 224 mmol/L) for non-cholera diarrhea.

To maintain hydration of children with "no signs of dehydration," WHO recommends giving extra fluid or oral rehydration solution after each loose stool. The suggested volume is 50-100 mL (quarter to half a large cup) for children under 2 years of age and a 100-200 mL (half to one large cup) for those above 2.[40] For children with "some signs of dehydration," WHO recommends correcting hydration over four hours with 75 mL/kg of solution.[40] However, a review of eight international guidelines showed that recommendations on the dose of oral rehydration solution were not evidence based and were inconsistent, reflecting the use of expert opinion and differences in how guidelines categorized dehydration.[37] The authors concluded that the optimal regimen was unclear.

It is important that breast feeding should continue throughout the rehydration and maintenance phases of treatment.[40] Feeding should be restarted as soon as possible because this will reduce the duration and severity of diarrhea, and there is no evidence that early refeeding increases the risk of unscheduled intravenous fluid use, episodes of vomiting, or development of persistent diarrhea.[22] Although lactose-free feeds may reduce the duration of diarrhea in children with mild to severe dehydration compared with feeds containing lactose, there is no evidence that lactose containing feeds are harmful for most children with acute gastroenteritis.[42]

Randomized controlled trials—including some that specifically assessed efficacy against rotavirus gastroenteritis—have shown that other treatments such as probiotics, zinc, ondansetron, nitazoxanide, and some biological compounds are effective in the management of acute gastroenteritis.[21] [23] [24] [40] [41] [42] [43] [44] [45] However, recommendations for the use of these treatments vary considerably between different developmental regions and different countries, and further discussion of their use is beyond the scope of this article.

How can rotavirus gastroenteritis be prevented?

Because rotavirus infects nearly all children in both industrialised and developing countries early in life, good hygiene and sanitation alone are considered inadequate for prevention. Observational studies have shown that breast feeding confers protection from rotavirus gastroenteritis, although one case-control study indicated that it may only postpone the occurrence of rotavirus gastroenteritis to the post-weaning period.[46]

Follow-up of birth cohorts indicates that, although children can be infected with rotavirus four to five times in the first two years of life, the incidence of severe rotavirus gastroenteritis is reduced with each repeat infection.[6] [7] Therefore, orally administered, live, attenuated rotavirus vaccines have been developed to mimic the effect of natural infection and prevent severe rotavirus disease.

A rhesus-human reassortant rotavirus vaccine (Rotashield, Wyeth) was licensed in the US in 1998 after showing high efficacy against severe rotavirus gastroenteritis in randomized clinical trials.[47] Rotashield was recommended for routine immunization of US infants the same year but was abruptly withdrawn a year later because post-licensure observational studies found that it was associated with a severe adverse event, intussusception.[48] [49] Intussusception is a form of bowel obstruction that often requires surgery and is associated with high fatality if not treated. It was

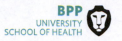

estimated that vaccination of 10 000 infants with Rotashield resulted in one excess case of intussusception.

Two other live oral rotavirus vaccines—a pentavalent bovine-human reassortant vaccine (RotaTeq, Merck) and a monovalent human vaccine (Rotarix, GSK Biologicals)—were in advanced stages of clinical testing when Rotashield was withdrawn (table 3). RotaTeq and Rotarix were each tested in randomized clinical trials of 60 000-70 000 infants to assess the risk of intussusception before licensure.[50 51] No increase in risk was found during the 42 and 30 days post-vaccination after the three doses of RotaTeq or two doses of Rotarix, respectively. The vaccines showed 85-98% efficacy against severe rotavirus gastroenteritis in these trials conducted in the Americas and Europe, with good protection against disease caused by rotavirus strains not included in the vaccines (heterotypic immunity). These findings supported vaccine licensure and recommendations for use by policy groups in the US and Europe and by WHO.[52]

As of December 2013, 51 countries include rotavirus vaccines in their national immunization programs. A systematic review of ecologic studies from eight countries reported a 49-89% decline in laboratory confirmed rotavirus hospital admissions and 17-55% reduction in all cause hospital admissions for gastroenteritis in children under 5 years within two years of vaccine introduction.[53] Unexpectedly, rotavirus vaccination of young infants has also resulted in decreases in rotavirus disease in children who missed vaccination, older children, and even adults who were not eligible for vaccination.[54] This phenomenon, known as herd protection, is probably related to reduced transmission of rotavirus in the community as a result of vaccination. Reductions in nosocomial rotavirus infections have also been seen since the introduction of the vaccine.[55] Lastly, ecologic studies from Mexico and Brazil have shown a 35% and 22% decline in childhood deaths from diarrhea, respectively, since the introduction of the vaccine,[56 57] and these reductions have been sustained for four years in Mexico. These findings are particularly noteworthy because vaccine efficacy against death from diarrhea was not evaluated in pre-licensure trials.

Post-licensure observational studies in several countries, including the US, Australia, Mexico, and Brazil, have also identified a low risk of intussusception with both rotavirus vaccines.[58 59 60 61 62 63 64 65] The evidence of risk for the two vaccines is difficult to compare directly because the study populations and designs differed. In general, the overall risk is one to five excess cases of intussusception per 100 000 vaccinated infants. Considering the substantial and well documented health benefits of vaccination against this low intussusception risk, policy makers in countries with documented risk, as well as global health authorities such as WHO, strongly support rotavirus vaccination of infants.

Live oral vaccines against many diseases, such as polio, typhoid, and cholera, have performed less well in developing countries than in industrialised ones. The reasons for this variability are not completely understood. Potential explanations include interference in vaccine uptake by greater levels of maternal antibody or concurrent enteric infections in developing countries, as well as reduced immune response in infants because of comorbidities or malnutrition, including micronutrient deficiencies.[66]

Because of these concerns, randomised efficacy trials of both RotaTeq and Rotarix were conducted in developing countries in Africa and Asia.[67 68 69] These trials showed modest vaccine efficacy (50-64%) against severe rotavirus gastroenteritis. Despite this reduced efficacy, the public health benefits of vaccination in terms of number of severe rotavirus gastroenteritis episodes prevented per 100 infants was greater in developing than in industrialised countries. This is because of the substantially greater rate of severe rotavirus gastroenteritis in developing countries. These considerations led WHO to issue a global recommendation for vaccination in 2009 and have prompted several low income countries to include rotavirus vaccination in their immunization programs.

As rotavirus vaccines are introduced into immunization programs of low income countries globally, it will be important to assess the real world impact of vaccination to gain a better understanding of vaccine effectiveness and safety in a range of settings. Although both of the licensed rotavirus vaccines have shown good protection against a range of circulating rotavirus strains, including strains with either or both G and P types not contained in the vaccine, further monitoring of the long term impact of vaccination on strain ecology is vital. Also, given the moderate efficacy of rotavirus vaccines in low income countries, interventions to improve vaccine performance (such as additional vaccine doses or different vaccination schedules) should be considered and evaluated. Finally, to sustain global implementation of vaccination, an adequate supply of affordable rotavirus vaccines must be assured. It is therefore encouraging that several manufacturers in emerging markets, including India, China, Indonesia, and Brazil, are developing candidate rotavirus vaccines that may be available within the next five years.

Contributors: UDP searched the literature and is guarantor. UDP, EASN, and GK each wrote different sections of the manuscript and revised the entire draft of the manuscript.

Competing interests: We have read and understood the BMJ Group policy on declaration of interests and declare the following interests: UDP and GK—none. EASN has participated in vaccine and disease surveillance studies funded by GlaxoSmithKline and Pfizer.

Provenance and peer review: Commissioned; externally peer reviewed.

The findings and conclusions in this report are those of the authors and do not necessarily represent the views of the Centers for Disease Control and Prevention (CDC).

AREAS FOR FUTURE RESEARCH

- Exploring the role of rotavirus in extraintestinal clinical syndromes (such as neurologic manifestations, necrotizing enterocolitis)
- Investigating the value of clinical signs and symptoms in assessing dehydration, particularly in general practice
- Defining the optimal dose of oral rehydration solution for each grade of dehydration, so that consistent recommendations can be made
- Identifying treatments (including antiviral agents) with clinical efficacy against rotavirus gastroenteritis
- Community based action research and sociocultural research on knowledge, attitudes, perceptions, cultural practices, and health seeking behaviours with regard to rotavirus infection
- Understanding the benefit-risk profile of routine rotavirus vaccination in a diverse range of geographic and socioeconomic settings
- Investigating the effectiveness and impact of rotavirus vaccination in low income settings
- Identifying interventions (such as additional vaccine doses or alternate schedules, supplementation with micronutrients) or alternative approaches (such as parenteral vaccines) that might improve the performance of rotavirus vaccines in low income settings

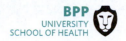

Table 3 Features of Rotarix and RotaTeq rotavirus vaccines

Feature	Rotarix	RotaTeq
Composition	Single human rotavirus strain (P1A[8], G1)	Five human G/P reassortants with bovine rotavirus strain WC3 (P7[5], G6): G1 × WC3; G2 × WC3; G3 × WC3; G3 × WC3; P1A[8] × WC3
Number of doses needed	2 oral doses	3 oral doses
Schedule*	Dose 1: minimum 6 weeks of age; dose 2: .4 weeks later; complete by 24 weeks of age	Dose 1: 6-12 weeks of age; doses 2 and 3: 4-10 week intervals; complete by 32 weeks of age
Dose	Each dose (1-1.5 mL) contains at least 10^6 median cell culture infectious doses	Each dose (2 mL) contains at least $2.0\text{-}2.8{\times}10^6$ infectious units per reassortant
Shelf life	36 months	24 months
Storage	2-8°C, protected from light	2-8°C, protected from light
Contraindications	History of hypersensitivity to the vaccine or any component of the vaccine; history of uncorrected congenital malformation of the gastrointestinal tract that would predispose to intussusception; history of severe combined immunodeficiency disease; history of intussusception	History of hypersensitivity to the vaccine or any component of the vaccine; history of severe combined immunodeficiency disease; history of intussusception

Ages for vaccine doses vary according to the recommendations of individual countries and vaccination schedules.

1 Parashar UD, Hummelman EG, Bresee JS, Miller MA, Glass RI. Global illness and deaths caused by rotavirus disease in children. *Emerg Infect Dis*2003;9:565-72.

2 Tate JE, Burton AH, Boschi-Pinto C, Steele AD, Duque J, Parashar UD, et al. 2008 estimate of worldwide rotavirus-associated mortality in children younger than 5 years before the introduction of universal rotavirus vaccination programmes: a systematic review and meta-analysis. *Lancet Infect Dis*2012;12:136-41.

3 Lanata CF, Fischer-Walker CL, Olascoaga AC, Torres CX, Aryee MJ, Black RE, et al. Global causes of diarrheal disease mortality in children <5 years of age: a systematic review. *PLoS One*2013;8:e72788.

4 Dickey M, Jamison L, Michaud L, Care M, Bernstein DI, Staat MA. Rotavirus meningoencephalitis in a previously healthy child and a review of the literature. *Pediatr Infect Dis J*2009;28:318-21.

5 Le Saux N, Bettinger JA, Halperin SA, Vaudry W, Scheifele DW. Substantial morbidity for hospitalized children with community-acquired rotavirus infections: 2005-2007 IMPACT surveillance in Canadian hospitals. *Pediatr Infect Dis J*2010;29:879-82.

6 Velazquez FR, Matson DO, Calva JJ, Guerrero L, Morrow AL, Carter-Campbell S, et al. Rotavirus infections in infants as protection against subsequent infections. *N Engl J Med*1996;335:1022-8.

7 Gladstone BP, Ramani S, Mukhopadhya I, Muliyil J, Sarkar R, Rehman AM, et al. Protective effect of natural rotavirus infection in an Indian birth cohort. *N Engl J Med*2011;365:337-46.

8 Anderson EJ, Weber SG. Rotavirus infection in adults. *Lancet Infect Dis*2004;4:91-9.

9 Newman RD, Grupp-Phelan J, Shay DK, Davis RL. Perinatal risk factors for infant hospitalization with viral gastroenteritis. *Pediatrics*1999;103:E3.

10 Dennehy PH, Cortese MM, Bégué RE, Jaeger JL, Roberts NE, Zhang R, et al. A case-control study to determine risk factors for hospitalization for rotavirus gastroenteritis in US children. *Pediatr Infect Dis J*2006;25:1123-31.

11 Patel MM, Pitzer VE, Alonso WJ, Vera D, Lopman B, Tate J, et al. Global seasonality of rotavirus disease. *Pediatr Infect Dis J*2013;32:e134-47.

12 Ward RL, Bernstein DI, Young EC, Sherwood JR, Knowlton DR, Schiff GM. Human rotavirus studies in volunteers: determination of infectious dose and serological response to infection. *J Infect Dis*1986;154:871-80.

13 Greenberg HB, Estes MK. Rotaviruses: from pathogenesis to vaccination. *Gastroenterology*2009;136:1939-51.

14 Richardson S, Grimwood K, Gorrell R, Palombo E, Barnes G, Bishop R. Extended excretion of rotavirus after severe diarrhoea in young children. *Lancet*1998;351:1844-8.

15 Boshuizen JA, Reimerink JH, Korteland-van Male AM, van Ham VJ, Koopmans MP, Büller HA, et al. Changes in small intestinal homeostasis, morphology, and gene expression during rotavirus infection of infant mice. *J Virol*2003;77:13005-16.

16 Blutt SE, Kirkwood CD, Parreño V, Warfield KL, Ciarlet M, Estes MK, et al. Rotavirus antigenaemia and viraemia: a common event? *Lancet*2003;362:1445-9.

17 Kang G, Iturriza-Gomara M, Wheeler JG, Crystal P, Monica B, Ramani S, et al. Quantitation of group A rotavirus by real-time reverse-transcription-polymerase chain reaction: correlation with clinical severity in children in South India. *J Med Virol*2004;73:118-22.

18 Herring AJ, Inglis NF, Ojeh CK, Snodgrass DR, Menzies JD. Rapid diagnosis of rotavirus infection by direct detection of viral nucleic acid in silver-stained polyacrylamide gels. *J Clin Microbiol*1982;16:473-7.

19 Thomas EE, Puterman ML, Kawano E, Curran M. Evaluation of seven immunoassays for detection of rotavirus in pediatric stool samples. *J Clin Microbiol*1988;26:1189-93.

20 Iturriza Gómara M, Kang G, Gray JJ. Rotavirus genotyping: keeping up with an evolving population of human rotaviruses. *J Clin Virol*2004;31:259-65.

21 Lazzerini M, Ronfani L. Oral zinc for treating diarrhoea in children. *Cochrane Database Syst Rev*2013;1:CD005436.

22 Gregorio GV, Dans LF, Silvestre MA. Early versus delayed refeeding for children with acute diarrhoea. *Cochrane Database Syst Rev*2011;7:CD007296.

23 Fedorowicz Z, Jagannath VA, Carter B. Antiemetics for reducing vomiting related to acute gastroenteritis in children and adolescents. *Cochrane Database Syst Rev*2011;9:CD005506.

24 Allen SJ, Martinez EG, Gregorio GV, Dans LF. Probiotics for treating acute infectious diarrhoea. *Cochrane Database Syst Rev*2010;11:CD003048.

25 Gregorio GV, Gonzales ML, Dans LF, Martinez EG. Polymer-based oral rehydration solution for treating acute watery diarrhoea. *Cochrane Database Syst Rev*2009;2:CD006519.

26 Guideline Development Group. Diarrhoea and vomiting caused by gastroenteritis: diagnosis, assessment and management in children younger than 5 years. National Collaborating Centre for Women's and Childrens Health, 2009. www.nice.org.uk/nicemedia/pdf/CG84FullGuideline.pdf.

27 Hartling L, Bellemare S, Wiebe N, Russell K, Klassen TP, Craig W. Oral versus intravenous rehydration for treating dehydration due to gastroenteritis in children. *Cochrane Database Syst Rev*2006;3:CD004390.

ADDITIONAL EDUCATIONAL RESOURCES

Resources for healthcare professionals

- Centers for Disease Control and Prevention. Prevention of rotavirus gastroenteritis among infants and children—recommendations of the Advisory Committee on Immunization Practices (ACIP). *MMWR* 2009;58(RR02):1-25. www.cdc.gov/mmwr/preview/mmwrhtml/rr5802a1.htm (free access)

- WHO. WHO position paper on rotavirus vaccines. *Wkly Epidemiol Rec* 2013;88:49-64. www.who.int/wer/2013/wer8805.pdf (free access)

- Soares-Weiser K, MacLehose H, Bergman H, Ben-Aharon I, Nagpal S, Goldberg E, et al. Vaccines for preventing rotavirus diarrhoea: vaccines in use. *Cochrane Database Syst Rev* 2012;11:CD008521 (subscription required)

- PATH (http://sites.path.org/rotavirusvaccine/rotavirus-advocacy-and-communications-toolkit/)—Free rotavirus disease and vaccine resources

- PATH (http://sites.path.org/rotavirusvaccine/current-issue-of-rotaflash-jpg/)—Breaking news and updates on rotavirus vaccines

Resources for patients and parents

- Centers for Disease Control and Prevention at (www.cdc.gov/rotavirus/index.html)—Basic information on the symptoms, treatment, and prevention of rotavirus gastroenteritis

TIPS FOR NON-SPECIALISTS

- All children are infected with rotavirus in the first 3-5 years of life, regardless of hygiene and sanitation conditions

- Vaccines are therefore the most effective way to prevent rotavirus diarrhea

- Treatment of rotavirus diarrhea relies on hydration therapy

- Rotavirus vaccines have performed well in countries where they are used routinely; in some settings, they have conferred additional benefits to unvaccinated children and adults through herd protection

- Although rotavirus vaccines work less well in developing countries, the potential to prevent severe disease and deaths is greater because of the high disease burden in these settings

- The documented health benefits of rotavirus vaccines far outweigh the small risk of intussusception that has been seen in some settings

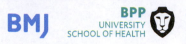

28 Hahn S, Kim S, Garner P. Reduced osmolarity oral rehydration solution for treating dehydration caused by acute diarrhoea in children. *Cochrane Database Syst Rev*2002;1:CD002847.

29 Nelson EA, Ko WK, Kwan E, Leung SF, Poon KH, Chow CB, et al. Guidelines for the management of acute diarrhoea in young children. *Hong Kong J Paediatr*2003;8:203-36.

30 Armon K, Stephenson T, MacFaul R, Eccleston P, Werneke U. An evidence and consensus based guideline for acute diarrhoea management. *Arch Dis Child*2001;85:132-42.

31 Murphy MS. Guidelines for managing acute gastroenteritis based on a systematic review of published research. *Arch Dis Child*1998;79:279-84.

32 Goldman RD, Friedman JN, Parkin PC. Validation of the clinical dehydration scale for children with acute gastroenteritis. *Pediatrics*2008;122:545-9.

33 Gorelick MH, Shaw KN, Murphy KO. Validity and reliability of clinical signs in the diagnosis of dehydration in children. *Pediatrics*1997;99:E6.

34 Alberta Health Service. Alberta Health Services acute childhood vomiting and diarrhea pathway. 2011. http://pert.ucalgary.ca/pathways/reference/Revised%20ED-UCC%20pathway%20Oct%2025%20 2011.pdf.

35 Lewis KDC, Dallas MJ, Victor JC, Ciarlet M, Mast TC, Ji M, et al. Comparison of two clinical severity scoring systems in two multi-center, developing country rotavirus vaccine trials in Africa and Asia. *Vaccine*2012;30(suppl 1):A159-66.

36 Freedman SB, Eltorky M, Gorelick M; Pediatric Emergency Research Canada Gastroenteritis Study Group. Evaluation of a gastroenteritis severity score for use in outpatient settings. *Pediatrics*2010;125 :e1278-85.

37 Van den Berg J, Berger MY. Guidelines on acute gastroenteritis in children: a critical appraisal of their quality and applicability in primary care. *BMC Fam Pract*2011;12:134.

38 Lo Vecchio A, Giannattasio A, Duggan C, De Masi S, Ortisi MT, Parola L, et al. Evaluation of the quality of guidelines for acute gastroenteritis in children with the AGREE instrument. *J Pediatr Gastroenterol Nutr*2011;52:183-9.

39 Pringle K, Shah SP, Umulisa I, Munyaneza RBM, Dushimiyimana JM, Stegmann K, et al. Comparing the accuracy of the three popular clinical dehydration scales in children with diarrhea. *Int J Emerg Med*2011;4:58.

40 WHO. The treatment of diarrhoea: a manual for physicians and other senior health workers. 4th ed. 2005. http://whqlibdoc.who.int/publications/2005/9241593180.pdf.

41 Lawson AL. Acute gastroenteritis and dehydration (child). Li STT, Ebell MH, eds. *Essential Evidence*2012. www.essentialevidenceplus.com/content/eee?class=GI.

42 Dalby-Payne J, Elliott E. Gastroenteritis in children. *Clin Evid*2011;07:314.

43 Rossignol JF, Abu-Zekry M, Hussein A, Santoro MG. Effect of nitazoxanide for treatment of severe rotavirus diarrhoea: randomised double-blind placebo-controlled trial. *Lancet*2006;368:124-9.

44 Sarker SA, Jäkel M, Sultana S, Alam NH, Bardhan PK, Chisti MJ, et al. Anti-rotavirus protein reduces stool output in infants with diarrhea: a randomized placebo-controlled trial. *Gastroenterology*2013;145:740-8.e8.

45 Sarker SA, Casswall TH, Juneja LR, Hoq E, Hossain I, Fuchs GJ, et al. Randomized, placebo-controlled, clinical trial of hyperimmunized chicken egg yolk immunoglobulin in children with rotavirus diarrhea. *J Pediatr Gastroenterol Nutr*2001;32:19-25.

46 Clemens J, Rao M, Ahmed F, Ward R, Huda S, Chakraborty J, et al. Breast-feeding and the risk of life-threatening rotavirus diarrhea: prevention or postponement? *Pediatrics*1993;92:680-5.

47 Centers for Disease Control and Prevention. Rotavirus vaccine for the prevention of rotavirus gastroenteritis among children. *Morb Mortal Wkly Rep*1999;48(RR-2).

48 Centers for Disease Control and Prevention. Intussusception among recipients of rotavirus vaccine—United States, 1998-1999. *Morb Mortal Wkly Rep*1999;48:577-81.

49 Murphy TV, Gargiullo PM, Massoudi MS, Nelson DB, Jumaan AO, Okoro CA, et al. Intussusception among infants given an oral rotavirus vaccine. *N Engl J Med*2001;344:564-72.

50 Ruiz-Palacios GM, Perez-Schael I, Velazquez FR, Abate H, Breuer T, Clemens SC, et al. Safety and efficacy of an attenuated vaccine against severe rotavirus gastroenteritis. *N Engl J Med*2006;354:11-22.

51 Vesikari T, Matson DO, Dennehy P, Van Damme P, Santosham M, Rodriguez Z, et al. Safety and efficacy of a pentavalent human-bovine (WC3) reassortant rotavirus vaccine. *N Engl J Med*2006;354:23-33.

52 WHO. Meeting of the strategic advisory group of experts on immunization, October 2009—conclusions and recommendations. *Wkly Epidemiol Rec*2009;84:518.

53 Patel MM, Glass R, Desai R, Tate JE, Parashar UD. Fulfilling the promise of rotavirus vaccines: how far have we come since licensure? *Lancet Infect Dis*2012;12:561-70.

54 Gastañaduy PA, Curns AT, Parashar UD, Lopman BA. Gastroenteritis hospitalizations in older children and adults in the United States before and after implementation of infant rotavirus vaccination. *JAMA*2013;310:851-3.

55 Zlamy M, Kofler S, Orth D, Würzner R, Heinz-Erian P, Streng A, et al. The impact of rotavirus mass vaccination on hospitalization rates, nosocomial rotavirus gastroenteritis and secondary blood stream infections. *BMC Infect Dis*2013;13:112.

56 De Carmo GM, Yen C, Cortes J, Siqueira AA, de Oliveira WK, Cortez-Escalante JJ, et al. Decline in diarrhea mortality and admissions after routine childhood rotavirus immunization in Brazil: a time-series analysis. *PLoS Med*2011;8:e1001024.

57 Richardson V, Hernandez-Pichardo J, Quintanar-Solares M, Esparza-Aguilar M, Johnson B, Gomez-Altamirano CM, et al. Effect of rotavirus vaccination on death from childhood diarrhea in Mexico. *N Engl J Med*2010;362:299-305.

58 Carlin JB, Macartney K, Lee KJ, Quinn HE, Buttery J, Lopert R, et al. Intussusception risk and disease prevention associated with rotavirus vaccines in Australia's national immunisation program. *Clin Infect Dis*2013; published online 30 Aug.

59 Buttery JP, Danchin MH, Lee KJ, Carlin JB, McIntyre PB, Elliott EJ, et al. Intussusception following rotavirus vaccine administration: post-marketing surveillance in the National Immunization Program in Australia. *Vaccine*2011;29:3061-6.

60 Patel M, López-Collada V, Bulhões M, De Oliveira LH, Bautista Márquez A, Flannery B, et al. Intussusception risk and health benefits of rotavirus vaccination in Mexico and Brazil. *N Engl J Med*2011;364:2283-92.

61 Velazquez FR, Colindres RE, Grajales C, Hernández MT, Mercadillo MG, Torres FJ, et al. Postmarketing surveillance of intussusception following mass introduction of the attenuated human rotavirus vaccine in Mexico. *Pediatr Infect Dis J*2012;31:736-44.

62 Haber P, Patel M, Pan Y, Baggs J, Haber M, Museru O, et al. Intussusception after rotavirus vaccines reported to US VAERS, 2006-2012. *Pediatrics*2013;131:1042-9.

63 Shui I, Baggs J, Patel M, Parashar UD, Rett M, Belongia EA, et al. Risk of intussusception following administration of a pentavalent rotavirus vaccine in US infants. *JAMA*2012;307:598-604.

64 Cortese M. Estimates of benefits and potential risks of rotavirus vaccination in the US presented at the Advisory Committee on Immunization Practices meeting, Atlanta, GA, USA, 20 June 2013. www.cdc.gov/vaccines/acip/meetings/downloads/slides-jun-2013/06-Rotavirus-Cortese.pdf.

65 Food and Drug Administration. Final study results of a mini-sentinel postlicensure observational study of rotavirus vaccines and intussusception. 2013. www.fda.gov/BiologicsBloodVaccines/SafetyAvailability/ucm356758.htm.

66 Glass RI, Parashar UD, Bresee JS, Turcios R, Fischer TK, Widdowson MA, et al. Rotavirus vaccines: current prospects and future challenges. *Lancet*2006;368:323-32.

67 Armah GE, Sow SO, Breiman RF, Dallas MJ, Tapia MD, Feikin DR, et al. Efficacy of pentavalent rotavirus vaccine against severe rotavirus gastroenteritis in infants in developing countries in sub-Saharan Africa: a randomised, double-blind, placebo-controlled trial. *Lancet*2010;376:606-14.

68 Zaman K, Dang DA, Victor JC, Shin S, Yunus M, Dallas MJ, et al. Efficacy of pentavalent rotavirus vaccine against severe rotavirus gastroenteritis in infants in developing countries in Asia: a randomised, double-blind, placebo-controlled trial. *Lancet*2010;376:615-23.

69 Madhi SA, Cunliffe NA, Steele D, Witte D, Kirsten M, Louw C, et al. Effect of human rotavirus vaccine on severe diarrhea in African infants. *N Engl J Med*2010;362:289-98.

Related links

bmj.com
- Gastroenterology updates from *BMJ* are at bmj.com/specialties/gastroenterology

bmj.com/archive
- Tick bite prevention and tick removal (BMJ 2013;347:f7123)
- Polymyalgia rheumatica (BMJ 2013;347:f6937)
- Diagnosis and management of hyperhidrosis (BMJ 2013;347:f6800)
- The diagnosis and management of erythrocytosis (BMJ 2013;347:f6667)
- Central venous catheters (BMJ 2013;347:f6570)
- The diagnosis and management of gastric cancer (BMJ 2013;347:f6367)

Cleveland Clinic CME
- Get Cleveland Clinic CME credits for this article

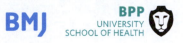

Managing gastro-oesophageal reflux in infants

Drug and Therapeutics Bulletin

[1]Drug and Therapeutics Bulletin Editorial Office, BMA House, London WC1H 9JR

Correspondence to:
dtb@bmjgroup.com

Cite this as: BMJ 2010;341:c4420

‹DOI› 10.1136/bmj.c4420
http://www.bmj.com/content/341/bmj.c4420

Transient, inappropriate relaxation of the lower oesophageal sphincter may permit contents of the stomach to pass into the oesophagus (gastro-oesophageal reflux).[1] This usually presents as regurgitation or vomiting and is common in infants, when it is usually mild and self limiting, and requires no specific treatment.[1] Gastro-oesophageal reflux disease (GORD) in infants describes reflux of gastric contents that causes troublesome symptoms or complications.[2] GORD is sometimes wrongly diagnosed in healthy infants with troublesome but harmless symptoms of "physiological" gastro-oesophageal reflux.[3] This has led to increasing, potentially inappropriate, use of acid reducing drugs.[3] [4] Furthermore, few of the drugs used to treat infants with GORD are licensed for this use, a situation that DTB criticised 12 years ago.[1] Here we consider GORD in infancy (that is, in those aged 0–12 months), the treatments available, and when these are needed.

About gastro-oesophageal reflux

Some reflux occurs in most infants, particularly in those who are preterm.[5] [6] The condition is more marked in those with slow gastric emptying or disorders of upper gastrointestinal motility due to severe neurodevelopmental impairment (such as cerebral palsy) or cows' milk hypersensitivity or allergy.[1] [7] [8] When reflux in infants causes troublesome symptoms (such as poor weight gain, unexplained crying, distressed behaviour) or complications (such as oesophagitis or respiratory problems), it is classified as GORD.[2] Oesophagitis may present with irritability, clinical features mimicking colic (crying, drawing the legs up towards the abdomen), features of pain after feeding, and, possibly, haematemesis or melaena.[9] [10] Sometimes, the oesophagitis disrupts oesophageal motility, reduces sphincter tone further, and so makes reflux even more likely.[1] Possible associations exist between GORD and asthma, pneumonia, bronchiectasis, and apparent life threatening events in infants, but causality has not been established.[2] [11] In preterm infants, reflux is associated with episodic apnoea resistant to standard treatment and with exacerbation of bronchopulmonary dysplasia.[1] [12]

Diagnosis of GORD

The diagnosis of GORD is often made clinically.[2] However, no symptom or cluster of symptoms reliably predicts complications or identifies infants likely to respond to treatment. Investigations are rarely needed, but they can be useful to document pathological reflux or its complications. However, there is a lack of reliable diagnostic tests.[13]

Intraluminal oesophageal pH monitoring is generally accepted as the optimal test for diagnosing GORD.[13] A probe is inserted into the oesophagus to measure the frequency and duration of oesophageal acid exposure.[2] The use of multiple intraluminal impedance—which shows the movement of fluids, solids, and gases—together with pH monitoring is superior to pH monitoring alone.[2] [14] Suspected oesophagitis is best confirmed by endoscopy with biopsy.[15] Barium swallow and meal studies and oesophageal manometry lack sensitivity and specificity for reflux in infants but can be used to detect underlying anatomical abnormalities or the mechanisms of GORD.[2] [16] [17] Scintigraphy with meals labelled with radioactive technetium-99 sulphur colloid, to assess aspiration into the lungs, and ultrasonography are not recommended for the routine diagnosis of GORD in infants.[2]

Treatment principles

For most infants with reflux, reassuring the parents that the condition will resolve without treatment is all that is needed.[1] Overfeeding is a common cause of reflux in infants, so this possibility needs to be explored, but with the caveat that prolonged severe reduction in feeding volume could cause nutritional problems. If regurgitation is frequent and other causes of vomiting have been excluded, growth should be monitored, ideally through the use of parent-held records. If there is clear evidence of faltering growth, intervention should be considered. The main aims of treatment are to alleviate symptoms, promote normal growth, and prevent complications.

Lifestyle and dietary changes

The prevalence of physiological gastro-oesophageal reflux is similar in breast fed and formula fed infants.[18] Some infants with allergy to cows' milk protein experience regurgitation and vomiting indistinguishable from that associated with primary gastro-oesophageal reflux.[7] [8] [19] [20] In these infants, vomiting frequency decreases substantially after the elimination of cows' milk protein from the diet (usually within two weeks), and reintroduction causes recurrence of symptoms.[2] Use of extensively hydrolysed or amino acid formula milks for up to four weeks may help to reduce troublesome symptoms.[8] [21] Since ingested cows' milk protein passes into human breast milk in small quantities, breast fed infants with regurgitation and vomiting may benefit

---

SUMMARY POINTS

- Gastro-oesophageal reflux is common in infants, particularly preterm babies, younger infants, and those with neurodevelopmental disorders

- Reflux is usually self limiting and without complications. Occasionally, it is associated with troublesome symptoms or complications (such as respiratory disorders or suspected oesophagitis), when it is known as gastro-oesophageal reflux disease (GORD)

- Parental education and reassurance, changes in feeds, thickening of fluids, or an alginate combination should be tried first for managing GORD. Infants whose symptoms are unresponsive, or those with complications, should be referred to specialist paediatric services for investigation

- An H_2 receptor antagonist to reduce acid secretion may be needed to control the condition, but there is little evidence to support such therapy. Ranitidine, which is licensed for use from 6 months of age, is now recommended by the BNF for Children as the most suitable such drug for infants

- If an H_2 receptor antagonist is unsuccessful, the next step is treatment with omeprazole (unlicensed in infants) or surgery

- No other drugs are licensed or recommended for GORD in infants

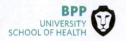

from a trial of withdrawal of cows' milk from the maternal diet.[19] However, the symptoms of infant gastro-oesophageal reflux are rarely severe enough to justify stopping breast feeding.[2]

Short-term (7–10 days) nasogastric feeding is sometimes used in infants with GORD (but no complicating disorders) who do not gain weight.[22] Nasojejunal feeding may be useful in infants with pneumonia related to gastro-oesophageal reflux to prevent recurrent aspiration.[2]

Thickening milk

A systematic review pooled data from 14 randomised controlled trials of thickened feeds involving a total of 877 otherwise healthy infants aged ‚2 years with gastro-oesophageal reflux.[23] It found that, compared with standard milk formulas, formulas thickened with carob bean gum, corn starch, rice starch, cereal, or soy fibre increased the percentage of infants with no regurgitation (risk ratio 2.91, 95% confidence interval 1.73 to 4.91), reduced the number of daily episodes of regurgitation and vomiting (weighted mean difference −1.37, −2.53 to −0.02), and increased daily weight gain (weighted mean difference 3.68, 1.55 to 5.81). No thickening agent seemed more effective than any other, and no serious unwanted effects were seen. The reviewers concluded that thickened food was "only moderately effective" for gastro-oesophageal reflux in healthy infants.

Some products can be used to thicken milk and are prescribable on the NHS as borderline substances (as detailed in Appendix 2 of the *BNF for Children*). These include the carob seed flour thickener Instant Carobel ("for thickening feeds in the treatment of vomiting") and the starch based thickeners Thick & Easy, Thixo-D, and Vitaquick ("for thickening of foods in dysphagia. Not suitable for children under 1 year except in cases of failure to thrive"). Parents should use teats with large holes and be shown how to increase feed viscosity without blocking the teat. Other drinks may also be thickened. Excessive calorie intake is a potential problem with starch based thickeners such as rice cereal and corn starch, which are not recommended unless there is accompanying faltering growth.[24] The allergenicity of commercial thickening agents is uncertain because of lack of data.[2]

Commercial anti-regurgitant formula feeds containing processed rice, corn or potato starch, guar gum, or locust bean gum are available. One potential advantage of these formulas over standard formulas with added thickener is that the former are designed to have a caloric density, osmolality, protein, calcium, and fatty acid content appropriate to an infant's nutritional needs. Also, they do not require teats with large holes nor substantially increased sucking effort. Two such formulas, Enfamil AR and SMA Staydown, are available on NHS prescription for "significant gastro-oesophageal reflux." However, according to Appendix 2 of the *BNF for Children*, they are not to be used "for a period of more than 6 months" or "in conjunction with any other feed thickener or antacid products."

Positioning of infants

One systematic review, including five randomised studies that assessed the effect of positioning infants with gastro-oesophageal reflux, found that the designs of the trials were too dissimilar to make any comparisons between positions.[25] The authors concluded that elevating the head of the crib so that the baby's head is always uppermost when lying supine is not justifiable, and that the prone position must not be used in infants because of the risk of sudden infant death syndrome. Placing premature infants in the left lateral position in the postprandial period can reduce gastro-oesophageal reflux.[26] [27] However, lying on the side is an unstable position for infants, and using pillows to maintain it is not recommended.[28]

Drug treatments for GORD

Many of the drugs used to treat GORD are not licensed for this use in infants. Furthermore, comparisons between drug treatments for GORD in children have been hampered by limited and heterogeneous evidence from small trials with inadequate controls.[29]

Alginate combinations

The aim of alginate combinations is to increase the viscosity of gastric contents and form a protective coating over the distal oesophagus.[30] In a double blind, randomised, placebo controlled trial involving 88 infants with gastro-oesophageal reflux, Gaviscon Infant (powder in sachets containing sodium alginate 225 mg and magnesium alginate 87.5 mg, but no aluminium) was effective in reducing the number of vomiting or regurgitation episodes at 14 days (the primary outcome measure) from a median of 8.5 to 3.0 (v from 7.0 to 5.0 with placebo, P=0.009), but not the severity of vomiting.[31] Another double blind, randomised, placebo controlled trial of Gaviscon Infant involving 20 infants with gastro-oesophageal reflux found no difference in the number of reflux events.[32]

Gaviscon Infant is licensed for use from birth.[33] However, the summary of product characteristics states that in premature infants or infants <1 year old it should be used only under medical supervision. It is contraindicated in those with known or suspected impairment of renal function, where excessive water loss is likely, or when there is intestinal obstruction. Also, it should not be given with other preparations that contain thickening agents. The licensed dose of Gaviscon Infant for children weighing <4.5 kg is one dose (half of a dual sachet) mixed with each feed (or water, for breastfed infants), and for those weighing .4.5 kg is two doses. It should not be administered more than six times in 24 hours.

Drugs to reduce gastric acid secretion

Infants with severe GORD—such as those who are unresponsive to dietary and lifestyle changes or to an alginate combination, or those with complications such as suspected oesophagitis or a respiratory disorder—need to be referred to a paediatrician for further investigation and possibly treatment to reduce gastric acid secretion (such as with H_2 receptor antagonists or proton pump inhibitors).[30]

H_2 receptor antagonists

In one non-blinded randomised controlled trial in 33 children aged 2–42 months with GORD and reflux oesophagitis, cimetidine (20 mg/kg/day) for 12 weeks was as effective as high doses of antacid in reducing reflux and oesophagitis as assessed clinically (P<0.05) and by pH monitoring and endoscopy.[34] In a randomised placebo controlled trial involving 35 infants aged 1.3–10.5 months with gastro-oesophageal reflux, oral famotidine 1.0 mg/kg reduced crying time (P=0.027) and regurgitation frequency (P=0.004) and volume (P=0.01), while famotidine 0.5 mg/kg reduced regurgitation frequency only (P=0.04).[35] We could find no randomised controlled trials of ranitidine for GORD in infants.

In the UK, the only two H$_2$ receptor antagonists licensed for treating GORD in children are cimetidine and ranitidine. The summary of product characteristics for cimetidine states that, for those aged <1 year, the drug has not been fully evaluated but that an oral dose of 20 mg/kg daily in divided doses "has been used."[36] However, cimetidine is not considered suitable for inclusion in the *BNF for Children* by the Paediatric Formulary Committee and is rarely used in practice.[30] The summary of product characteristics for ranitidine gives an intravenous infusion regimen for infants aged >6 months.[37] The *BNF for Children* recommends an oral dose of ranitidine of 1 mg/kg three times daily (up to a maximum of 3 mg/kg three times daily) for infants aged 1–6 months and 2–4 mg/kg twice daily for those aged 6–12 months, or a slow intravenous injection dose of 0.5–1 mg/kg every 6–8 hours for neonates and 1 mg/kg every 6–8 hours for infants aged .1 month.[30] Unwanted effects of H$_2$ receptor antagonists in infants include gastrointestinal disturbances such as diarrhoea, rash, agitation and irritability, head rubbing and headache, and somnolence.[30] [35] Reassessment is necessary if symptoms persist after four to six weeks of treatment with ranitidine.[30]

Proton pump inhibitors

In one double blind, randomised, placebo controlled trial including 10 preterm infants with gastro-oesophageal reflux, oral omeprazole 0.7 mg/kg daily for seven days reduced gastric acidity (P<0.0005), oesophageal acid exposure (P<0.01), and the number and duration of acid gastro-oesophageal reflux episodes (P<0.05 and P<0.01, respectively).[38] In another such trial including 162 infants with clinically diagnosed GORD, oral lansoprazole (0.2–0.3 mg/kg daily for infants aged ,10 weeks and 1.0–1.5 mg daily for those aged >10 weeks) was no more effective than placebo for GORD symptoms. However, more of the infants given lansoprazole developed serious unwanted effects, particularly lower respiratory tract infections (10 v 2 infants with placebo, P=0.032).[39]

Omeprazole is licensed for children aged >1 year with GORD with severe symptoms.[30] However, no marketed proton pump inhibitors are licensed for GORD in infants. For omeprazole, the *BNF for Children* recommends an oral dose of 0.7 mg/kg once daily for infants, which can be increased if necessary after 7–14 days to 1.4 mg/kg (maximum 2.8 mg/kg) in neonates (aged <1 month) and to 3 mg/kg (maximum 20 mg) in infants aged .1 month. The *BNF for Children* states that lansoprazole may be considered when the available formulations of omeprazole are unsuitable and recommends an oral dose of 0.5–1 mg/kg (maximum 15 mg) once daily in the morning for children weighing under 30 kg. Unwanted effects have been reported in around 2–15% of children taking proton pump inhibitors[40] [41] and include gastrointestinal disturbances and headache.[30]

Increasing evidence suggests that acid suppression with proton pump inhibitors or H$_2$ receptor antagonists may increase rates of gastroenteritis (in infants aged >4 months), candidaemia (in infants in neonatal intensive care), and necrotising enterocolitis (in very low birthweight infants).[42] [43] [44]

Other drugs

Antacids directly buffer gastric contents, thereby potentially reducing heartburn and healing oesophagitis. However, evidence of benefit in infants is unclear, and antacids containing aluminium should not be used in infants aged <1 year because accumulation may lead to increased plasma aluminium concentrations.[30] Neither simeticone (activated dimeticone) nor sucralfate (a complex of aluminium hydroxide and sulphated sucrose) has a place in treating GORD in infants.[30]

Motility stimulants increase oesophageal sphincter pressure and stimulate gastric emptying. Cisapride is an example of a motility stimulant that was widely used for infant gastro-oesophageal reflux.[1] However, it has been withdrawn from the market in most countries, including the UK, because it prolongs the QTc interval, increasing the likelihood of sudden death.[45] Domperidone and metoclopramide are dopamine receptor antagonists that have been used to treat GORD, but neither is licensed for this use in infants and both can cause acute dystonic reactions.[1] [30] Furthermore, an association between domperidone and prolongation of QTc interval in infants has been reported,[46] and metoclopramide has caused tardive dyskinesia.[30] A systematic review of domperidone identified only four randomised controlled trials in children, which provided "very little evidence" for the drug's efficacy in paediatric GORD.[47] A recent randomised controlled trial found a paradoxical increase in the number of gastro-oesophageal reflux episodes in newborns given domperidone.[48] A systematic review, which included 12 studies of metoclopramide (five blinded and randomised) involving a total of 343 children (aged 0–23 months) with symptoms of gastro-oesophageal reflux, found that the available evidence did not show a clinically significant benefit or any harm with the drug.[49] By contrast, another systematic review (described above) found evidence that metoclopramide reduced the number of daily symptoms (standard mean difference 0.72, 0.98 to 0.45) and reflux index (0.43, 0.72 to 0.14) compared with placebo in infants with GORD.[25]

Surgery

Surgery may help selected children with severe GORD for whom optimum medical therapy has failed or who have life threatening complications. However, it is thought to have a relatively high failure rate and some complications.[50] [51]

1 Managing childhood gastro-oesophageal reflux. *DTB*1997;35:77–80.
2 Vandenplas Y, Rudolph CD, Di Lorenzo C, Hassall E, Liptak G, Mazur L, et al. Pediatric gastroesophageal reflux clinical practice guidelines: joint recommendations of the North American Society of Pediatric Gastroenterology, Hepatology, and Nutrition and the European Society of Pediatric Gastroenterology, Hepatology, and Nutrition. *J Pediatr Gastroenterol Nutr*2009;49:498–547.
3 Khoshoo V, Edell D, Thompson A, Rubin M. Are we overprescribing antireflux medications for infants with regurgitation? *Pediatrics*2007;120:946–9.
4 Barron JJ, Tan H, Spalding J, Bakst AW, Singer J. Proton pump inhibitor utilization patterns in infants. *J Pediatr Gastroenterol Nutr*2007;45:421–7.
5 Newell SJ, Booth IW, Morgan ME, Durbin GM, McNeish AS. Gastro-oesophageal reflux in preterm infants. *Arch Dis Child*1989;64:780–6.
6 Nelson SP, Chen EH, Syniar GM, Kaufer Christoffel K. Prevalence of symptoms of gastroesophageal reflux during infancy. A pediatric practice-based survey. *Arch Pediatr Adolesc Med*1997;151:569–72.
7 Nielsen RG, Bindslev-Jensen C, Kruse-Andersen S, Husby S. Severe gastroesophageal reflux disease and cow milk hypersensitivity in infants and children: disease association and evaluation of a new challenge procedure. *J Pediatr Gastroenterol Nutr*2004;39:383–91.

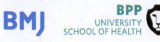

8   Iacono G, Carroccio A, Cavataio F, Montalto G, Kazmierska I, Lorello D, et al. Gastroesophageal reflux and cow's milk allergy in infants: a prospective study. *J Allergy Clin Immunol*1996;97:822–7.

9   Davies AEM, Sandhu BK. Diagnosis and treatment of gastro-oesophageal reflux. *Arch Dis Child*1995;73:82–6.

10 Vandenplas Y. Reflux esophagitis in infants and children: a report from the working group on gastro-oesophageal reflux disease of the European Society of Paediatric Gastroenterology and Nutrition. *J Pediatr Gastroenterol Nutr*1994;18:413–22.

11 Tolia V, Vandenplas Y. Systematic review: the extra-oesophageal symptoms of gastro-oesophageal reflux disease in children. *Aliment Pharmacol Ther*2009;29:258–72.

12 Hrabovsky EE, Mullett MD. Gastroesophageal reflux and the premature infant. *J Pediatr Surg*1986;21:583–7.

13 Birch JL, Newell SJ. Gastroesophageal reflux disease in preterm infants—current management and diagnostic dilemmas. *Arch Dis Child Fetal Neonatal Ed*2009 published online doi:10.1136/adc.2008.149112.

14 Wenzl TG. Evaluation of gastroesophageal reflux events in children using multichannel intraluminal electrical impedance. *Am J Med*2003;115:161–5S.

15 Dahms BB. Reflux oesophagitis: sequelae and differential diagnosis in infants and children including eosinophilic esophagitis. *Pediatr Dev Pathol*2004;7:5–16.

16 Meyers WF, Roberts CC, Johnson DG, Herbst JJ. Value of tests for evaluation of gastroesophageal reflux in children. *J Pediatr Surg*1985;20:515–20.

17 Simanovsky N, Buonomo C, Nurko S. The infant with chronic vomiting: the value of the upper GI series. *Pediatr Radiol*2002;32:549–50.

18 Barak M, Lahav S, Mimouni FB, Dollberg S. The prevalence of regurgitations in the first 2 days of life in human milk- and formula-fed term infants. *Breastfeed Med*2006;1:168–71.

19 Cavataio F, Iacono G, Montalto G, Soresi M, Tumminello M, Carroccio A. Clinical and pH-metric characteristics of gastro-oesophageal reflux secondary to cows' milk protein allergy. *Arch Dis Child*1996;75:51–6.

20 Semeniuk J, Kaczmarski M. Gastroesophageal reflux in children and adolescents. Clinical aspects with special respect to food hypersensitivity. *Adv Med Sci*2006;51:327–35.

21 Hill DJ, Heine RG, Cameron DJ, Catto-Smith AG, Chow CW, Francis DE, et al. Role of food protein intolerance in infants with persistent distress attributed to reflux oesophagitis. *J Pediatr*2000;136:641–7.

22 Ferry GD, Selby M, Pietro TJ. Clinical response to short-term nasogastric feeding in infants with gastroesophageal reflux and growth failure. *J Pediatr Gastroenterol Nutr*1983;2:57–61.

23 Horvath A, Dziechciarz P, Szajewska H.The effect of thickened-feed interventions on gastroesophageal reflux in infants: systematic review and meta-analysis of randomized, controlled trials. *Pediatrics*2008;122:e1268–77.

24 Chao HC, Vandenplas Y. Comparison of the effect of a cornstarch thickened formula and strengthened regular formula on regurgitation, gastric emptying and weight gain in infantile regurgitation. *Dis Esophagus*2007;20:155–60.

25 Craig WR, Hanlon-Dearman A, Sinclair C, Taback SP, Moffatt M. Metoclopramide, thickened feedings, and positioning for gastro-oesophageal reflux in children under two years. *Cochrane Database Syst Rev*2004;(3):CD003502.

26 Corvaglia L, Rotatori R, Ferlini M, Aceti A, Ancora G, Faldella G. The effect of body positioning on gastroesophageal reflux in premature infants: evaluation by combined impedance and pH monitoring. *J Pediatr*2007;151:591–6.

27 Van Wijk MP, Benninga MA, Dent J, Lontis R, Goodchild L, McCall LM, et al. Effect of body position changes on postprandial gastroesophageal reflux and gastric emptying in the healthy premature neonate. *J Pediatr*2007;151:585–90.

28 American Academy of Pediatrics Task Force on Sudden Infant Death Syndrome. The changing concept of sudden infant death syndrome: diagnostic coding shifts, controversies regarding the sleeping environment, and new variables to consider in reducing risk. *Pediatrics*2005;116:1245–55.

29 Tighe MP, Afzal NA, Bevan A, Beattie RM. Current pharmacological management of gastro-esophageal reflux in children: an evidence-based systematic review. *Paediatr Drugs*2009;11:185–202.

30 Paediatric Formulary Committee. *BNF for children 2009*. BMJ Group, RPS Publishing, 2009.

31 Miller S. Comparison of the efficacy and safety of a new aluminium-free paediatric alginate preparation and placebo in infants with recurrent gastro-oesophageal reflux. *Curr Med Res Opin*1999;15:160–8.

32 Del Buono R, Wenzl TG, Ball G, Keady S, Thomson M. Effect of Gaviscon Infant on gastro-oesophageal reflux in infants assessed by combined intraluminal impedance/pH. *Arch Dis Child*2005;90:460–3.

33 *Gaviscon Infant. Summary of product characteristics, UK.* Reckitt Benckiser Healthcare (UK), August 2003.

34 Cucchiara S, Staiano A, Romaniello G, Capobianco S, Auricchio S. Antacids and cimetidine treatment for gastro-oesophageal reflux and peptic oesophagitis. *Arch Dis Child*1984;59:842–7.

35 Orenstein SR, Shalaby TM, Devandry SN, Liacouras CA, Czinn SJ, Dice JE, et al. Famotidine for infant gastro-oesophageal reflux: a multi-centre, randomized, placebo-controlled, withdrawal trial. *Aliment Pharmacol Ther*2003;17:1097–107.

36 *Tagamet syrup. Summary of product characteristics, UK.* Chemidex Pharma, February 2009.

37 *Zantac injection 50mg/2mL. Summary of product characteristics, UK.* Glaxo Wellcome UK, March 2009.

38 Omari TI, Haslam RR, Lundborg P, Davidson GP. Effect of omeprazole on acid gastroesophageal reflux and gastric acidity in preterm infants with pathological acid reflux. *J Pediatr Gastroenterol Nutr*2007;44:41–4.

39 Orenstein SR, Hassall E, Furmaga-Jablonska W, Atkinson S, Raanan M. Multicenter, double-blind, randomized, placebo-controlled trial assessing the efficacy and safety of proton pump inhibitor lansoprazole in infants with symptoms of gastroesophageal reflux disease. *J Pediatr*2009;154:514–20.

40 Hassall E, Kerr W, El-Serag HB. Characteristics of children receiving proton pump inhibitors continuously for up to 11 years duration. *J Pediatr*2007;150:262–7.

41 Tolia V, Fitzgerald J, Hassall E, Huang B, Pilmer B, Kane R 3rd. Safety of lansoprazole in the treatment of gastroesophageal reflux disease in children. *J Pediatr Gastroenterol Nutr*2002;35:S300–7.

42 Canani RB, Cirillo P, Roggero P, Romano C, Malamisura B, Terrin G, et al. Therapy with gastric acidity inhibitors increases the risk of acute gastroenteritis and community-acquired pneumonia in children. *Pediatrics*2006;117:e817–20.

43 Guillet R, Stoll BJ, Cotten CM, Gantz M, McDonald S, Poole WK, et al. Association of H2-blocker therapy and higher incidence of necrotizing enterocolitis in very low birth weight infants. *Pediatrics*2006;117:137–42.

44 Saiman L, Ludington E, Dawson JD, Patterson JE, Rangel-Frausto S, Wiblin RT, et al. Risk factors for candida species colonization of neonatal intensive care unit patients. *Pediatr Infect Dis J*2001;20:1119–24.

45 Perrio M, Voss S, Shakir SA. Application of the Bradford Hill criteria to assess the causality of cisapride-induced arrhythmia: a model for assessing causal association in pharmacovigilance. *Drug Saf*2007;30:333–46.

46 Djeddi D, Kongolo G, Lefaix C, Mounard J, Léké A. Effect of domperidone on QT interval in neonates. *J Pediatr*2008;153:663–6.

47 Pritchard DS, Baber N, Stephenson T. Should domperidone be used for the treatment of gastro-oesophageal reflux in children? Systematic review of randomized controlled trials in children aged 1 month to 11 years old. *Br J Clin Pharmacol*2005;59:725–9.

48 Cresi F, Marinaccio C, Russo MC, Miniero R, Silvestro L. Short-term effect of domperidone on gastroesophageal reflux in newborns assessed by combined intraluminal impedance and pH monitoring. *J Perinatol*2008;28:766–70.

49 Hibbs AM, Lorch SA. Metoclopramide for the treatment of gastroesophageal reflux disease in infants: a systematic review. *Pediatrics*2006;118:746–52.

50 Hassall E. Outcomes of fundoplication: causes for concern, newer options. *Arch Dis Child*2005;90:1047–52.

51 Lobe TE. The current role of laparoscopic surgery for gastroesophageal reflux disease in infants and children. *Surg Endosc*2007;21:167–74.

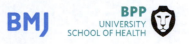

Weight faltering and failure to thrive in infancy and early childhood

Brian Shields paediatric specialty registrar[1], Ian Wacogne consultant paediatrician[1],
Charlotte M Wright professor of community child health/consultant paediatrician[2]

[1]Department of General Paediatrics,
Birmingham Children's Hospital,
Birmingham B4 6NH, UK

[2]Paediatric Epidemiology and
Community Health Unit, School
of Medicine, College of Medical,
Veterinary, and Life Sciences,
University of Glasgow, Glasgow, UK

Correspondence to: I Wacogne
Ian.wacogne@bch.nhs.uk

Cite this as: BMJ 2012;345:e5931

‹DOI› 10.1136/bmj.e5931
http://www.bmj.com/content/345/
bmj.e5931

Weight faltering, or failure to thrive, is a childhood condition that provokes concern about possible neglect, deprivation, and organic illness. However, research over the past 20 years has brought the validity of this concern into question, leading to the proposal that management should be less aggressive.[1] We summarise the evidence base, discuss new developments, and provide a practical approach to management. Failure to thrive has been defined in a range of ways, with no overall accepted definition[2] but an essential element is subnormal growth or weight gain, hence the increasing use in recent years of the term weight faltering.

What is normal growth?

Growth charts rank a child's measurements against children of the same age and sex. If a child gains weight more slowly than their peers, their measurement moves to a lower centile (crosses centiles). The World Health Organization has proposed that its growth standards, based on healthy, relatively affluent, breastfed infants from six countries, should be used to represent healthy growth for babies internationally.[3] These standards, along with UK birth and preterm growth data, have been incorporated into the UK-WHO growth charts[4] as well as being adopted in other countries worldwide. Studies that assessed the growth pattern of representative samples of European children compared with these new charts found that these children tended to gain weight more rapidly.[5] As a result, for example, only around 0.5% of UK children will be below the 2nd centile at 12 months.[6] Previous epidemiological studies have shown that while healthy children will usually roughly progress along the same centile, moderate movements up and down the chart are common.[7] The weights of larger babies tend to fall towards the average over time, while those of smaller babies move upwards: the phenomenon of regression to the mean.[8]

SOURCES AND SELECTION CRITERIA

We searched Pubmed, Medline, Embase, and the Cochrane Database of Systemic Reviews with key reference terms "failure to thrive," "growth faltering," and "weight faltering." We reviewed citations from key articles. We also used our personal archive of references.

SUMMARY

- Weight faltering is not a disease, but rather a description of a relatively common growth pattern
- It is most commonly caused by undernutrition relative to a child's specific energy requirements
- Causes tend to be multifactorial and often involve problems with diet and feeding behaviour that usually respond to simple targeted advice
- More rarely, weight faltering may be associated with neglect or maternal mental health problems or addiction
- The health visitor (public health nurse) is often best placed to assess and advise in the first instance
- Organic disease is rare in otherwise asymptomatic children, but it is reasonable to rule out organic disease if dietary and behavioural interventions are unsuccessful

What is weight faltering?

Weight faltering describes a weight gain pattern rather than a diagnosis. It represents a spectrum from what may simply be a normal variant to children with serious problems. In clinical practice, a weight that crosses more than two major centile spaces downwards is often the recommended threshold for concern[1] (a centile space is the distance between two major centile lines). On UK growth charts from 1990 this pattern would be seen in around 5% children, but on the new UK-WHO charts, centile crossing is much less common; a recent analysis of UK population based data suggest that after the first four months as few as 0.5% average children will cross two centile spaces.[9] Regression to the mean describes how smaller babies will grow faster than larger babies and both will move towards the mean weight. Research assessment of weight gain uses a calculation of "conditional weight gain" to allow for regression to the mean automatically, but it is not feasible to use this approach in clinical practice.

What causes weight faltering?

It is plausible that weight faltering will occur as a consequence of inadequate nutrition, since energy requirements in infancy are very high.[10] Observational studies of children with weight faltering have found that they eat less at test meals.[11] [12] There is also evidence that children with weight faltering show growth patterns suggesting chronic undernutrition. A study of children with weight faltering identified by population screening found that on average they had low body mass index and showed subsequent catch up weight gain,[13] [14] while a more recent cohort study found that children with both slow conditional weight gain and low body mass index went on to be relatively stunted in later childhood.[9]

Explaining why these children become undernourished is complex and the cause is usually multifactorial. Here we review the evidence for and against the roles of several factors that have been associated with weight faltering.

Organic disease

The traditional model of classifying causes of weight faltering as organic or non-organic is overly simplistic and places too much emphasis on organic causes. Major organic causes of weight faltering are rare, while weight faltering itself is common. Two UK population based studies found substantial organic disease in only 5-10% of children with slow weight gain.[13] [15] The conditions found were heterogeneous but all featured clear symptoms or signs suggesting underlying disease. Two earlier hospital based studies in the United States[16] [17] found that investigation in asymptomatic children with failure to thrive yielded no substantial new diagnoses of organic disease. This evidence suggests that organic disease is unlikely in children who are asymptomatic and well on examination, so that investigations should be

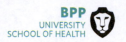

planned to rule out rare major conditions (table) rather than to identify a cause of the weight faltering.

Socioeconomic and educational status

Weight faltering has traditionally been seen as a manifestation of poverty. While this is still likely to be true in poorer societies, there is good evidence from three large, population based studies that in the United Kingdom there is no significant association between low socioeconomic status, poor educational attainment, and weight faltering.[18] [19] [20] All three studies identified children with slow conditional weight gain in infancy. One study[18] found no association with either social class or educational status, while the other two found weak U shaped associations, with slightly higher prevalence in the most and least deprived groups.[19] [20] This lack of association probably reflects the safety net of modern welfare systems, which prioritise support to families with young children.

Neglect

A cohort study of 97 children with weight faltering identified by population screening found evidence of neglect in only 5%.[13] However, another population based study found that the risk of being placed on the child protection register was four times higher in weight faltering children than in controls.[21] Thus, as neglect and abuse are rare and weight faltering common, so neglect may be seen more commonly in association with weight faltering, but most children with weight faltering are not neglected.

Feeding and eating difficulties

Several observational studies have shown that feeding difficulties such as low appetite, weak suck, and weaning difficulties are associated with weight faltering.[18] [20] [22] [23] Two observational case-control studies found associated differences in maternal feeding behaviour.[12] [24] For example, infants with weight faltering had significantly fewer positive interactions (where parents anticipate and support a child's needs) during meals than controls. It is not clear whether this association is causal or simply a maternal adaptive response to their child's eating behaviour.[24]

Maternal depression

One case-control study found an association between weight faltering and maternal depression; significantly more mothers in the weight faltering group scored above the threshold for depression on the Edinburgh Postnatal Depression Scale.[25] However, in three medium to large cohort studies one found no link,[26] another found an association that had disappeared by 12 months,[20] and a third it was only seen in later onset weight faltering.[27]

Variation with age

The population study of children with weight faltering described above found that although children were identified at a mean age of 15.5 months, the slowing of their weight gain began in the early weeks and 50% had already crossed the screening threshold by age 6 months.[13] A large whole population study found that weight faltering seen in the first 2 weeks of life was associated with perinatal factors such as preterm birth and maternal smoking, while later onset was associated with organic disease and feeding problems.[27]

What are the potential consequences of weight faltering?

A number of consequences have been postulated, including impaired growth, cognition, and behaviour. Early studies suggested major long term cognitive effects.[28] A systematic review and a meta-analysis both found only small effects (3-5 IQ points)[29] [30] and a similar result was found in a more recent cohort study.[31]

Weight faltering children in two population based studies followed up at age 6-9 years were found to be significantly shorter and lighter and to have smaller heads than controls.[15] [32] A randomised control trial found that children receiving a primary care based intervention for weight faltering were heavier and taller at age 4 years than untreated controls,[14] suggesting that growth outcomes are potentially reversible. One systematic review, which included studies from developing countries, concluded that immune, gastrointestinal, and cardiac dysfunction recovered with correction of malnutrition, but other effects, such as impairment in cognition, attention, and behaviour, were permanent.[33]

In summary, current evidence suggests that weight faltering in infancy does have an effect on long term growth and may have a small effect on cognition.

How can a child with weight faltering be identified?

Concerns about weight faltering tend to arise as a result of routine weighing. All babies should be weighed during the first week as part of the assessment of feeding (usually around the time of immunisations) and at eight weeks, 12 weeks, 16 weeks, one year, and whenever concerns are raised.[34] The study described above suggested that a useful threshold for closer assessment is a fall through two centile spaces on the UK-WHO charts—although for infants with birth weights below the ninth centile, a fall through one centile space should trigger concern, while infants above the 91st centile could be allowed to cross three centile spaces.[9] Weighing alone does not distinguish slow growth from thinness, so where there is concern length should also be measured.[4] The UK department of health guidance on the UK-WHO growth charts also suggests that children below the

Possible investigations to be undertaken in secondary care		
Investigation	**Indication**	**Condition being sought**
Full blood count	Any persistent weight faltering	Anaemia, leukaemia
Ferritin	Any persistent weight faltering	Iron deficiency
Urea and electrolytes	Any persistent weight faltering	Renal failure, electrolyte abnormalities
Thyroid function tests	Any persistent weight faltering	Thyroid disorders
Coeliac blood tests	Any persistent weight faltering	Coeliac disease
Midstream urine	Any persistent weight faltering	Urinary tract infection
Chromosome analysis	Girls	Turner's syndrome
Chest radiograph	Infants under 3 months; history of respiratory infection	Cardiac anomalies; cystic fibrosis
Sweat test	History of respiratory infection	Cystic fibrosis
Vitamin D levels	Solid diet is limited, dark skin colour	Rickets

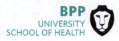
o.4th centile for weight or with a body mass index below the second centile should be carefully assessed,[34] but children with low weight, length, or body mass index along with weight faltering are probably most at risk.[9]

What history and examination are required?

The first necessity is to confirm that weight faltering is truly persistent and substantial: weight may dip sharply after minor illnesses, or a plotting error may have occurred. Measure and plot current weight and length, with re-plotting of previous measurements on an appropriate centile chart. Adjust for prematurity in infants born before 37 completed weeks, up to age 2 years. If both the weight and length centiles are low this suggests slow growth, rather than weight faltering, so measuring parental heights may also be informative.

If weight faltering is confirmed, exclude underlying medical problems by history and medical examination, including auscultation of the chest and assessment of whether neurodelopment is appropriate for age. Assuming this is normal, a thorough dietary history should then be taken by the member of the primary care team with most access to the family. In the United Kingdom this would be the health visitor, a public health nurse with responsibility to monitor all pre-school children, as they have good contextual family knowledge and can offer non-stigmatising advice. Some key areas that should be covered are:

- history of milk feeding
- age of weaning
- range and types of food now taken
- mealtime routine and eating and feeding behaviour
- ask the family to complete a three day food diary for a fuller and more accurate picture
- if possible observe a meal being taken

It is also important to probe for evidence of psychosocial factors such as maternal depression.

What investigations are required?

Investigations should not usually be undertaken in primary care, but should be deferred until paediatric assessment has taken place. Undertake investigations only if signs or symptoms of disease are present, or where weight faltering is persistent or severe. There is no formal evidence to suggest an ideal routine set of investigations, but the table shows a suggested schedule of tests to rule out possible pathology, which should usually be undertaken all at once to avoid multiple blood tests.

What management options are available for children with weight faltering?

Figure 1 shows a graded response to weight faltering.

Community-based management

Early studies of failure to thrive were hospital based, but in recent years structured ambulatory management has been recognised as more cost-effective.[35] It may also benefit development,[36] is more acceptable to patients and their families, and is more likely to succeed.[14] With appropriate training in mealtime observations and food diaries, health visitors can make wide ranging and effective assessments, and can support families to improve feeding and increase calorie intake (see box).

A trial in the United Kingdom of structured health visitor intervention, including basic dietetics training and regular follow-up, showed better growth in the trial group.[14] A US intervention trial of weekly home visits by trained lay home visitors versus follow-up in a multidisciplinary nutrition clinic showed similar improvements in weight and height for age in both groups, but the intervention group also showed better receptive language and cognitive development.[36] Another UK study comparing specialist health visitor intervention with conventional care showed no difference in weight outcomes, but the intervention group had 50% less hospital admissions and defaulted fewer hospital and health visitor appointments.[35] If such programmes are to succeed it is important for health visitors to be able to access specialist support, particularly for more complex or severe cases. Dietetic input is likely to be most commonly accessed.

Monitoring progress

The key measure of improvement should be recovery in the weight gain pattern—a rise up through the centiles (catch-up) that usually begins within four to eight weeks of a successful intervention such as dietary advice. Plotting on the neonatal and infant close monitoring chart allows detailed assessment of change over time and allows for gestation if the child was preterm.[37] It is still important not to measure too frequently. Optimal intervals and timings for measurement have not been formally established, but the Royal College of Paediatrics and Child Health suggest weighing no more than monthly

---

POSSIBLE STRATEGIES FOR INCREASING ENERGY INTAKE IN CHILDREN AGED OVER 9 MONTHS[33]

Dietary
- Three meals and two snacks each day
- Increase number and variety of foods offered
- Increase energy density of usual foods (for example, add cheese, margarine, cream)
- Limit milk intake to 500 mL per day
- Avoid excessive intake of fruit juice and squash

Behavioural
- Offer meals at regular times with other family members
- Praise when food is eaten, ignore when not
- Limit meal time to 30 minutes
- Eat at same time as child
- Avoid meal time conflict
- Never force feed

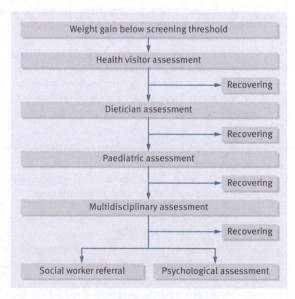

Fig 1 Graded response to weight faltering

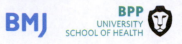

before age 6 months, every two months aged 6-12 months, and every three months after that.[34] A child can be said to have recovered once their current centile is within 1-2 centile spaces of their earlier position, which may take several months. Some children may show only partial recovery while others may remain within the same low centile. If such children are not markedly underweight for their height and their growth in length is steady and proportionate to their parental heights, it may have to be accepted that they are showing a variant pattern of normal growth.[9]

The role of specialist input

Dietician assessment

For confirmed weight faltering without medical features, refer initially to a paediatric trained dietician in most cases. Referral can usually only be done by the primary care doctor, but some pathways allow direct access through specialist health visitors. The primary role of the dietician is to optimise the existing diet and advise on meal time management, rather than to identify deficiencies. For this purpose a single home visit may be more effective than clinic review.[1] The dietician can assess the adequacy of the current diet to supply essential nutrients and offer targeted advice about enhancing the diet. Paediatric dieticians can also advise effectively on the management of basic feeding behavioural problems. Although high energy supplement drinks are often suggested for weight faltering, evidence from older children suggests that they do not improve weight gain[38] and may even depress solid food intake.[39 40]

Paediatrician

Given the value of community based management, infants need only be referred to a secondary care paediatrician if they show features suggesting an associated illness or have severe weight faltering (a fall through two or more centile spaces on the UK-WHO chart) that has persisted despite community and dietetic interventions. In practice all a paediatrician will to do is reassess the growth data, undertake investigations to exclude organic pathology, and then usually reinforce previous dietary advice.

Inpatient monitoring is not advisable, except in very extreme circumstances. Hospitals are an unnatural place in which to assess feeding and mother-child interaction and the risk of hospital acquired infection is present.

Social work

Weight faltering on its own, even if it is severe, does not require a social work referral. Referral is only appropriate in cases where the family has major social problems, such as drug or alcohol abuse, or where direct evidence suggests abuse or neglect. Families may lack adequate resources to ensure that a child is well nourished, and engagement of social services, treating these as "children in need," can enable families to access appropriate support.

Psychology

Indications for involvement from psychology include pronounced food refusal or very anxious, stressful mealtimes. A meal time video observation has been suggested as the basis for structured supportive feedback and advice as well as for working with the parents to control anxiety.[41]

Competing interests: All authors have completed the Unified Competing Interest form at http://www.icmje.org/coi_disclosure.pdf (available on request from the corresponding author) and declare: no support from any organisation for the submitted work; no financial relationships with any organisations that might have an interest in the submitted work in the previous three years, no other relationships or activities that could appear to have influenced the submitted work.

Provenance and peer review: Commissioned; externally peer reviewed.

TIPS FOR NON-SPECIALISTS

- Look at the weight gain pattern over time rather than single measurements
- Measure length in addition to weight whenever weight faltering is suspected
- Weight faltering is common in infancy and mostly occurs in otherwise healthy children living in non-neglecting environments
- Weight faltering can cause long term stunting and developmental delay if not reversed
- Involve the health visitor (public health nurse) before considering specialist referral
- A dietary assessment often reveals problems that respond well to simple advice
- High energy milks or supplement drinks are not likely to be helpful and should not be started in primary care

---

ADDITIONAL EDUCATIONAL RESOURCES

For clinicians

- UK-WHO 0-4 years growth chart resources (www.rcpch.ac.uk/child-health/research-projects/uk-who-growth-charts-early-years/uk-who-0-4-years-growth-charts-initi)—guidance from the Royal College of Paediatrics and Child Health
- Maternal and child nutrition (www.nice.org.uk/PH011)—NICE guidance for midwives, health visitors, pharmacists, and other primary care services to improve the nutrition of pregnant and breastfeeding mothers and children in low income households
- Faltering growth (www.gp-training.net/training/tutorials/clinical/paediatrics/pgrowth2.htm)—guidance on managing weight faltering in primary care

For patients

- Healthy eating (www.eatwell.gov.uk)—NHS guidance on healthy eating and nutrition for children, parents and families
- Your baby's first solid foods (www.nhs.uk/Conditions/pregnancy-and-baby/Pages/solid-foods-weaning.aspx)—NHS guidance on weaning infants

---

BOX: QUESTIONS FOR FUTURE RESEARCH:

- Do any behavioural interventions prevent weight faltering—for example, a baby led weaning approach to reduce the risk of force feeding by mothers and avoidant eating behaviours in the child?
- Are children with weight faltering more or less likely to go on to be obese as adults or to have long term health effects?

1 Wright CM. Identification and management of failure to thrive: a community perspective. *Arch Dis Child* 2000;82:5-9.
2 Olsen EM, Petersen J, Skovgaard AM, Weile B, Jørgensen T, Wright CM. Failure to thrive: the prevalence and concurrence of anthropometric criteria in a general infant population, *Arch Dis Child* 2007;92:109-114.
3 World Health Organization. The WHO child growth standards. 2009. www.who.int/childgrowth/en.
4 Wright CM, Williams AF, Elliman D, Bedford H, Birks E, Butler G, et al. Using the new UK-WHO growth charts *BMJ* 2010;340:c1140.
5 Juliusson PB, Roelants M, Hoppenbrouwers K, Hauspie R, Bjerknes R. Growth of Belgian and Norwegian children compared to the WHO growth standards: prevalence below -2 and above +2 SD and the effect of breastfeeding. *Arch Dis Child* 2011;96:916-21.
6 Wright C, Lakshman R, Emmett P, Ong KK. Implications of adopting the WHO 2006 Child Growth Standard in the UK: two prospective cohort studies. *Arch Dis Child* 2008;93:566-9.
7 Wright CM, Matthews JN, Waterston A, Aynsley-Green A. 1994a. What is a normal rate of weight gain in infancy? *Acta Paediatr* 1994;83:351-6.
8 Cole TJ. Conditional reference charts to assess weight gain in British infants. *Arch Dis Child* 1995;73:8-16.
9 Wright CM, Garcia A. 2012. Child under-nutrition in affluent societies: what are we talking about? *Proc Nutrition Soc* (forthcoming).
10 Committee on the medical aspects of food policy. Dietary reference values for food energy and nutrients for the UK. HMSO, 1991.
11 Parkinson KN, Wright CM, Drewett RF. Feeding behaviour and energy intake in children who fail to thrive. *J Reprod Infant Psychol* 2002;20:173.
12 Heptinstall E, Puckering C, Skuse D, Start K, Zur-Szpiro S, Dowdney I. Nutrition and meal time behaviour in families of growth-retarded children. *Hum Nutr Appl Nutr* 1987;41A:390-402.

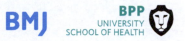

13 Wright C, Birks E. Risk factors for failure to thrive: a population-based survey. *Child Care Health Dev*2000;26:5-16.

14 Wright CM, Callum J, Birks E, Jarvis S. Effect of community based management in failure to thrive: randomised controlled trial. *BMJ*1998;317:571-4.

15 Drewett R, Corbett S, Wright C. Cognitive and educational attainments at school age of children failed to thrive in infancy: a population based study. *J Child Psychol Psychiatr*1999;40:551-61.

16 Homer C, Ludwig S. 1981. Categorization of etiology of failure to thrive. *Am J Dis Child* 135:848-51.

17 Sills RH.. Failure to thrive. The role of clinical and laboratory evaluation. *Am J Dis Child*1978;132:967-9.

18 Emond A, Drewett R, Blair P, Emmett P. Postnatal factors associated with failure to thrive in term infants in the Avon Longitudinal Study of Parents and Children. *Arch Dis Child*2007;92:115-9.

19 Wright CM, Waterston A, Aynsley-Green A. 1994b. The effect of deprivation on weight gain in infancy. *Acta Paediatrica*1994;83:357-9.

20 Wright CM, Parkinson KN, Drewett RF. The influence of maternal socioeconomic and emotional factors on infant weight gain and weight faltering (failure to thrive): data from a prospective birth cohort. *Arch Dis Child*2006;91:312-7.

21 Skuse DH, Gill D, Reilly S, Wolke D, Lynch MA. Failure to thrive and the risk of child abuse: a prospective population survey. *J Med Screen*1995;2:145-9.

22 McDougall P, Drewett RF, Hungin AP, Wright CM. The detection of early weight faltering at the 6-8-week check and its association with family factors, feeding and behavioural development. *Arch Dis Child*2009;94:549-52.

23 Reilly SM, Skuse DH, Wolke D, Stevenson J. Oral-motor dysfunction in children who fail to thrive: organic or non-organic? *Dev Med Child Neurol*1999;41:115-22.

24 Robertson J, Puckering C, Parkinson K, Corlett L, Wright C. Mother-child feeding interactions in children with and without weight faltering; nested case control study. *Appetite*2011;56:753-9.

25 O'Brien LM, Heycock EG, Hanna M, Jones PW, Cox JL. Postnatal depression and faltering growth: a community study. *Pediatrics* 200;113:1242-7.

26 Drewett R, Blair P, Emmett P, Emond A. Failure to thrive in the term and preterm infants of mothers depressed in the postnatal period: a population-based birth cohort study. *J Child Psychol Psychiatry*2004;45:359-66.

27 Olsen EM, Skovgaard AM, Weile B, Petersen J, Jørgensen T. Risk factors for weight faltering in infancy according to age at onset. *Paediatr Perinat Epidemiol*2010;24:370-82.

28 Dowdney l, Skuse D, Heptinstall E, Puckering C, Zur-Szpiro S. Growth retardation and developmental delay among inner-city children. *J Child Psychol Psychiatr*1987;28:529-41.

29 Rudolf MCJ, Logan S. What is the long term outcome for children who fail to thrive? A systematic review. *Arch Dis Child*2005;90:925-31.

30 Corbett SS, Drewett RF. To what extent is failure to thrive in infancy associated with poorer cognitive development? A review and meta-analysis. *J Child Psychol Psychiatry*2004;45:641-54.

31 Emond AM, Blair PS, Emmett PM, Drewett RF. Weight faltering in infancy and IQ levels at 8 years in the Avon Longitudinal Study of Parents and Children. *Pediatrics*2007;120:e1051-8.

32 Boddy J, Skuse D, Andrews B. The developmental sequelae of nonorganic failure to thrive. *J Child Psychol Psychiatry*2000;41:1003-14.

33 Perrin EC, Frank DA, Cole CH. Criteria for determining disability in infants and children: failure to thrive. Evidence reports/technology assessments, no 72. Agency for Healthcare Research and Quality (US), 2003.

34 UK Department of Health. Using the new UK-World Health Organization 0-4 years growth charts: information for healthcare professionals about the use and interpretation of growth charts. Department of Health, 2009.

35 Raynor P, Rudolf M, Cooper K, Marchant P, Cottrell D. A randomised controlled trial of specialist health visitor intervention for failure to thrive. *Arch Dis Child*1999;80:500-05.

36 Black MM, Dubowitz H, Hutcheson J, Berenson-Howard J, Starr RH Jr. A randomized clinical trial of home intervention for children with failure to thrive *Pediatrics*1995;95:807-14.

37 Cole TJ, Wright CM, Williams AF, RCPCH Growth Chart Expert Group. Designing the new UK-WHO growth charts to enhance assessment of growth around birth. *Arch Dis Child Fetal Neonatal Ed*2012;97:F219-22.

38 Poustie VJ, Russell JE, Watling RM, Ashby D, Smyth RL. Oral protein energy supplements for children with cystic fibrosis: CALICO multicentre randomised controlled trial. *BMJ*2006;332:632-6.

39 Kasese-Hara M, Wright C, Drewett R. Energy compensation in young children who fail to thrive. *J Child Psychol Psychiatry*2002;43:449-56.

40 Parkinson KN, Wright CM, Drewett RF. Mealtime energy intake and feeding behaviour in children who fail to thrive: a population-based case-control study. *J Child Psychol Psychiatry*2004;45:1030-5.

41 Skuse D. Identification and management of problem eaters. *Arch Dis Child*1993;69:604-8.

Related links

bmj.com/archive
Previous articles in this series
- Preimplantation genetic testing (2012;345:e5908)
- Early fluid resuscitation in severe trauma (2012;345:e5752)
- Irritable bowel syndrome (2012;345:e5836)
- Management of renal colic (2012;345:e5499)
- Diagnosis and management of peripheral arterial disease (2012;345:e5208)Tips for non-specialists

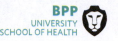

Managing cows' milk allergy in children

Sian Ludman paediatric allergy registrar[1], Neil Shah consultant paediatric gastroenterologist[23], Adam T Fox consultant paediatric allergist[14]

[1]Children's Allergy Service, Guy's and St Thomas' NHS Foundation Trust, London SE1 9RT, UK

[2]Paediatric Gastroenterology Department, Great Ormond Street Hospital, London, UK

[3]TARGID, KU Leuven University, Belgium

[4]Division of Asthma, Allergy and Lung Biology, MRC and Asthma UK Centre in Allergic Mechanisms of Asthma, King's College London, UK

Correspondence to: T Fox adam_fox@btinternet.com

Cite this as: BMJ 2013;347:f5424

<DOI> 10.1136/bmj.f5424
http://www.bmj.com/content/347/bmj.f5424

Cows' milk allergy mainly affects young children and because it is often outgrown is less commonly seen in older children and adults. It is one of the most common childhood food allergies in the developed world, second to egg allergy,[1] affecting 2-7.5% of children under 1 year of age.[2] The mainstay of treatment is to remove cows' milk protein from the diet while ensuring the nutritional adequacy of any alternative.

Cows' milk allergy can often be recognised and managed in primary care. Patients warranting a referral to specialist care include those with severe reactions, faltering growth, atopic comorbidities, multiple food allergies, complex symptoms, diagnostic uncertainty, and incomplete resolution after cows' milk protein has been excluded.

Although there are non-immune reactions to cows' milk, such as primary lactose intolerance (when malabsorption of sugar can cause bloating and diarrhoea), these are extremely rare in very young children. Except after a gastrointestinal infection, infants with gastrointestinal symptoms on exposure to cows' milk are more likely to have cows' milk allergy than lactose intolerance. This article focuses on immune mediated reactions to cows' milk in children and reviews the evidence on how to diagnose and manage the condition

What is cows' milk allergy?

Cows' milk allergy is an immune mediated reaction to proteins within milk.[3] Milk contains casein and whey fractions, each of which have five protein components. Patients can be sensitised to one or more components within either group.

Cows' milk allergies are classified according to the underlying mechanism, which affects the presentation, diagnosis, treatment, and prognosis. IgE mediated allergy is an immediate type (type 1) hypersensitivity reaction that occurs rapidly after exposure, usually within 20 minutes.

One of the main causes of symptoms is histamine release, and the symptoms are highlighted in table 1.

Non-IgE mediated allergy is a delayed type (type 4) hypersensitivity reaction that seems to be equally common but less well described than IgE mediated cows' milk allergy. Non-IgE mediated milk allergy can occasionally cause a severe form of allergic reaction with acute gastrointestinal symptoms that can mimic sepsis (food protein induced enterocolitis syndrome). However, the T cell mediated reactions are usually more delayed and are often chronic because of continued milk exposure during infancy. Typical symptoms are largely gastrointestinal or cutaneous (table 1).[4] The high frequency of such symptoms in infants without cows' milk allergy, combined with the lack of an immediate temporal relation with milk exposure or any clinical tests, can make non-IgE mediated allergy difficult to diagnose.

How does it present?

IgE mediated allergy usually manifests within minutes but no longer than 2 hours after ingestion of cows' milk protein. Symptoms include angioedema of the oropharynx, oral pruritus, urticaria, and rhinorrhoea. Although most reactions are mild, around 15% may be more severe with features of anaphylaxis such as stridor or wheeze.[5]

Non-IgE mediated allergy presents with more non-specific symptoms that are often chronic because of regular consumption. The most common presentations are treatment resistant gastro-oesophageal reflux, eczema, colic or persistent crying, diarrhoea (sometimes with mucous or blood), food aversion, and, less commonly, constipation. Gastrointestinal symptoms are thought to be due to gastrointestinal inflammation and associated dysmotility.

Who is affected?

Cows' milk allergy affects all ages but is most prevalent in infancy, affecting 2-7% of formula fed infants.[2] It can present in the first month of life and is one of the most common food allergies. Exclusively breast fed babies can also develop cows' milk allergy as a result of protein in the maternal diet transferring through breast milk.[6]

Predicting which children will develop a food allergy is difficult, but the presence of atopic dermatitis is a risk factor for developing sensitisation to common food allergens. The earlier the atopic dermatitis starts and the more severe it is, the higher the risk of food allergy. Hence there should be the highest index of suspicion of IgE mediated allergy in infants with moderate to severe atopic dermatitis that starts in the first six months of life.[7][8][9]

A family history of atopy is a risk factor for developing food allergies, although only an allergic predisposition is inherited not specific allergies.[10] Associated atopic comorbidities, especially asthma, are a risk factor for more severe reactions to milk.[5] The frequency of severe reactions is higher in asthmatic children, especially those with poorly controlled asthma, than in those without asthma.[5] The

SOURCES AND SELECTION CRITERIA

Our search included PubMed, the Cochrane Collaboration using the search terms "Cow's milk allergy," "milk allergy," "natural history," "management," and "treatment." When possible, evidence from randomised controlled trials and systematic reviews were used, although case series and observational studies were also included. We referenced expert review articles and used expert clinical opinion.

SUMMARY POINTS

- Cows' milk allergy is common, occurring in up to 7% of children and usually presents in infancy
- Allergy may be IgE mediated with rapid onset of symptoms such as urticaria or angioedema or non-IgE mediated, producing more delayed symptoms such as eczema, gastro-oesophageal reflux, or diarrhoea
- Management is by exclusion of cows' milk protein from the diet (including from the diet of a breastfeeding mother) under dietetic supervision
- Most children with milk allergy outgrow it (average age 5 years for IgE mediated and majority by age 3 years for uncomplicated non-IgE mediated allergy)

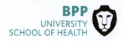

Table 1 Symptoms and signs of IgE and non-IgE mediated cows' milk allergy[4]

IgE mediated	Non-IgE mediated
Skin	
Pruritus	Pruritus
Erythema	Erythema
Acute urticaria—localised or generalised	Atopic eczema
Acute angioedema—most commonly lips, face, and around eyes	
Gastrointestinal system	
Angioedema of the lips, tongue, and palate	Gastro-oesophageal reflux disease
Oral pruritus	Loose or frequent stools
Nausea	Blood or mucus in stools
Colicky abdominal pain	Abdominal pain
Vomiting	Infantile colic
Diarrhoea	Food refusal or aversion
	Constipation
	Perianal redness
	Pallor or tiredness
	Faltering growth in conjunction with at least one of above gastrointestinal symptoms (with or without atopic eczema)
Respiratory system (usually in combination with one or more of above symptoms and signs)	
Upper respiratory tract symptoms (nasal itching, sneezing, rhinorrhoea, stridor, or congestion ± conjunctivitis)	Lower respiratory tract symptoms (cough, chest tightness, wheezing, or shortness of breath)
Lower respiratory tract symptoms (cough, chest tightness, wheezing, or shortness of breath)	
Other	
Signs or symptoms of anaphylaxis or other systemic allergic reactions	

underlying mechanisms that cause initial sensitisation to milk remain unclear.

What are the symptoms?

An allergy focused history is vital in establishing whether cows' milk allergy is a potential diagnosis in patients presenting with suggestive symptoms. The investigations depend on whether the clinician suspects an IgE or non-IgE mediated allergy. The history should elicit the symptoms and how quickly they occur after ingestion of cows' milk protein, how long they last, their severity, and which treatments were implemented and their effects.

It is important to distinguish children with non-IgE mediated cows' milk allergy from those who have gastro-oesophageal reflux or eczema with other causes. Clinical clues lie in the severity of the symptoms and treatment resistance, both of which make underlying milk allergy more likely. A dose dependent relation to any change in milk protein consumption—for example, when moving from breast to bottle feeding—may also provide useful insight. The presence of symptoms in more than one system also suggests a possible unifying underlying cause—for example, gastro-oesophageal reflux or diarrhoea in infants with atopic dermatitis.[11]

As well as exploring the symptoms in table 1,[4] doctors should ask about other symptoms of atopy such as atopic dermatitis or seasonal allergic rhinitis (hay fever) and asthma in older children. Any family history of atopy should also be documented, as well as the foods that the parents have already removed from the child's diet, and the effect of exclusions and subsequent food challenges.

How is cows' milk allergy investigated?

Once clinical suspicion has guided the clinician towards a diagnosis, appropriate investigation can be undertaken (fig 1). If IgE mediated allergy is suspected, then confirmation is by either a skin prick test or measurement of specific immunoglobulin E in the blood (spIgE, previously known as RAST). Skin prick testing is ideally done using fresh milk as commercial extracts can be less sensitive.[W1] It should be carried out only where there are the facilities and expertise to manage anaphylactic reactions as 0.12% of patients having skin prick tests develop systemic allergic reactions.[W2] Specific immunoglobulin E testing is therefore usually more suitable in primary care.

Although a larger wheal diameter on skin prick test or a higher IgE concentration gives a higher probability of clinical allergy, an appropriate clinical history on exposure to the allergen is required for diagnosis. An observational study showed that 5.6% of infants had a positive skin prick test response to milk but only 2.7% had clinical cows' milk allergy, showing that a positive test result in isolation is not enough for a conclusive diagnosis.[12] The size of the response to testing does not relate to the severity of the clinical response to exposure.

When the allergy tests fail to confirm the history, the gold standard for investigating cows' milk allergy is a double blind placebo controlled food challenge. These can be expensive and time consuming so an open oral food challenge can be used to elicit reproducible, objective symptoms. Like skin prick tests, food challenges must be carried out in a safe environment with resuscitation facilities and experience, such as an allergy clinic or hospital day case unit.

Skin prick tests and specific IgE measurement are of little use if non-IgE mediated cows' milk allergy is suspected. The only reliable diagnostic test is a strict elimination diet.[13] If symptoms do not improve within two to eight weeks, cows' milk allergy is unlikely and milk should be reintroduced. Improvement of symptoms on milk exclusion coupled with recurrence of symptoms on reintroduction is strongly indicative of non-IgE mediated allergy. In a breast fed baby, the cows' milk protein can be removed from the mother's diet under dietetic advice.

No evidence supports the use of investigations such as serum IgG testing, Vega testing, kinesiology, or hair analysis.[4]

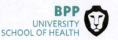

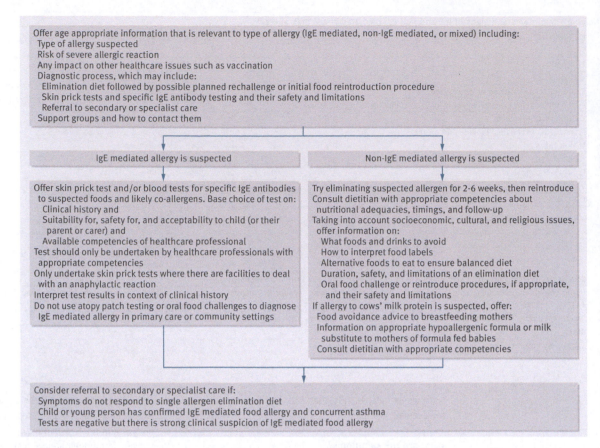

Fig 1 National Institute for Health and Care Excellence recommendations for diagnosis and management of cows' milk allergy[4]

How do we manage cows' milk allergy?

IgE mediated cows' milk allergy is managed by exclusion of cows' milk protein from the diet. For non-IgE mediated allergy both cows' milk protein and soya (if applicable) should be removed from the diet in the first instance because of the risk of cross reactivity.[13] For exclusively breast fed babies, the mother should be put on an exclusion diet under supervision to ensure she maintains adequate nutrition. Mothers should be given a supplement of 1000 mg of calcium and 10 μg of vitamin D every day.[14] In formula fed infants, cows' milk based formula can be replaced by hypoallergenic infant formulas such as extensively hydrolysed (tolerated by 90% of children with cows' milk allergy) or amino acid formulas.

Most symptoms will usually resolve within two to four weeks of a cows' milk elimination diet. Once it has been instituted and shown to help, milk must be reintroduced into the diet to prove it is the causal agent. Once the diagnosis is confirmed, the child should remain on the elimination diet for at least five months or until 1 year of age, when reintroduction can be tried, usually at home.

The input of a dietitian is highly recommended to maintain optimal nutrition and guide choice of milk substitute.

Observational and cohort data show malnutrition in children on exclusion diets as well as those with newly diagnosed food allergies.[15w4 w5] These patients require dietetic input to ensure that this is managed or averted. Obesity can also be present in children on exclusion diets.[w6] If access to a dietitian is not possible in primary care, the child's height and weight should be measured regularly to assess growth and nutrition and appropriate calcium supplements should be initiated. The child should be referred to a hospital dietitian or allergy clinic if concerns arise.

Once cows' milk protein is excluded from the diet, the family must be counselled on how to both avoid and manage accidental exposures to milk. This requires education on reading and understanding food labels. Management of IgE mediated reactions may require the use of antihistamines, or in rare cases of anaphylaxis, an adrenaline autoinjector. Autoinjectors are indicated for patients who meet the criteria in the European Academy of Allergy and Clinical Immunology management of anaphylaxis guideline (box 1).[w7]

Any children who also have asthma should be identified and well controlled because of the increased risk of severe reactions. For IgE mediated allergy, a written emergency management plan should be provided for the families' reference and for nursery or school. Examples of these can be found on the British Society for Allergy and Clinical Immunology website (www.bsaci.org).

Which milk should be recommended?

In most cases, first line treatment would be with an extensively hydrolysed formula—these are based on cows' milk but are extensively broken down into smaller peptides that are less well recognised by the immune system. If symptoms do not fully resolve after two to eight weeks,

---

BOX 1: INDICATIONS FOR PRESCRIBING SELF INJECTABLE ADRENALINE IN COWS' MILK ALLERGY

Absolute indications

- Previous cardiovascular or respiratory reactions to any food
- Child with food allergy and coexistent persistent asthma

Relative indications

- Any reaction to small amounts of a food (eg airborne food allergen or contact only through skin)
- Remoteness of home from medical facilities
- Food allergic reaction in a teenager

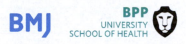

infants should be changed to an amino acid formula,[16] which contains no peptides to be bound by IgE.

Amino acid formula should be the first choice in infants with severe reactions such as anaphylaxis or severe delayed gut (unresponsive bleeding per rectum leading to a haematological disturbance) or skin symptoms as well as those with faltering growth. Children who exhibited symptoms when exclusively breast fed should also have an amino acid formula in the first instance.

Soya based formula milks should be avoided in children aged under 6 months because they contain isoflavins, which have a weak oestrogen effect.[17] Further advice is available in the milk allergy in primary care guideline (see supplementary material on bmj.com). [18]

Other mammalian milks, such as goat, mare, or sheep, are not recommended because of the high species cross reactivity.[18] [19] Children over 6 months can be tried on a soy formula if this is more palatable,[13] but clinicians also need to consider the cross reactivity between cows' milk and soya; up to 60% of patients with non-IgE mediated cows' milk allergy and up to 14% with IgE mediated allergy also react to soya.[w3] In older children there are a range of supplemental milks such as oat, or in the over 5 year olds, rice milk. These should be calcium fortified, but it is important to note that organic milks under governmental legislation cannot be fortified with calcium. Children should be eating three portions of calcium rich foods per day to obtain adequate calcium; this should be titrated to the recommended daily allowances for particular age groups (table 2).[w8]

When to refer on to specialist care

Uncomplicated cows' milk allergy can be managed in primary or secondary care as long as dietetic support is available. Referral to a paediatric allergy specialist is indicated if cows' milk is:

- Not the only allergen suspected of causing a reaction (other than cross reaction to soya in non-IgE mediated allergies)
- Thought to be causing gastrointestinal symptoms or faltering growth
- Thought to have caused severe IgE or non-IgE mediated reactions (box 2)[4]

In addition, review by a paediatric allergist is prudent in children with IgE mediated allergies and asthma because of the risk of more severe reaction.[w9]

A prospective parental survey has shown that children attending specialist allergy clinics are more likely to be able to manage a reaction as well as being less likely to have one.[w9] However, provision of specialist allergy services is relatively limited. The British Society for Allergy and Clinical Immunology website has a tool to identify the nearest allergy clinic in the UK (www.bsaci.org).

What is the prognosis?

Recent prospective longitudinal studies[20] [21] following children with IgE mediated cows' milk allergy found that 53-57% outgrow their milk allergy by 5 years of age. Tolerance is assessed by intermittent allergy tests to detect a fall in either specific IgE level or skin prick wheal diameter with a hospital based oral food challenge when tolerance is suspected. The Consortium of Food Allergy Research website has a tool to help predict when tolerance will develop (www.cofargroup.org). Observational and cohort studies have shown that IgE mediated cows' milk allergy is more likely to persist in children with asthma or allergic rhinitis, those who have more severe reactions, and those with larger allergy test results at diagnosis.[3] [21] [22] [23] [24]

The natural course of non-IgE mediated cows' milk allergy is less well defined, but one large prospective population based study and a large retrospective study suggest that most children will be milk tolerant by 2.5 years of age.[22] [25] The development of tolerance can be assessed by a carefully planned home challenge, which can be undertaken every six months from the age of 1 year. If a child has a history of severe non-IgE mediated reactions (such as food protein induced enterocolitis syndrome), the challenges should be supervised in hospital.

A recent well designed prospective study of 100 children has established that up to 70% of children with IgE mediated milk allergy are able to tolerate baked milk.[26] In these children, the IgE binds predominantly to milk proteins that alter when milk is extensively heated, making them unrecognisable to the patients' immune system. Such children tend to have milder reactions, smaller allergy test responses, and outgrow their allergy earlier.[w10-w12] Introducing baked milk to the diet may also speed up the acquisition of tolerance to unheated milk.[27] However, testing to identify children who are tolerant to baked milk is limited and requires challenge testing best directed by a paediatric allergist.

What new therapies are on the horizon?

Much research interest exists in the use of oral immunotherapy to induce tolerance in patients with cows' milk allergy. Oral immunotherapy is the controlled introduction of small but increasing volumes of cows' milk to allergic patients. A recent Cochrane review of four randomised controlled trials and five observational studies in children with IgE mediated allergy concluded that the chances of achieving full tolerance (>150 ml of milk a day) was 10 times higher in the oral immunotherapy treatment group than the control group.[28] However, the authors commented on the possibility of bias in these small trials and also the safety as 90% of patients experienced adverse reactions. This approach is not currently advocated in any national or international guidelines.

Another area of interest is the addition of prebiotics and probiotics to hypoallergenic milk formulas as a means to speed up the development of tolerance.[w13] Also under

---

BOX 2 INDICATIONS FOR REFERRAL TO SECONDARY CARE OR SPECIALIST CARE

Symptoms

- Systemic reactions, including immediate referral for anaphylaxis
- Gastrointestinal symptoms—eg faltering growth, diarrhoea (particularly with blood), vomiting, protein losing enteropathy, and blood
- Respiratory symptoms—eg acute laryngoedema, bronchial obstruction, or difficulty breathing
- Other related conditions (suspected or diagnosed)—gastro-oesophageal reflux or food induced enterocolitis syndrome

Comorbidity (especially when unresponsive to treatment)

- Asthma when assessing for environmental allergens
- Atopic dermatitis and eczema, especially when widespread and severe
- Other related conditions such as rhinoconjunctivitis

Other reasons

- Diet—including children with restricted diet or in whom diet may become too limited because of perceived reactions to food
- Parental suspicion of food allergy, especially in infants with perplexing or difficult symptoms

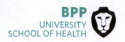

Table 2 British Dietetic Association recommended calcium requirements for different age groups[w8]

Age (years)	Calcium/ day (mg)
<1	525
1-3	350
4-6	450
7-10	550
11-18	800 (girls) 1000 (boys)

AREAS FOR FUTURE RESEARCH

- What is the initial event causing sensitisation to cows' milk protein?
- What intervention could prevent the acquisition of cows' milk protein allergy in children?
- Can a biomarker be developed to diagnose non-IgE mediated cows' milk allergy?
- Is there a role for oral tolerance induction?

ADDITIONAL EDUCATIONAL RESOURCES

Resources for health professionals

- NICE guideline 116: Assessment and diagnosis of food allergy in young children and young people in a community setting. (www.nice.org.uk/nicemedia/live/13348/53214/53214.pdf)
- Diagnostic approach and management of cow's-milk protein allergy in infants and children: ESPGHAN GI Committee practical guidelines. *J Paedlatr Gastrointest Nutr* 2012;55:221-9
- Consortium of Food Allergy Group online milk allergy calculator (www.cofargroup.org)—Tool to help predict likely age of milk tolerance development in IgE mediated allergy based on clinical features and allergy test results
- Venter C, Brown T, Walsh J, Shah N, Fox AT. Diagnosis and management of non-IgE mediated cow's milk allergy in infancy—a UK primary care practical guide. *Clin Translational Allergy* 2013;3:23. A practical primary care focused guideline

Resources for patients and carers

- Allergy UK (www.allergyuk.org)—Day to day tips and support
- NHS Choices (www.nhs.uk/conditions/food-allergy/pages/intro1.aspx)—Clear guidance on symptoms and how to access help
- Food Allergy Research and Education (www.foodallergy.org)—US resource for people with food allergies
- Food Standards Agency allergy alerts (http://food.gov.uk/policy-advice/allergyintol/alerts/#.UbYDf_lllHc)—Provides text message alerts of incorrect food labelling

TIPS FOR NON-SPECIALISTS

- Most formula fed infants can be started on an extensively hydrolysed formula, but if symptoms persist, an amino acid formula may be required
- Infants with severe reactions, faltering growth, or who developed symptoms when exclusively breast fed should be started on an amino acid formula
- Soya milk is not suitable for children under 6 months old
- Other mammalian milks (goat, sheep, etc) should not be substituted for cows' milk because of the risk of allergic cross reactivity
- In older children milk substitutes such as soya, oat, and in children over 5 years, rice milk may be used. These should be fortified with calcium
- Ensure parents are aware of all the terms in ingredients lists that can be substituted for milk and provide dietetic support to ensure nutritional adequacy
- Patients should be referred to specialist care if they have multiple food allergies, severe allergic reactions, faltering growth, or complex symptoms or if they fail to respond to an exclusion diet

investigation is the possibility that the type of formula milk chosen for treatment could affect outcome.[w14]

Contributors: SL wrote first draft and reviews, NS reviewed drafts and references, and ATF reviewed drafts and had final input on completed manuscript. ATF is guarantor.

We have read and understood the BMJ Group policy on declaration of interests and declare the following interests: ATF has done consultancy work for Mead Johnson Nutrition, Danone, Nestle Nutrition, and Abbot. He has received fees for lectures or producing educational material from Mead Johnson Nutrition and Danone. He is site principal investigator for a Danone sponsored study funded through Guy's and St Thomas' NHS Hospitals NHS Foundation Trust and King's College London.

Provenance and peer review: Commissioned; externally peer reviewed.

1 Venter C, Pereira B, Voigt K, Grundy J, Clayton CB, Higgins B, et al. Prevalence and cumulative incidence of food hypersensitivity in the first 3 years of life. *Allergy* 2008;63:354-9.
2 Agostoni C, Braegger C, Decsi T, Kolacek S, Koletzko B, Michaelsen KF, et al. Breast-feeding: a commentary by the ESPGHAN committee on nutrition. *J Pediatr Gastroenterol Nutr* 2009;49:112-25.
3 Fiocchi A, Schünemann HJ, Brozek J, Restani P, Beyer K, Troncone R, et al. Diagnosis and Rationale for Action Against Cow's Milk Allergy (DRACMA): a summary report. *J Allergy Clin Immunol* 2010;126:1119-1128.e12.
4 National Institute for Health and Care Excellence. NICE clinical guideline 116. Food allergy in children and young people. 2011 www.nice.org.uk/guidance/CG116.
5 Boyano-Martínez T, García-Ara C, Pedrosa M, Díaz-Pena JM, Quirce S. Accidental allergic reactions in children allergic to cow's milk proteins. *J Allergy Clin Immunol* 2009;123:883-8.
6 Høst A, Husby S, Osterballe O. A prospective study of cow's milk allergy in exclusively breast-fed infants. Incidence, pathogenetic role of early inadvertent exposure to cow's milk formula, and characterization of bovine milk protein in human milk. *Acta Paediatr Scand* 1988;77:663-70.
7 Hill DJ, Hosking CS, De Benedictis FM, Oranje AP, Diepgen TL, Bauchau V, et al. Confirmation of the association between high levels of immunoglobulin E food sensitization and eczema in infancy: an international study. *Clin Exp Allergy* 2008;38:161-8.
8 Hill DJ, Heine RG, Hosking CS, Brown J, Thiele L, Allen KJ, et al. IgE food sensitization in infants with eczema attending a dermatology department. *J Pediatr* 2007;151:359-63.
9 Hill DJ, Hosking CS. Food allergy and atopic dermatitis in infancy: an epidemiologic study. *Pediatr Allergy Immunol* 2004;15:421-7.
10 Goldberg M, Eisenberg E, Elizur A, Rajuan N, Rachmiel M, Cohen A, et al. Role of parental atopy in cow's milk allergy: a population-based study. *Ann Allergy Asthma Immunol* 2013;110:279-83.
11 National Institute for Health and Care Excellence. NICE guideline 57. Atopic eczema in children. Management of atopic eczema in children from birth up to the age of 12 years. 2007. http://guidance.nice.org.uk/CG57/NICEGuidance/pdf/English.
12 Osborne NJ, Koplin JJ, Martin PE, Gurrin LC, Lowe AJ, Matheson MC, et al. Prevalence of challenge-proven IgE-mediated food allergy using population-based sampling and predetermined challenge criteria in infants. *J Allergy Clin.Immunol* 2011;127:668-76.
13 Koletzko S, Niggemann B, Arato A, Dias JA, Heuschkel R, Husby S, et al. Diagnostic approach and management of cow's-milk protein allergy in infants and children: ESPGHAN GI committee practical guidelines. *J Pediatr Gastroenterol Nutr* 2012;55:221-9.
14 Vandenplas Y, Koletzko S, Isolauri E, Hill D, Oranje AP, Brueton M, et al. Guidelines for the diagnosis and management of cow's milk protein allergy in infants. *Arch Dis Child* 2007;92:902-8.
15 Meyer R, Venter C, Fox AT, Shah N. Practical dietary management of protein energy malnutrition in young children with cow's milk protein allergy. *Pediatr Allergy Immunol* 2012;23:307-14.
16 Järvinen KM, Chatchatee P. Mammalian milk allergy: clinical suspicion, cross-reactivities and diagnosis. *Curr Opin Allergy Clin Immunol* 2009;9:251-8.
17 Setchell KD, Zimmer-Nechemias L, Cai J, Heubi JE. Isoflavone content of infant formulas and the metabolic fate of these phytoestrogens in early life. *Am J Clin Nutr* 1998;68(6 suppl):1453-1461S.
18 Venter C, Brown T, Walsh J, Shah N, Fox AT. Diagnosis and management of non -IgE mediated cow's milk allergy in infancy—a UK primary care practical guide. *Clin Translational Allergy* 2013;3:23.
19 Host A, Koletzko B, Dreborg S, Muraro A, Wahn U, Aggett P, et al. Dietary products used in infants for treatment and prevention of food allergy. Joint statement of the European Society for Paediatric Allergology and Clinical Immunology (ESPACI) Committee on Hypoallergenic Formulas and the European Society for Paediatric Gastroenterology, Hepatology and Nutrition (ESPGHAN) Committee on Nutrition. *Arch Dis Child* 1999;81:80-4.
20 Elizur A, Rajuan N, Goldberg MR, Leshno M, Cohen A, Katz Y. Natural course and risk factors for persistence of IgE-mediated cow's milk allergy. *J Pediatr* 2012;161482-487.e1.
21 Sicherer SH, Wood RA, Stablein D, Burks AW, Liu AH, Jones SM, et al. Immunologic features of infants with milk or egg allergy enrolled in an observational study (Consortium of Food Allergy Research) of food allergy. *J Allergy Clin Immunol* 2010;125:1077-1083.e8.
22 Saarinen KM, Pelkonen AS, Mäkelä MJ, Savilahti E. Clinical course and prognosis of cow's milk allergy are dependent on milk-specific IgE status. *J. Allergy Clin Immunol* 2005;116:869-75.
23 Fiocchi A, Terracciano L, Bouygue GR, Veglia F, Sarratud T, Martelli A, et al. Incremental prognostic factors associated with cow's milk allergy outcomes in infant and child referrals: the Milan Cow's Milk Allergy Cohort study. *Ann Allergy Asthma Immunol* 2008;101:166-73.
24 Skripak JM, Matsui EC, Mudd K, Wood RA. The natural history of IgE-mediated cow's milk allergy. *J Allergy Clin Immunol* 2007;120:1172-7.
25 Sicherer SH, Eigenmann PA, Sampson HA. Clinical features of food protein-induced enterocolitis syndrome. *J Pediatr* 1998;133:214-9.
26 Nowak-Wegrzyn A, Bloom KA, Sicherer SH, Shreffler WG, Noone S, Wanich N, et al. Tolerance to extensively heated milk in children with cow's milk allergy. *J Allergy Clin Immunol* 2008;122:342-347, 347.e1-2.
27 Kim JS, Nowak-Wegrzyn A, Sicherer SH, Noone S, Moshier EL, Sampson HA. Dietary baked milk accelerates the resolution of cow's milk allergy in children. *J Allergy Clin Immunol* 2011;128:125-131.e2.

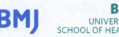

28 Brożek JL, Terracciano L, Hsu J, Kreis J, Compalati E, Santesso N, et al. Oral immunotherapy for IgE-mediated cow's milk allergy: a systematic review and meta-analysis. *Clin Exp Allergy* 2012;42:363-74.

Related links

bmj.com
- Get Cleveland clinic CME points for this article

bmj.com/archive

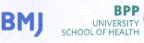

Developmental assessment of children

Martin Bellman consultant paediatrician[1], Orlaith Byrne consultant community paediatrician[2], Robert Sege professor of pediatrics[3]

[1]Department of Paediatrics, Royal Free Hospital, London NW3 2QG, UK

[2]Department of Child Health, Birmingham Community Healthcare NHS Trust, Birmingham, UK

[3]Department of Pediatrics, Boston University, Boston, MA, USA

Correspondence to: M Bellman m.bellman@nhs.net

Cite this as: BMJ 2013;346:e8687

‹DOI› 10.1136/bmj.e8687
http://www.bmj.com/content/346/bmj.e8687

Developmental assessment is the process of mapping a child's performance compared with children of similar age. The comparison group is obtained from a representative sample of the population that the child comes from. Several factors contribute to performance varying greatly between different population groups.[1] In a multicultural society it can be challenging to find appropriate benchmarks for these standards.

This article reviews the literature on the assessment of child development. It aims to highlight what normal developmental parameters are, when and how to assess a child, and when to refer for specialist assessment.

We have extensive clinical experience in developmental paediatrics in the United Kingdom and United States, which we drew on to comment on the extensive and potentially confusing technology currently used for developmental assessment.

What is child development?

Development is the process by which each child evolves from helpless infancy to independent adulthood.

Growth and development of the brain and central nervous system is often termed psychomotor development and is usually divided into four main domains:

- Gross and fine motor skills
- Speech and language

SOURCES AND SELECTION CRITERIA

We searched PubMed, the *Cochrane Database of Systematic Reviews*, and reference lists of relevant publications using the subject headings and key words "development", "developmental assessment", "developmental delay", "disability", "mental retardation", "developmental screening tools", "screening", and "diagnosis". We also reviewed guidelines from the American Academy of Pediatrics[2] and the UK Healthy Child Programme.[3]

- Social and personal and activities of daily living
- Performance and cognition.

Fetal brain development starts by the fourth week of gestation and progresses rapidly throughout intrauterine life and early childhood. Brain development—the target of developmental surveillance and screening—reflects neurological maturation. It consists of a complex process of cell growth, migration, connection, pruning, and myelination, and it persists through at least the second decade. This fundamental phenomenon, which determines brain development, is a preprogrammed process that occurs in all children.

What is normal development?

The pattern of development is remarkably constant, within fairly broad limits, but the rate at which goals are achieved varies from child to child. Skills are acquired sequentially, with one goal acquired after another. Later goals often depend on achievement of earlier goals within the same field—for example, children must learn to sit independently before they can stand and then walk.

Descriptions of normal development, linked to the ability to perform a particular task at a particular age, relate to the performance of the average child. The acquisition of a key performance skill, such as walking, is referred to as a milestone. For each skill, the normal age range for attainment of the milestone varies widely. A median age is the age at which half a population of children acquire a skill. A limit age is the age at which a skill should have been achieved and is two standard deviations from the mean. It is important to know which milestones are most consistent. Smiling socially by the age of 8 weeks is a consistent milestone, whereas crawling is not. Crawling occurs at a widely varying time point, and some children with normal development never learn to crawl.

Genetic factors may determine the fundamental developmental potential, but environmental factors have crucial influences on the profile achieved. Positive experiences during early childhood may enhance brain development, particularly in the area of linguistic and social skills. Unfortunately, however, the brain is also vulnerable to various insults, particularly in the early embryonic stages, but also in later life (box 1). Studies on abandoned Romanian children provide good evidence of how an adverse environment affects brain growth. Children who were institutionalised have smaller brains than those who were adopted abroad or brought up in a family environment,

---

BOX 1 ENVIRONMENTAL CAUSES OF DAMAGE TO BRAIN DEVELOPMENT

Antenatal

- Early maternal infections, such as rubella, toxoplasma, cytomegalovirus
- Late maternal infections, such as varicella, malaria, HIV
- Toxins—for example, alcohol, pesticides, radiation, smoking
- Drugs—for example, cytotoxics, antiepileptics

Postnatal

- Infections—for example, meningitis, encephalitis, cytomegalovirus
- Metabolic disorders, such as hypoglycaemia, hyponatraemia or hypernatraemia, dehydration
- Toxins—for example, lead, mercury, arsenic, chlorinated organic compounds, solvents
- Trauma, especially head injury
- Severe understimulation, maltreatment, or domestic violence
- Malnutrition, especially deficiency of iron, folate, and vitamin D
- Maternal mental health disorders, most commonly depression

SUMMARY POINTS

- Every consultation is an opportunity to ask flexible questions about a child's development as part of comprehensive medical care
- Parents who voice concerns about their child's development are usually right
- Loss of previously acquired skills (regression) is a red flag and should prompt rapid referral for detailed assessment and investigation
- Parents and carers are usually more aware of norms for gross motor milestones, such as walking independently, than for milestones and patterns of normal speech, language acquisition, and play skills; consider targeted questioning
- Consider use of developmental screening questionnaires and measurement tools to supplement clinical judgment

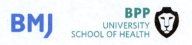

including foster care in Romania.[4] Other studies showed significant gains in cognitive and language skills after abandoned children are taken into care.[5] [6]

What is developmental delay?

Many clinicians use the term "global developmental delay" to mean a significant delay in two or more of the four main developmental domains listed above. Significant delay is defined as performance two or more standard deviations below the mean on age appropriate standardised norm-referenced testing (usually a secondary care procedure). In the United Kingdom and the United States, the term global developmental delay is usually reserved for younger children (typically under 5 years of age). In the UK learning disability is usually applied to older children, when IQ testing is more valid and reliable (although formal testing of IQ is rarely performed in clinical practice and the child's assessment is based on functional abilities). In the US, the term developmental disability or mental retardation is used in the over 5 age group.

The term developmental impairment or disorder covers a heterogeneous group of conditions that start early in life and present with delay or an abnormal pattern of progression in one or more developmental domain. Children with autism spectrum disorder fall into this category. In this context, the use of the term developmental delay has been challenged because it conveys a message that the child may "catch up," which is often not true.[7] Nevertheless, it remains in common use because it is well understood by professionals and parents.

How common are developmental problems?

Global developmental delay affects 1-3% of children. About 1% (95% confidence interval 90-141 per 10 000) of children have an autism spectrum disorder,[8] 1-2% a mild learning disability, 0.3-0.5% a severe learning disability, and 5-10% have a specific learning disability in a single domain.[9] [10]

Structured assessment of a child's development aims mainly to clarify the quantity and quality of the child's developmental status. However, the procedure also offers several advantages in terms of health promotion (box 2).

Children develop at different rates, and it is important to distinguish those who are within the "normal" range from those who are following a pathological course. We now have good evidence that early identification and early intervention improve the outcomes of children with developmental impairments.[11] [12]

A persuasive body of work, which reviewed evidence from neurosciences, developmental psychology, social sciences, epidemiology (including animal and human studies), longitudinal studies, case series, and case reports,[13] [14] [15] describes the importance of the early years in promoting healthy brain development. This literature builds on the scientific understanding of brain development and finds that environments that do not promote healthy development have a cumulative and ongoing negative impact on a range of social, economic, and learning outcomes over the life course. This body of work emphasises that early interventions are an effective way to improve children's outcomes than later remediation.

Given the importance of the early years, early intervention is crucial. Early intervention seems to be even more important for children with developmental disabilities than for children more generally, because learning is cumulative, and barriers to healthy development early in life impede development at each subsequent stage.[16] [17]

Obviously, identification of abnormality must be followed by further action. Children develop relentlessly, and if they are on a deviant path the course becomes more difficult to change as time goes by. Early child health promotion, which includes support for parenting and treatment, is an effective investment that may prevent the need for more intensive, costly, and often less effective intervention later on. A series of systematic reviews of strategies for improving child development in 13 relatively deprived countries, published in the *Lancet*, found good evidence that interventions at pre-school age are highly cost effective.[18] A linked editorial stated that "Neglect of young children most in need is an outrage—and a huge strategic mistake."[19]

How do children present with developmental problems?

Children with developmental problems may present in several ways:

- In countries with routine child health surveillance or developmental screening practices, concerns may be raised at scheduled contacts
- In children with identified risk factors (such as prematurity) who have undergone developmental surveillance, developmental problems may be detected early
- Parents may recognise a delay or be worried about a child's behaviour or social skills and seek professional advice (either through their health visitor, public health nurse, or general practitioner)
- Professionals in a nursery or day care setting may recognise deviant patterns of development and highlight their concerns to the family, thus prompting referral
- Concerns may be detected opportunistically at health contacts for other reasons, such as childhood illnesses, if questions are asked about development.

Development can be assessed at several levels, depending on the circumstances. Screening is a process to identify children at increased risk of having developmental difficulties that uses relatively brief and simple techniques, according to well recognised criteria.[20] Screening tests are inherently imperfect assessments because they have to balance the risk of missing a child with delays (sensitivity) versus erroneously identifying children without true delays (specificity).[21] Repeating the test after an appropriate time interval, or conducting a secondary screening with a more accurate and specific test, may improve test accuracy. The inherent trade-off of sensitivity and specificity makes screening controversial—it is promoted universally in some countries,[2] whereas others have a selective policy.[22]

BOX 2 BENEFITS OF DEVELOPMENTAL ASSESSMENT

- Early diagnosis and intervention
- Early diagnosis of conditions with a genetic basis, such as Duchene muscular dystrophy and fragile X syndrome, facilitates genetic counselling for families
- Provides carers with reliable information before a developmental problem becomes obvious and gives them more time to adjust to the child's difficulty and make appropriate management plans for their family
- Carers are reassured and relieved of anxiety if assessment shows that the child is within the normal range
- Early assessments can be compared with later ones, allowing the practitioner to follow a child's individual developmental trajectory
- Provides an opportunity to encourage good parenting and developmental stimulation

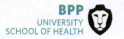

The practice of child health surveillance and screening has changed in the UK since the introduction of the Healthy Child Programme (HCP) which supersedes Health for all Children IV. In the UK, the HCP offers every child and family a programme that includes developmental reviews to facilitate early detection of, and action to deal with, developmental delay.[3] The emphasis is on a review at 2.5 years. The HCP is based on a model of "progressive universalism"—in other words, standard services that are available to everyone (universal) and extra services available to those who need them or are at risk (progressively more services provided according to need). It is basically a child health promotion programme that includes opportunities for developmental surveillance and screening or case finding. It is a flexible and non-prescriptive programme that can be adapted locally according to population needs. Primary care practitioners should opportunistically ask flexible questions about a child's development at every visit where possible, as part of comprehensive medical care (box 3). Children identified as at risk (often by a health visitor) may be referred for further assessment in primary or secondary care. Currently, standardised developmental screening tools are not routinely used in primary care in the UK.

By contrast, in the US the American Academy of Pediatrics (AAP) and many American state Medicaid programmes recommend the use of standardised developmental screening tools during each routine healthcare visit. The AAP guideline for health supervision, *Bright Futures*,[23] suggests the use of structured developmental screens from the age of 18 months. The 2009 Affordable Care Act requires health insurance plans to cover preventive care,[24] as described in *Bright Futures*. Despite these federal protocols, strategy and implementation vary greatly between individual states.

How to assess a child's development

A good starting point is to believe parents and carers who are worried about their child.

Box 4 lists factors that can result in a deviant pattern of development. It is important that these are elicited through appropriate history and examination. Ask about prenatal, perinatal, and postnatal events, including maternal health during pregnancy. Ask about the child's acquisition of developmental milestones (table 1). The personal child health record ("red book" in the UK) is often a valuable source of information because it contains details of pregnancy, mode of delivery, condition at birth, Apgar scores, birth weight, birth head circumference, and newborn hearing screen results. A sensitive but thorough environmental, social, and family history is essential, particularly asking about consanguinity and a family history of developmental problems or learning difficulties, which may point to metabolic problems or recessive conditions.

Many parents make video recordings of their child on a camera or mobile telephone and these may be invaluable for illustrating the past and present developmental profile. Table 2 lists the main physical examination features pertinent to developmental assessment. Always consider difficulties of hearing and vision when there are concerns about development.

Much information can be gained by observing the child entering and moving around the clinic while playing with a few age appropriate toys, such as blocks, toy cars, pull-along toys, paper, and crayons. Observation of the child at home or nursery can also prove invaluable, as can reports from other carers, such as nursery workers or school teachers. For those interested in further reading about developmental assessment and examination, we recommend a comprehensive review of methods and interpretation by Sharma.[25]

In primary care, when time is limited, clinicians with paediatric experience should base their assessment on clinical judgment and knowledge of the broadly normal range of child development. Table 1 contains normal milestones and gives some indicators of when to worry and

---

BOX 3 SUGGESTED OPPORTUNISTIC SCREENING QUESTIONS[35]

- Do you have any concerns about the way your child is behaving, learning, or developing?
- Do you have any concerns about the way he or she moves or uses his or her arms or legs?
- Do you have any concerns about how your child talks and understands what you say?
- Does your child enjoy playing with toys? Describe what he or she does while playing
- Has your child ever stopped doing something he or she could previously do?
- Does your child get along with others?
- Do you have any concerns about how your child is learning to do things for himself or herself?

BOX 4 DEVELOPMENTAL VARIATION

Normal patterns

- Late talking or walking (including bottom shuffling) may be familial
- Language development may seem delayed at first in children of bilingual families, but counting total words in both languages typically compensates for perceived delay. Receptive language precedes language expression
- Black and Indian infants are more likely than white ones to have advanced motor skills[1]

Correctable causes of slow development

- Undernutrition (failure to thrive)
- Iron deficiency anaemia
- Social isolation of the family or maternal depression
- Hypothyroidism

BOX 5 RED FLAGS

These indicators suggest that development is seriously disordered and that the child should be promptly referred to a developmental or community paediatrician[10]

Positive indicators (the presence of any of the following)

- Loss of developmental skills at any age
- Parental or professional concerns about vision, fixing, or following an object or a confirmed visual impairment at any age (simultaneous referral to paediatric ophthalmology)
- Hearing loss at any age (simultaneous referral for expert audiological or ear, nose, and throat assessment)
- Persistently low muscle tone or floppiness
- No speech by 18 months, especially if the child does not try to communicate by other means such as gestures (simultaneous referral for urgent hearing test)
- Asymmetry of movements or other features suggestive of cerebral palsy, such as increased muscle tone
- Persistent toe walking
- Complex disabilities
- Head circumference above the 99.6th centile or below 0.4th centile. Also, if circumference has crossed two centiles (up or down) on the appropriate chart or is disproportionate to parental head circumference
- An assessing clinician who is uncertain about any aspect of assessment but thinks that development may be disordered

Negative indicators (activities that the child cannot do)

- Sit unsupported by 12 months
- Walk by 18 months (boys) or 2 years (girls) (check creatine kinase urgently)
- Walk other than on tiptoes
- Run by 2.5 years
- Hold object placed in hand by 5 months (corrected for gestation)
- Reach for objects by 6 months (corrected for gestation)
- Point at objects to share interest with others by 2 years

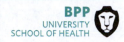

Table 1 Normal developmental milestones

Age	Skills				
	Gross motor	Fine motor and vision	Hearing, speech, and language	Social, emotional, and behavioural	Red flags
6 weeks	Head level with body in ventral suspension	Fixes and follows	Becomes still in response to sound	Smiles	Unresponsive to sound or visual stimuli
3 months	Holds head at 90° in ventral suspension	Holds an object placed in the hand	Turns to sound	Hand regard, laughs, and squeals	Lack of social response or vocalisation
6 months	No head lag on pull to sit; sits with support; in prone position lifts up on forearms	Palmar grasp of objects; transfers objects hand to hand	Vocalisations	May finger feed self	Poor head control, floppiness, not reaching
9 months	Crawls; sits steadily when unsupported and pivots around	Pincer grasp; index finger approach; bangs two cubes together	2 syllable babble, non-specific—consonant-vowel, such as "mama"	Waves bye bye, plays pat-a-cake; indicates wants; stranger anxiety emerging	Can't sit unsupported; no babble
12 months	Pulls to stand; cruises; may stand alone briefly; may walk alone	Puts block in cup; casts about	One or two words; imitates adults' sounds	Imitates activities; object permanence (the understanding that objects still exist when they cannot be seen) established; stranger anxiety established; points to indicate wants	Not communicating by gestures, such as pointing; not weight bearing through legs
18 months	Walks well; runs	Builds tower of 2-4 cubes; hand preference emerges	6-12 words	Uses spoon; symbolic play—"talking" on telephone; domestic mimicry—"helps" in household chores like sweeping, wiping surfaces	Not walking; no symbolic play; no words
2 years	Kicks ball; climbs stairs two feet per step	Builds tower of 6-7 cubes; does circular scribbles	Joins 2-3 words; knows some body parts; identifies objects in pictures	Can remove some clothes	Not joining two words; cannot run
3 years	Stands briefly on one foot; climbs stairs one foot per step	Builds tower of 9 cubes; copies a circle	Talks in short sentences that a stranger can understand	Eats with fork and spoon; puts on clothing; may be toilet trained	Not communicating with words; cannot climb stairs

box 5 contains some important red flags for significantly disordered development, which should prompt early referral to secondary care for diagnostic assessment.

In children presenting with mild developmental delay in the absence of any red flags, primary care practitioners may consider basic investigations such as full blood count, bone profile, thyroid function tests, and measurement of vitamin D and creatine kinase. Some causes of mild developmental delay such as iron deficiency anaemia can be easily treated. However, to avoid multiple venepuncture, investigations should be deferred in children with moderate or serious delay, or red flags, because they will require a battery of tests in secondary care.

What tools are available for developmental assessment in primary care?

Professionals who work with children learn to recognise deviant patterns of development, but screening questionnaires and developmental screening tools can improve accuracy.[26 27]

Examples of screening questionnaires include: the ages and stages questionnaire (ASQ),[28] the parents ' evaluation of developmental status (PEDS),[29 30] and the modified checklist for autism in toddlers (M-CHAT).[31] These surveys can be self administered and can be answered by parents in the waiting room or during the consultation itself. These tools can help focus the consultation and increase the confidence of primary care practitioners in their referral decisions.

Several short (10-20 minutes) standardised assessment tools can be used to complement clinical impressions in primary care. Examples include the Denver developmental screening test, which is completed by an observer and gives "pass or fail" results in the four major developmental fields,[32] and the schedule of growing skills II. This last test is based on the standardised Sheridan stycar sequences,[33] and it objectively assesses the child's developmental level in nine subfields of development.[34] Both give visual maps of a child's developmental skills with clear cut-off points to guide referral to secondary care (table 3).

When should a child be referred for specialist assessment?

The presence of a red flag (table 1 and box 5) is a clear indication for referral to secondary care. Referral is also recommended if there are concerns about the extent of developmental delay or the lack of response to primary care interventions, such as health visitor advice or speech and language therapy.

What happens when a child is referred to a specialist?

Children with developmental concerns are most often seen by community paediatricians who work as part of a multidisciplinary team, often in child development centres. Members of the team may include a nursery nurse, preschool teacher, speech and language therapist, physiotherapist, occupational therapist, and psychologist. The child usually has an initial consultation to clarify the nature of the developmental difficulties.

Investigations (blood and urine tests, cranial imaging) may be arranged at this stage or later. The child may then undergo a multidisciplinary team assessment and intervention package of care over several weeks, after which a diagnosis will be reached, a report issued, and recommendations for ongoing support made.

Examples of developmental instruments used in secondary care that are more accurate, sophisticated, and time consuming (2-3 hours) than those used in primary care include the Griffiths mental development scales, Bayley scales of infant development, and the Wechsler preschool and primary scale of intelligence. Specific instruments are also available for the diagnosis of developmental disorders such as autism spectrum disorder. Standardised structured parental interviews, such as the developmental, dimensional, and diagnostic interview and autism diagnostic interview-revised, complement objective assessments of the child, such as the autism diagnostic observation schedule.

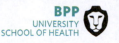

Table 2 Key features of the developmental examination

Key features on examination	Possible diagnosis
Head circumference measured and plotted on centile chart and interpreted in context of height and weight centiles; consider measurement of parental occipitofrontal head circumference	Microcephaly or macrocephaly
Dysmorphic features: does the child look like other family members? Are there any unusual features?	Genetic, metabolic, or syndromic conditions, such as fragile X syndrome
Skin abnormalities: café au lait patches, axillary freckling, neurofibromas, or hypopigmented patches (ash leaf macules)	Suggestive of neurocutaneous syndromes, such as neurofibromatosis or tuberous sclerosis
Observation of child's movements to look for signs of unsteadiness, weakness, or spasticity; check tone, power, and reflexes where possible	Underlying neurological disorder
Child's ability to sit up and to stand up from lying down supine and to clear the floor on jumping from a standing position	Muscle weakness suggestive of a muscular dystrophy
Observation of eye movements and examination of eyes looking for cataracts, nystagmus, or wobbly eye movements	Disorder of vision; underlying neurological condition
General examination of respiratory and cardiovascular systems	Underlying systemic disease
Abdominal examination for hepatomegaly	Metabolic disorder

EDUCATIONAL RESOURCES FOR PARENTS AND CARERS

- Contact a Family (www.cafamily.org.uk)—A directory of support organisations for a wide range of disabling conditions in childhood

- Mencap (www.mencap.org.uk)—Information and advice for lay and professional carers of people with learning disabilities

- Department of Education (www.education.gov.uk/publications/standard/earlysupport/page1)—Useful information for parents and carers regarding developmental delay and more specific diagnoses, such as Down's syndrome

Contributors: All authors contributed sections of the manuscript, reviewed the complete article, and are guarantors.

Competing interests: All authors have completed the ICMJE uniform disclosure form at www.icmje.org/coi_disclosure.pdf (available on request from the corresponding author) and declare: no support from any organisation for the submitted work; MB is joint author of one of the screening tools mentioned in the article (Schedule of Growing Skills); OB is currently working as a junior coauthor updating the Schedule of Growing Skills; no other relationships or activities that could appear to have influenced the submitted work.

Provenance and peer review: Commissioned; externally peer reviewed.

1 Kelly Y, Sacker A, Schoon I, Nazroo J. Ethnic differences in achievement of developmental milestones by 9 months of age: The Millennium Cohort Study. *Dev Med Child Neurol*2006;48:824-30.

2 American Academy of Pediatrics, Council on Children with Disabilities, Section on Developmental and Behavioral Pediatrics. Identifying infants and young children with developmental disorder in the medical home: an algorithm for developmental surveillance and screening. *Pediatrics*2006;118:405-20.

3 Department of Health. The Healthy Child Programme. 2009. www.dh.gov.uk/en/Publicationsandstatistics/Publications/PublicationsPolicyAndGuidance/DH_107563.

4 Sheridan MA, Fox NA, Zeanah CH, McLaughlin K, Nelson CA. Variation in neural development as a result of exposure to institutionalization early in childhood. *Proc Natl Acad Sci USA*2012;109:12927-32.

5 Windsor J, Wing CA, Koga SF, Fox NA, Benigno JP, Carroll PJ, et al. Effect of foster care on young children's language learning. *Child Dev* 2011;82:1040-6.

6 Nelson CA, Zeanah CH, Fox NA, Marshall PJ, Smyke AT, Guthrie D. Cognitive recovery in socially deprived young children: the Bucharest Early Intervention Project. *Science*2007;318:1937-40.

7 Williams AN, Essex C. Developmental delay or failure to arrive? *Dev Med Child Neurol*2004;46:502.

8 Baird G, Simonoff E, Pickles A, Chandler S, Loucas T, Meldrum D, Charman T. Prevalence of disorders of the autism spectrum in a population cohort of children in South Thames: the special needs and autism project (SNAP). *Lancet*2006;368:210-5.

9 Blanchard LT, Gurka MJ, Blackman JA. Emotional, developmental, and behavioural health of American children and their families: a report from the 2003 national survey of children's health. *Paediatrics*2006;117:e1202-12.

10 Horridge KA. Assessment and investigation of the child with disordered development. *Arch Dis Child Educ Pract Ed*2011;96:9-20.

11 Guralnik M. The effectiveness of early intervention. Paul H Brookes, 1997.

12 Gomby DS, Larner MB, Stevenson CS, Lewit EM, Behrman RE. Long term outcomes of early childhood programs: analysis and recommendations. *Future Child*1995;5:6-24.

13 Shonkoff J, Phillips D, eds. From neurons to neighborhoods: the science of early childhood development. National Academies Press, 2000.

14 Perry B. Childhood experience and the expression of genetic potential: what childhood neglect tells us about nature and nurture. *Brain Mind*2002;3:79-100.

15 McCain M, Mustard F. Reversing the real brain drain. Early Years study final report, Ontario Children's Secretariat Toronto. Academy Press, 1999.

16 Heckman J, Masterov D. The productivity argument for investing in young children. *Rev Agricult Econ*2007;29:446-93

17 KPMG. Reviewing the evidence on the effectiveness of early childhood intervention. Report to Department of Families, Housing, Community Services and Indigenous Affairs, Australia. 2011. www.fahcsia.gov.au/sites/default/files/documents/05_2012/childhood_int_effectiveness_report_0.pdf.

18 Engle PL, Fernald LC, Alderman H, Behrman J, O'Gara C, Yousafzai A, et al. Strategies for reducing inequalities and improving developmental outcomes for young children in low-income and middle-income countries. *Lancet* 2011;378:1339-53.

19 Lake A. Early childhood development—global action is overdue. *Lancet* 2011;378:1277.

20 Wilson JMG, Jungner G. Principles and practice of screening for disease. *WHO Bull*1968;22:473.

21 Cochrane AL, Holland WW. Validation of screening procedures. *Br Med Bull* 1971;27:3-8.

22 Köhler L, Rigby M. Indicators of children's development: considerations when constructing a set of national child health indicators for the European Union. *Child Care Health Dev*2003;29:551-8.

23 Hagan JF, Shaw JS, Duncan PM, eds. Bright futures: guidelines for health supervision of infants, children, and adolescents. 3rd ed. American Academy of Pediatrics, 2008. http://brightfutures.aap.org/pdfs/guidelines_pdf/1-bf-introduction.pdf.

24 HR 3962. To provide affordable, quality health care for all Americans and reduce the growth in health care spending, and for other purposes. 2009. http://housedocs.house.gov/rules/health/111_ahcaa.pdf.

25 Sharma A. Developmental examination: birth to 5 years. *Arch Dis Child Educ Pract Ed*2011;96:162-75.

26 Bax M, Whitmore K. The medical examination of children on entry to school. The results and use of neurodevelopmental assessment. *Dev Med Child Neurol*1987;29:40-55.

27 Voight RG, Llorente AM, Jensen CL, Fraley JK, Barbaresr WJ, Heird WC. Comparison of the validity of direct pediatric developmental evaluation versus developmental screening by parental report. *Clin Pediatr*2007;46:523-9.

28 Klamer A, Lando A, Pinborg A, Greisen G. Ages and stages questionnaire used to measure cognitive deficit in children born extremely preterm. *Acta Paediatr*2005;94:1327-9.

29 Glascoe FP. Parents' concerns about children's development: prescreening technique or screening test? *Pediatrics*1997;99:522-8.

30 Glascoe FP. Evidence-based approach to developmental and behavioural surveillance using parents' concerns. *Child Care Health Dev*2000,26:137-49.

31 Robins D, Fein D, Barton M, Green J. The modified checklist for autism in toddlers: an initial study investigating the early detection of autism and pervasive developmental disorders. *J Autism Dev Disord*2001;31:131-4.

32 Glascoe FP, Byrne KE, Ashford LG, Johnson KL, Chang B, Strickland B. Accuracy of the Denver II in developmental screening. *Pediatrics* 1992;89:1221-5.

33 Sheridan M, Sharma A, Cockerill H. From birth to five years: children's developmental progress. Routledge, 2007.

34 Bellman M, Lingam S, Aukett A. Schedule of growing skills II. NFER-Nelson, 1997.

35 Glascoe FP. A method for deciding how to respond to parents' concerns about development and behavior. *Ambul Child Health*1999;5:197-208.

36 Glascoe FP, Byrne KE. The accuracy of developmental screening tests. *J Early Interv*1993;17:368-78.

37 Squires J, Bricker D, Potter L. Revision of a parent-completed developmental screening tool: ages and stages questionnaire. *J Pediatr Psychol*1996;22:313-28.

38 Bellman MH, Rawson NS, Wadsworth J, Ross EM, Cameron S, Miller DL. A developmental test based on the Stycar sequences used in the National Childhood Encephalopathy Study. *Child Care Health Dev*1985;11:309-23.

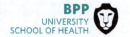

Table 3 Developmental screening questionnaires

Instrument	Method	Age range	Outcome	Availability	Validation, sensitivity, specificity data
Parents' evaluation of developmental status (PEDS)	A parent reported questionnaire used to identify general developmental delay in primary care; takes 5 minutes to complete, 2 minutes to score	0-8 years	High, moderate, or low risk for developmental or behavioural problems	Purchase from publisher (www.pedstest.com)	Validated in a large diverse standardisation sample; sensitivity of 74-79% and specificity of 70-80% in ages 0-8 years for detection of developmental delays and behavioural problems[36]
Ages and stages questionnaire (ASQ)	A parent reported questionnaire of 30 developmental items used to identify general developmental delay in primary care; takes 10-15 minutes to complete	4-60 months	Cut-off point guides need for further assessment	Purchase from publisher (www.brookespublishing.com)	Validated in a large diverse standardisation sample; specificity ranges from 81% (16 months) to 92% (36 months), and 86% overall; sensitivity averages 72%; published validation studies[37]
Modified checklist for autism in toddlers (M-CHAT)	A parent report of 23 items used to screen for autism in primary care population; takes 2 minutes to complete	16-30 months	Cut-off point for further assessment	Freely available online (www.firstsigns.org/downloads/m-chat.PDF)	Published validation study[31]
Schedule of growing skills	Professional scores items in 9 developmental fields; takes 10-15 minutes to complete	0-59 months	Graphic profile of developmental age compared with chronological age; guidelines to aid professional judgment of next action	Purchase from publisher (www.gl-assessment.co.uk)	Original data validation study showed specificity of 94-100% and sensitivity of 44-82% in different fields[38]; validation of revised schedule showed high reliability (Cronbach α 0.91)[33]
Denver developmental screening test	Professional scores items in 4 developmental fields	2-71 months	Graphic display of developmental age with "pass/fail" score compared with "normal" centiles	Purchase from publisher (www.denverii.com)	Originally validated in Colorado, US; later statistical study showed specificity of 43% and sensitivity of 83%[32]

Cite this as: *BMJ* 2013;346: e8687

Related links

bmj.com/archive
Previous articles in this series
- Thunderclap headache (2013;346:e8557)
- Bipolar disorder (2012;345:e8508)
- Diagnosis and management of supraventricular tachycardia (2012;345:e7769)
- Advances in radiotherapy (2012;345:e7765)
- Generalized anxiety disorder: diagnosis and treatment (2012;345:e7500)

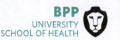

Managing wheeze in preschool children

Andrew Bush professor of paediatrics and head of section (paediatrics)[1] professor of paediatric respirology[2] consultant paediatric chest physician[3], Jonathan Grigg professor of paediatric respiratory and environmental medicine[4], Sejal Saglani reader in paediatric respiratory medicine[35]

[1]Imperial College, London UK

[2]National Heart and Lung Institute, Imperial College, London, UK

[3]Respiratory Paediatrics, Royal Brompton Harefield NHS Foundation Trust, London, UK

[4]Blizzard Institute, Barts and the London Hospital, London, UK

[5]Leukocyte Biology, NHLI, Imperial College London, UK

Correspondence to: A Bush, Department of Paediatric Respiratory Medicine, Royal Brompton Hospital, London SW3 6NP, UK a.bush@ imperial.ac.uk

Cite this as: *BMJ* 2014;348:g15

‹DOI› 10.1136/bmj.g15
http://www.bmj.com/content/348/bmj.g15

Lower respiratory tract illnesses with wheeze are common, occurring in around a third of all preschool children (here defined as aged between 1 and 5 years). They are a major source of morbidity and healthcare costs, including time off work for carers, and are often difficult to treat. This review focuses on the two areas in which there have been recent developments. The first is the classification of these children by symptom pattern into "episodic viral" and "multiple trigger" wheezers.[1] These phenotypes can change within an individual over time,[2] but they are a useful guide to current treatment, and there are also physiological and pathological rationales for their use.[3] [4] The second area is the recent series of large randomised controlled trials of treatment, specifically related to the roles of intermittent montelukast and inhaled and oral corticosteroids. These trials have shown clearly that inhaled corticosteroids and prednisolone in particular have been misused and overused in the past, mandating a reappraisal of treatment algorithms.

What is wheeze?

Wheeze is a term that is often used imprecisely, as has been shown in studies with a video questionnaire and direct quantification of wheeze.[5] [6] [7] [8] Indeed, some European languages do not even have a word for wheeze. Our definition is high pitched whistling sounds usually in expiration and associated with increased work of breathing, but which can also sometimes be heard in inspiration. In research studies, wheeze can be quantified directly by using surface microphones, which is the ideal. With this technique, it was shown that physicians auscultating the chest accurately identify wheeze[8]; parents and nurses were much less reliable.

How common is wheeze in preschool children?

Preschool wheeze is common. In the Avon Longitudinal Study of Parents and Children (ALSPAC) study, a prospective longitudinal observational study, 26% of 6265 infants reported on had had at least one episode of wheeze by the age of 18 months.[9]

What is the best clinical approach to the preschool wheezer?

Once it is established that the child has actual wheeze, history and a careful physical examination should be used to place the child in one of four categories (table). History and physical examination are used to categorise the child and to decide whether further investigation is needed. In general, there are three reasons for a referral: if diagnosis is in doubt, if treatment is not working, and if any party (general practitioner, parent) is unhappy with progress. A report of two cross sectional, community based observational studies found that isolated dry cough in a community setting, without wheeze or breathlessness, is most unlikely to be caused by any form of asthma.[9] Most preschool wheezers do not require any additional tests.

Confusion arises from the different uses of the term "bronchiolitis." In the United Kingdom, this is an illness characterised by respiratory distress and showers of fine crackles in a child aged under 1 year; though wheeze can be present as well, it is the crackles that define the illness. It should be emphasised that any rigid definitions based on age are likely, to some extent, to be artificial. In the United States and elsewhere, "bronchiolitis" is used synonymously with wheezing illness. We have not discussed the approach to bronchiolitis as defined in the UK; interested readers are referred elsewhere.[10] [11] [12]

Should preschool wheezers be subdivided (phenotyped)?

Several approaches have been used to categorise preschool wheezers. The first two are mentioned because they are of scientific importance and are widely quoted in the literature, but they are not useful in guiding treatment.

- Epidemiological: patterns such as transient early (wheeze only in the first three years of life) and persistent (wheeze throughout the first six years of life).[9] [13] These studies have led to many insights into the evolution of symptoms and lung function, but the categories can be determined only retrospectively and give no guide to treatment, so are not useful for the clinician
- Atopic versus non-atopic: early aeroallergen sensitisation is certainly predictive of ongoing symptoms and loss of lung function at school age,[14] but does not predict the response to treatment with inhaled corticosteroids[15]
- Symptom pattern: the European Respiratory Society Task Force[1] suggested that preschool wheezers should be

SOURCES AND SELECTION CRITERIA

We performed a PubMed search using the terms (("asthma" or "wheeze") and preschool), with the filters "clinical trial", "published in the last 5 years", "humans", "English" activated, with the subject age range "infant" (0-23 months) and "preschool" (2-5 years). Additionally, we separately searched the Cochrane database and Clinical Evidence, as well as our personal archives of references, extending beyond the previous five years, and also checked the reference lists in all manuscripts.

We selected only those manuscripts that either related to practical phenotyping of preschool wheezers or contributed to the evidence base for treatment. We eliminated all manuscripts that also included children of school age and above unless we could differentiate data from pre-schoolers aged 5 and under from data from older children because the pathophysiology of wheeze and the treatment algorithms are different in these two age spans. We also eliminated small trials and case series if the findings had been subsumed into a meta-analysis or Cochrane review.

SUMMARY POINTS

- Preschool wheeze should be divided into "episodic viral" and "multiple trigger" according to the history, and these categories, which can change over time, should be used to guide treatment
- No treatment has been shown to prevent progression of preschool wheeze to school age asthma, so treatment is driven solely by current symptoms
- In all but the most severe cases, episodic symptoms should be treated with episodic treatment
- If trials of prophylactic treatment are contemplated, they should be discontinued at the end of a strictly defined time period because many respiratory symptoms remit spontaneously in preschool children
- Prednisolone is not indicated in preschool children with attacks of wheeze who are well enough to remain at home and in many such children, especially those with episodic viral wheeze, who are admitted to hospital

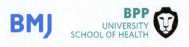

placed into one of two pragmatic categories. This is our favoured categorisation for planning treatment:

- Episodic viral wheeze (EVW): the child wheezes only with usually clinically diagnosed viral upper respiratory infections and is otherwise totally symptom free
- Multiple trigger wheeze (MTW): the child wheezes with clinically diagnosed upper respiratory infections but also with other triggers, such as exercise and smoke and allergen exposure.

This last classification is used to guide treatment (see below). It has been criticised because children might change between categories over time,[2] but in that event pharmacological treatment should also change. This is analogous to the situation in school age children with asthma; treatment is not left fixed over time but is increased or decreased depending on symptom pattern and severity. Unfortunately, few studies adopt this classification; most randomised controlled trials and genetic and epidemiological studies combine children with both symptom patterns.

Is it asthma?

This question is commonly asked by parents who want to know whether their child will continue to have symptoms and require drug treatment into school age and beyond. The answer, however, depends on what definition of asthma is being used by the questioner. If a purely symptomatic definition is used (symptoms of wheeze and breathlessness fluctuating over time and with treatment), then the answer is affirmative. If, however, the definition includes evidence of airway eosinophilic inflammation, the answer is more difficult as few if any have the ability to measure this in preschool children. What most parents actually want to know is whether their child will go on with symptoms and the need for treatment into school age and beyond. The evidence from cross sectional physiological work and studies of endobronchial biopsies in children with severe preschool wheeze is that multiple trigger wheeze is associated with more airflow obstruction than episodic viral wheeze, and the airway pathology (eosinophilic inflammation and remodelling) is similar to childhood and adult asthma.[16]

By contrast, episodic viral wheeze is not associated with evidence of eosinophilic inflammation, so the use of inhaled corticosteroids in this group is questionable.

Does preschool wheeze lead to asthma?

Several clinical predictive indices for future risk of asthma have been developed based on combinations of the presence of atopic manifestations, indirect evidence of airway inflammation, such as peripheral blood eosinophil count, and severity of preschool wheeze.[17] [18] [19] They all have a high negative predictive value and a poor positive predictive value (typically positive predictive values 44-54, negative 81-88[17] [18] [19]). Children who have episodic viral wheeze only have no increased risk of atopy or respiratory symptoms in the long term once they reach the age of 14.[20]

Can we prevent preschool wheeze progressing to school age asthma?

The clear cut evidence from good randomised controlled trials is that early use of inhaled corticosteroids, whether continuously or intermittently with viral colds, does not affect progression of disease.[21] [22] [23] A trial of oral cetirizine in high risk children seemed to show benefit in preventing symptoms in subgroups sensitised to particular aeroallergens,[24] but a subsequent trial with L-cetirizine did not replicate these findings (J Warner, personal communication, 2013). This means that we have no disease modifying drug treatments, and treatment should solely be focused on current symptoms.

What are the broad treatment strategies for children with preschool wheeze?

Before any drugs are prescribed for either episodic viral wheeze or multiple trigger wheeze, it is essential to ensure that the home environment is optimal, particularly that the child is not exposed to tobacco smoke; parental smoking "not in front of the children" does not protect them from harm.[25] A birth cohort study found that air pollution can increase vulnerability to preschool wheeze,[26] but to date we have no specific advice based on individual exposure profiles. Drugs might reasonably be targeted at prevention of future complications such as airway remodelling and persistent airflow obstruction, and, additionally, to treat present symptoms. In practice, we have no drug strategies to reduce future risk of asthma; neither early use of continuous[21] [22] nor intermittent[23] inhaled corticosteroids reduces the risk of progression to school age asthma. If inhaled drugs are prescribed, repeated education of the parents in the correct use of spacers is essential. If inhaled drugs in particular do not seem to be working, check that they are being properly administered rather than escalate treatment. The use of a skilled respiratory nurse to help carers give inhaled drugs to children is invaluable.

How to treat episodic viral wheeze?

Intermittent symptoms should be treated with intermittent therapy (and in practice this is likely to be what parents do anyway). Failure to instigate regular inhaled treatment will not prejudice future respiratory health. It is important to consider whether the child needs treatment at all. The use of inhaled therapy to treat mild respiratory noises with minimal respiratory distress might be more problematic than the disease. If treatment is required, then initial treatment should be with an intermittent bronchodilator (either short acting β2 agonist or anticholinergic).

If treatment needs to be escalated beyond intermittent β2 agonist or anticholinergic because of failure to control symptoms, the next options are intermittent leucotriene receptor antagonist (montelukast), intermittent inhaled corticosteroids, or both. There have been important recent randomised controlled trials of intermittent therapy.

The PREEMPT study examined intermittent montelukast compared with placebo in 220 children aged 2-14.[27] Treatment was initiated at the onset of symptoms of a respiratory tract infection and continued for a minimum of a week or until symptoms had disappeared for 48 hours. The montelukast group had fewer unscheduled consultations for asthma (odds ratio 0.65, 95% confidence interval 0.47 to 0.89) and fewer days away from school or childcare and less time off work for parents (37% and 33%, respectively; P<0.001 for both). In a predefined subgroup analysis, the benefits were greater in children aged 2-5 (about 80% of the study group). These findings were not confirmed in a much larger three way comparison of intermittent montelukast, continuous montelukast, and placebo (nearly 600 children in each group).[28] A three way comparison between standard treatment, intermittent montelukast, and intermittent nebulised budesonide (the only aerosolised steroid permitted by the FDA in preschool children) in 238 children aged 12-59 months showed minor and equivalent benefits

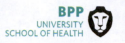

Four groups of childhood wheezing disorders, based on personal practice		
Wheeze category	Suggestive features	Suggested actions
Normal child—commonest and also the hardest diagnosis to make (includes those with postviral cough, pertussis, and parents who are overanxious about minor symptoms or do not appreciate the number of viral infections a normal preschooler will acquire)	Child well and thriving, with no other features on history or examination to raise concerns	Reassurance
Serious condition (such as immunodeficiency)—rare but essential to diagnose or refer	Suspect if history of symptoms from first day of life, chronic wet cough, sudden onset of symptoms, continuous unremitting symptoms, systemic illness; physical examination shows digital clubbing, unusually severe chest deformity, stridor, fixed wheeze, or asymmetric signs on auscultation, anything to suggest systemic disease	Refer for investigation (by telephone if sudden onset of signs suggesting endobronchial foreign body)
Minor conditions that might may exacerbate or mimic wheezing syndrome—for example, gastro-oesophageal reflux, chronic rhinitis	Otherwise well and thriving child with history of easy vomiting, arching away from breast, poor feeder (gastro-oesophageal reflux), or prominent upper airway disease, inflamed nose, adenotonsillar hypertrophy	Initial empirical trials of treatment; refer if no response and symptoms troublesome. Child with prominent snoring should be considered for referral for sleep study
True wheezing syndrome: episodic viral wheeze (EVW); multiple trigger wheeze (MTW)	An otherwise well and thriving child with wheeze only at time of viral cold, often but not invariably with no personal or family history of atopic disorders (EVW); wheeze with viral colds and also between colds with typical asthma triggers such as exertion and excitement, cold air, allergens (MTW). There is often but not invariably a personal or family history of atopic disorders	Treatment options discussed in text. Refer if child is not responding

for the two active treatments compared with standard treatment.[29] Benefits were greater in the subgroup with a modified asthma predictive index. Taken together, these studies suggest that a trial of montelukast in preschool children with troublesome viral induced wheeze is worth attempting. We recommend starting treatment at the first sign of a viral cold and discontinuing it when the child is clearly better, rather than for a fixed period of days.

The Cochrane review identified use of intermittent inhaled corticosteroids as a partially effective strategy for episodic wheeze in preschool children.[30] A proof of concept study in 129 children aged 1-6 years showed that the pre-emptive use of 750 µg twice a day (compared with the maximum licensed dose of 200 µg twice daily in children aged 4 and above; not licensed in any dose below age 4) of fluticasone dipropionate for up to 10 days, starting at the first sign of a viral upper respiratory tract infection, led to a reduction in dose of rescue prednisolone (8% of upper respiratory tract infections in the fluticasone group v 18% in the placebo group; odds ratio 0.49, 95% confidence interval 0.30 to 0.83).[31] This huge dose, however, was unsurprisingly associated with side effects and cannot be recommended. Another study looked at regular twice daily nebulised budesonide 0.5 mg compared with intermittent nebulised budesonide 1 mg twice a day at the time of viral respiratory illnesses. This was a randomised double blind controlled trial in 278 children aged between 12 and 53 months who had a positive modified asthma predictive index.[32] There was no difference in any respiratory outcome, but in the absence of a placebo group it is not possible to state that either strategy was beneficial. What this study definitely shows is that regular nebulised budesonide does not prevent viral exacerbations of wheeze. Smaller older trials of inhaled beclometasone also failed to show a preventive effect.[33] There is currently no evidence to support the use of inhaled corticosteroids at licensed doses in children with episodic viral wheeze. As some studies suggest that intermittent inhaled corticosteroids might be a useful approach in children with viral induced wheeze at higher than licensed doses, further studies are required to clarify the dose and duration that might be beneficial in this setting. In practice, however, it would be unwise to go above a fluticasone dose of 150 µg twice a day, given the number and duration of viral colds in normal preschool children and the risk of side effects including growth suppression and adrenal failure with higher doses. There are currently no studies that have combined intermittent inhaled corticosteroids with intermittent montelukast to treat episodic viral wheeze.

Is there any role for prophylactic continuous inhaled corticosteroids in episodic viral wheeze?

There is no evidence to support the use of regular inhaled corticosteroids in preschool children who do not wheeze between viral colds. In those children with really severe episodic wheeze who require repeated admission to hospital or have prolonged disruptive symptoms managed at home, however, a trial of prophylactic inhaled corticosteroids can be given. In some cases it might become apparent that in fact there were interval symptoms that were underappreciated. In any event, the clinical trials of inhaled corticosteroids in episodic viral wheeze were carried out in relatively mildly affected children, so the evidence in severely affected children is less robust. Treatment should be reviewed and discontinued if there is no benefit; there is no evidence to suggest the optimal duration of the therapeutic trial, but six to eight weeks would seem a reasonable time period. If the viral wheezing improves on treatment, regular attempts should still be made to reduce the dose. It should be noted that, in a small study, even really severe episodic viral wheeze was not associated with eosinophilic airway inflammation[4] and that inhaled corticosteroids (fluticasone 100 µg twice a day) led to growth suppression in the PEAK trial,[21] so trials of inhaled corticosteroids in this context should be deployed only exceptionally. If there is a suspicion that the child might in fact have symptoms between colds, which are underappreciated by the carers, a trial of inhaled steroids can reveal that the child was previously much more symptomatic than was thought.

Whatever the context of therapeutic trials in preschool children, they should be for a fixed time period (such as six to eight weeks, see above) and discontinued at the end of the agreed period to see if symptoms recur or in fact have resolved and treatment has become unnecessary (see the three stage trial proposal below).

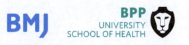

Is there a role for oral prednisolone in primary care for preschool wheeze?

Recent evidence has questioned the role of prednisolone in acute episodes of episodic viral preschool wheeze. In a home based study, 217 preschool children who had at least one admission to hospital were randomised to a parent initiated course of prednisolone or placebo at the next wheezing episode. No benefit was observed in the treatment group.[34] A hospital study that randomised 687 preschool children admitted with wheeze to prednisolone or placebo in addition to bronchodilator therapy found there was no benefit in the prednisolone group.[35]

The implication of these two studies, involving more than 900 children, is that any preschool child with viral induced wheeze who is well enough to stay in the community should not be prescribed oral prednisolone, and many children admitted to hospital also should not be prescribed oral prednisolone.[36] These studies, however, were undertaken in children with relatively mild symptoms and most were discharged from hospital in less than 24 hours, so what these studies do not tell us is whether prednisolone is indicated in really severe preschool viral wheeze. In the absence of evidence, it is likely that prednisolone will continue to be prescribed in this small subgroup of children in hospital.

How should I treat multiple trigger wheeze?

Preschool children who have wheeze or cough responsive to bronchodilator treatment and breathlessness on most days even when they do not have a viral cold should be considered for a trial of preventive drug treatment, either inhaled corticosteroids or a leucotriene receptor antagonist (montelukast). As airway inflammation cannot routinely be measured in this age group, and many children will become asymptomatic before school age, it would be incorrect to assume the pathophysiology of the disease is the same as school age asthma. Furthermore, the younger the child, the less likely there is to be any eosinophilic inflammation[37] and therefore more reluctance to use inhaled corticosteroids.

There is a dearth of evidence, but the box shows a pragmatic three stage trial of treatment, which is recommended in our practice.

QUESTIONS FOR FUTURE RESEARCH AND ONGOING STUDIES

- Is nebulised hypertonic saline an effective strategy to contemplate in children with acute preschool wheeze needing admission to hospital?
- What is the minimum effective dose of inhaled corticosteroids for intermittent use in preschool children with episodic viral wheeze?
- Would fine particle inhaled corticosteroids, which might be expected to deposit in the peripheral airways, offer additional benefit?
- Is intermittent high dose inhaled corticosteroid safe and beneficial in children with acute preschool wheeze who need admitting to hospital?
- How can we predict which children with preschool wheeze will go on to develop asthma, and how can we prevent this?
- Does prevention of respiratory syncytial virus infection with palivizumab lead to a reduction in prevalence of school age asthma?
- Parent-determined oral montelukast therapy for preschool wheeze with stratification for arachidonate-5-lipoxygenase (ALOX5) promoter genotype (http://clinicaltrials.gov/show/NCT01142505). This is a randomised controlled trial of intermittent therapy with montelukast started at the first sign of a viral cold or wheeze by parents. Both phenotypes of wheeze were recruited and analysis is due January 2014

PRAGMATIC REGIMEN FOR TRIAL OF TREATMENT

Step 1: Trial of inhaled corticosteroids or montelukast in standard dose for a defined period, usually four to eight weeks

Step 2: Stop treatment; either there has been no improvement, in which case further escalation is not valuable, or symptoms have disappeared; in the latter case, it is not possible to know if this was spontaneous or as a result of treatment. If there is no benefit and the symptoms are troublesome, referral for consideration of further investigation is recommended

Step 3: Restart treatment only if symptoms recur; then reduce treatment to the lowest level that controls symptoms

The aim of this three step approach is to prevent children being falsely labelled and inappropriately treated because someone has started a drug when the child was about to get better spontaneously. Long acting β2 agonists are not licensed for use in preschool children.

Are there any other new treatments around?

In a small double blind trial, a total of 41 children aged 1-6 years were randomised to nebulised hypertonic (7%) or normal (0.9%) saline, in each case combined with salbutamol twice 20 minutes apart in the emergency department and then, if the child was admitted to hospital, four times a day thereafter.[38] Admission rates and lengths of stay were significantly reduced in the hypertonic saline group, but there was no significant change in severity score, possibly because of the small size of the study. Further work in larger numbers of children is needed to define the role of hypertonic saline in acute preschool wheeze. Given the possibility of bronchoconstriction being induced by hypertonic saline, this treatment should be given only in a hospital setting.

Palivizumab has been used to prevent infection with respiratory syncytial virus in high risk infants—for example, survivors of extreme prematurity. The cost and inconvenience of monthly injections means this has never been, and is still not, a treatment strategy for all babies. A recent double blind study, however, randomised 429 infants born at 33-35 weeks' gestation to palivizumab or placebo.[39] Palivizumab reduced the number of days with wheeze in the first year of life by 61% and the proportion of infants with recurrent wheeze from 21% to 10%. The more interesting question, which this trial could answer, is the vexed one as to whether early respiratory syncytial virus infection causes asthma or is merely a sign that the child was previously predisposed to asthma, provided the infants are followed up to school age. The current position is that this is work in progress, rather than an indication for a change in public policy.

What about treatment plans?

Treatment plans outlining self management actions to be taken depending on the severity of symptoms and peak flow measurements are widely recommended in school age children. In a randomised controlled trial in which 200 children age 18 months to 5 years who had an unscheduled hospital visit or admission with wheezing were allocated either to standard care or to receive a package consisting of a booklet, a written guided self management plan, and two structured educational sessions, there were no differences in any outcomes.[40] Despite this, many will use educational sessions and plans, but there is no evidence of efficacy.

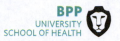

13 Martinez FD, Wright AL, Taussig LM, Holberg CJ, Halonen M, Morgan WJ. Asthma and wheezing in the first six years of life: the Group Health Medical Associates. *N Engl J Med*1995;332:133-8.

14 Illi S, von Mutius E, Lau S, Niggemann B, Grüber C, Wahn U; Multicentre Allergy Study (MAS) group. Perennial allergen sensitisation early in life and chronic asthma in children: a birth cohort study. *Lancet*2006;368:763-70.

15 Castro-Rodriguez JA, Rodrigo GJ. Efficacy of inhaled corticosteroids in infants and preschoolers with recurrent wheezing and asthma: a systematic review with meta-analysis. *Pediatrics*2009;123:e519-25.

16 Saglani S, Payne DN, Zhu J, Wang Z, Nicholson AG, Bush A, et al. Early detection of airway wall remodelling and eosinophilic inflammation in preschool wheezers. *Am J Respir Crit Care Med*2007;176:858-64.

17 Savenije OE, Kerkhof M, Koppelman GH, Postma DS. Predicting who will have asthma at school age among preschool children. *J Allergy Clin Immunol*2012;130:325-31.

18 Guilbert TW, Morgan WJ, Zeiger RS, Bacharier LB, Boehmer SJ, Krawiec M, et al. Atopic characteristics of children with recurrent wheezing at high risk for the development of childhood asthma. *J Allergy Clin Immunol*2004;114:1282-7.

19 Devulapalli CS, Carlsen KC, Håland G, Munthe-Kaas MC, Pettersen M, Mowinckel P, et al. Severity of obstructive airways disease by age 2 years predicts asthma at 10 years of age. *Thorax*2008;63:8-13.

20 Harris JM, Bush A, Wilson N, Mills P, White C, Moffat S, et al. Preschool wheezing phenotypes in a representative school cohort. *Thorax*2010;65(suppl 4):A37.

21 Guilbert TW, Morgan WJ, Zeiger RS, Mauger DT, Boehmer SJ, Szefler SJ, et al. Long-term inhaled corticosteroids in preschool children at high risk for asthma. *N Engl J Med*2006;354:1985-97.

22 Murray CS, Woodcock A, Langley SJ, Morris J, Custovic A; IFWIN study team. Secondary prevention of asthma by the use of inhaled fluticasone dipropionate in wheezy infants (IWWIN): double-blind, randomised controlled study. *Lancet*2006;368:754-62.

23 Bisgaard H, Hermansen MN, Loland L, Halkjaer LB, Buchvald F. Intermittent inhaled corticosteroids in infants with episodic wheezing. *N Engl J Med*2006;354:1998-2005.

24 Pool J, Petrova N, Russell RR. Exposing children to secondhand smoke. *Thorax*2012;67:926.

25 Warner JO; ETAC Study Group. Early treatment of the atopic child. A double-blinded, randomized, placebo-controlled trial of cetirizine in preventing the onset of asthma in children with atopic dermatitis: 18 months' treatment and 18 months' posttreatment follow-up. *J Allergy Clin Immunol*2001;108:929-37.

26 Andersen ZJ, Loft S, Ketzel M, Stage M, Scheike T, Hermansen MN, et al. Ambient air pollution triggers wheezing symptoms in infants. *Thorax*2008;63:710-6.

27 Robertson CF, Price D, Henry R, Mellis C, Glasgow N, Fitzgerald D, et al. Short-course montelukast for intermittent asthma in children: a randomized controlled trial. *Am J Respir Crit Care Med*2007;175:323-9.

28 Valovirta E, Boza ML, Robertson CF, Verbruggen N, Smugar SS, Nelsen LM, et al. Intermittent or daily montelukast versus placebo for episodic asthma in children. *Ann Allergy Asthma Immunol*2011;106:518-26.

29 Bacharier LB, Phillips BR, Zeiger RS, Szefler SJ, Martinez FD, Lemanske RF Jr; CARE Network. Episodic use of an inhaled corticosteroid or leukotriene receptor antagonist in preschool children with moderate-to-severe intermittent wheezing. *J Allergy Clin Immunol*2008;122:1127-35.

30 McKean M, Ducharme F. Inhaled steroids for episodic viral wheeze of childhood. *Cochrane Database Syst Rev*2000;2:CD001107.

31 Ducharme FM, Lemire C, Noya FJ, Davis GM, Alos N, Leblond H, et al. Preemptive use of high-dose fluticasone for virus-induced wheezing in young children. *N Engl J Med*2009;360:339-53.

32 Zeiger RS, Mauger D, Bacharier LB, Giobert TW, Martinez FD, Lemanske RF Jr et al; CARE Network of the National Heart, Lung, and Blood Institute. Daily or intermittent budesonide in preschool children with recurrent wheezing. *N Engl J Med*2011;365:1990-2001.

33 Wilson N, Sloper K, Silverman M. Effect of continuous treatment with topical corticosteroid on episodic viral wheeze in preschool children. *Arch Dis Child*1995;72:317-20.

34 Oommen A, Lambert PC, Grigg J. Efficacy of a short course of parent-initiated oral prednisolone for viral wheeze in children aged 1-5 years: randomised controlled trial. *Lancet*2003;362:1433-8.

35 Panickar J, Lakhanpaul M, Lambert PC, Kenia P, Stephenson T, Smyth A, et al. Oral prednisolone for preschool children with acute virus-induced wheezing. *N Engl J Med*2009;360:329-38.

36 Bush A. Practice imperfect—treatment for wheezing in preschoolers. *N Engl J Med*2009;360:409-10.

37 Saglani S, Malmstrom K, Pelkonen AS, Malmberg LP, Lindahl H, Kajosaari M, et al. Airway remodeling and inflammation in symptomatic infants with reversible airflow obstruction. *Am J Respir Crit Care Med*2005;171:722-7.

38 Ater D, Shai H, Bar B-E, Fireman N, Tasher D, Dalal I, et al. Hypertonic saline and acute wheezing in preschool children. *Pediatrics*2012;129:e1397.

39 Blanken MO, Rovers MM, Molenaar JM, Winkler-Seinstra PL, Meijer A, Kimpen JL, et al; Dutch RSV Neonatal Network. Respiratory syncytial virus and recurrent wheeze in healthy preterm infants. *N Engl J Med*2013;368:1791-9.

40 Stevens CA, Wesseldine LJ, Couriel JM, Dyer AJ, Osman LM, Silverman M. Parental education and guided self-management of asthma and

What is the role of nebulised therapy?

There is no role for nebulised therapy to deliver bronchodilator apart from in children too sick to use inhalers. For all other purposes, the evidence is clear that metered dose inhalers and spacers are at least as good as nebuliser.

Contributors: AB wrote the initial draft of the manuscript and is guarantor. The manuscript was reviewed and edited by SS and JG; all authors agreed the final version.

Competing interests: We have read and understood the BMJ Group policy on declaration of interests and declare the following interests: AB was supported by the NIHR Respiratory Disease Biomedical Research Unit at the Royal Brompton and Harefield NHS Foundation Trust and Imperial College London.

Provenance and peer review: Not commissioned; externally peer reviewed.

1 Brand PL, Baraldi E, Bisgaard H, Boner AL, Castro-Rodriguez JA, Custovic A, et al. Definition, assessment and treatment of wheezing disorders in preschool children: an evidence-based approach. *Eur Respir J*2008;32:1096-110.

2 Schultz A, Devadason SG, Savenije OE, Sly PD, Le Souef PN, Brand PL. The transient value of classifying preschool wheeze into episodic viral wheeze and multiple trigger wheeze. *Acta Paediatr*2010;99:56-60.

3 Sonnappa S, Bastardo CM, Wade A, Saglani S, McKenzie SA, Bush A, et al. Symptom-pattern and pulmonary function in preschool wheezers. *J Allergy Clin Immunol*2010;126:519-26.

4 Sonnappa S, Bastardo CM, Saglani S, Bush A, Aurora P. Relationship between past airway pathology and current lung function in preschool wheezers. *Eur Respir J*2011;38:1431-6.

5 Cane RS, Ranganathan SC, McKenzie SA. What do parents of wheezy children understand by "wheeze"? *Arch Dis Child*2000;82:327-32.

6 Elphick HE, Ritson S, Rodgers H, Everard ML. When a "wheeze" is not a wheeze: acoustic analysis of breath sounds in infants. *Eur Respir J*2000;16:593-7.

7 Saglani S, McKenzie SA, Bush A, Payne DN. A video questionnaire identifies upper airway abnormalities in pre-school children with reported wheeze. *Arch Dis Child*2005;90:961-4.

8 Levy ML, Godfrey S, Irving CS, Sheikh A, Hanekom W, Bush A, et al. Wheeze detection: recordings vs assessment of physician and parent. *J Asthma*2004;41:845-53.

9 Henderson J, Granell R, Heron J, Sherriff A, Simpson A, Woodcock A, et al. Associations of wheezing phenotypes in the first 6 years of life with atopy, lung function and airway responsiveness in mid-childhood. *Thorax*2008;63:974-80.

10 Kelly YJ, Brabin BJ, Milligan PJ, Reid JA, Heaf D, Pearson MG. Clinical significance of cough and wheeze in the diagnosis of asthma. *Arch Dis Child*1996;75:489-93.

11 British Guideline on the Management of Asthma (2012 update). www.brit-thoracic.org.uk/guidelines/asthma-guidelines.aspx.

12 Bush A, Thomson AH. Acute bronchiolitis. *BMJ*2007;335:1037-41.

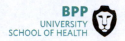

wheezing in the pre-school child: a randomised controlled trial.
*Thorax*2002;57:39-44.

Related links

bmj.com/videos
- Watch a collection of videos on this topic at bmj.com/content/348/
  bmj.g15

bmj.com/
Previous articles in this series
- Erectile dysfunction (BMJ 2014;348:g129)
- Acute haematogenous osteomyelitis in children (BMJ 2014;348:g66)
- Supporting smoking cessation (BMJ 2014;348:f7535)
- Abortion (BMJ 2014;348:f7553)
- Diagnosis, management, and prevention of rotavirus gastroenteritis
  in children (BMJ 2013;347:f7204)
- Tick bite prevention and tick removal (BMJ 2013;347:f7123)Tips for
  non-specialists

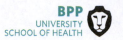

Managing common symptoms of cerebral palsy in children

Mathew D Sewell paediatric spinal fellow[1], Deborah M Eastwood paediatric orthopaedic consultant[1], Neil Wimalasundera consultant in paediatric neurodisability[2]

[1]Royal National Orthopaedic Hospital, Catterall Unit, Stanmore, UK

[2]Wolfson Neurodisability Service, Great Ormond Street, London, UK

Correspondence to: M D Sewell
matbuzz1@hotmail.com

Cite this as: BMJ 2014;349:g5474

‹DOI› 10.1136/bmj.g5474
http://www.bmj.com/content/349/bmj.g5474

Cerebral palsy describes a heterogeneous group of permanent disorders of movement and posture which are attributed to non-progressive disturbances in the developing fetal or infant brain and cause limitations in activity. The motor disorders of cerebral palsy are often accompanied by disturbances of sensation, perception, cognition, communication, and behavior; epilepsy; and secondary musculoskeletal problems.[1] Worldwide, cerebral palsy is the commonest cause of motor disability in childhood, with an incidence of 2-3 per 1000 live births,[2 3 4] increasing to 40-100 per 1000 live births in premature babies and those of very low or low birth weight.[5] As cerebral palsy is a permanent disabling condition it is a major consumer of healthcare resources in developed countries. The motor disorder results from centrally mediated abnormal muscle tone: spasticity ("high tone") is the commonest abnormality. Multiple impairments can limit involvement in life situations in childhood and place great strains on the family. Thirty per cent of affected children are unable to walk, 30% have a severe intellectual impairment, 28% have impaired or no speech, and 12% are blind.[4 5 6] Family doctors can and should play a pivotal role in coordinating care, identifying associated problems early, and providing lifelong support. This article presents an overview of cerebral palsy but focuses on the common problems of spasticity, pain, and feeding difficulties that affect a substantial number of children.

What are the risk factors and causes of cerebral palsy?

Registry data from large multicentre collaborative studies have shown that 50% of children with cerebral palsy are born at term (.37 weeks' gestation), 20% at 32-36 weeks, and 25% before 32 weeks.[5] Large observational studies have shown that despite advances in perinatal care, the prevalence of cerebral palsy has not changed, mainly because of the increased survival of preterm babies.[3] Preterm and very low birthweight babies are at greatest risk; large multicentre cohort studies found that the risk of cerebral palsy in babies born weighing less than 1500 g is 70-fold greater than in those weighing 2500 g or more, although recent registry data from Australia suggest that this risk is decreasing.[3 7 8] Interestingly, smaller cohort studies have shown that babies with a birth weight above the 97th centile are also at greater risk; it is unclear whether excessively low or high intrauterine growth is a cause or consequence of the disability.[7] Recently, the risk of cerebral palsy in very low birthweight babies has declined, which may be related to the use of prenatal corticosteroids in mothers.[9 10] Some causal pathways have been identified, thus cerebral palsy caused by maternal iodine deficiency or kernicterus associated with rhesus isoimmunisation can be prevented.[11] Box 1 lists the risk factors for cerebral palsy.[9 12 13 14] Historically only small numbers of cases of cerebral palsy were related to genetic factors,[15 16] however, more genes are being identified for congenital brain malformations, and a recent registry based cohort study suggested that a genetic component might be more common than previously thought, acting as part

---

SOURCES AND SELECTION CRITERIA

We conducted a Medline search using the key words "cerebral palsy", "tone", "spasticity", "pain", "quality of life", and "feeding". We also searched the Cochrane and Clinical Evidence databases. Well conducted prospective randomised controlled trials on this topic are lacking, and the evidence mainly comes from systematic reviews, meta-analyses, and large multicentre prospective cohort studies.

SUMMARY POINTS

- Cerebral palsy is a disorder of movement and posture secondary to abnormal muscle tone, spasticity being the most common abnormality of tone
- The majority of cerebral palsy is not related to birth asphyxia
- Cerebral palsy is most reliably diagnosed by assessing general movements and neurological examination
- The management of spasticity includes physiotherapy, orthotics, botulinum toxin injections, oral drugs, and surgery (orthopaedic and neurosurgical)
- Cerebral palsy is often accompanied by disturbances in sensation, cognition, communication, behaviour, and epilepsy, which should be looked for continuously, as these problems may be more functionally disabling than the motor problems
- Cerebral palsy is a chronic condition with no cure and as such the overall goal of treatment is to improve quality of life and participation in life situations
- Pain is a common problem and is increasingly recognised as a major determinant of quality of life
- Most children with cerebral palsy have the potential to gain a similar quality of life to their peers and this should guide social and educational policy to ensure that children with disability participate fully in society

BOX 1 CAUSES AND RISK FACTORS FOR CEREBRAL PALSY[9 12 13 14]

Prenatal (80%)
- Prematurity (<37 weeks' gestation)
- Low birth weight (<2500 g)
- Intrauterine growth restriction
- Multiple births
- Intracranial haemorrhage, white matter injury, and cerebral malformations
- Maternal age >35 years
- Severe maternal iodine deficiency
- Associated birth defects
- Maternal infection—for example, cytomegalovirus

Perinatal (10%)
- Peripartum asphyxia
- Maternal infection

Postnatal (10%)
- Head trauma and hypoxia within the first two years of life
- Meningitis
- Intentional injury

These patterns reflect the developed world; other problems, such as cerebral malaria and lack of access to obstetric services, are major causes in many developing countries

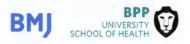

BOX 2 ASSOCIATED FEATURES OF CEREBRAL PALSY AND RECOMMENDED MANAGEMENT[3]

Feeding difficulties

- Related to GMFCS level: >90% in those with GMFCS level 4 or 5 cerebral palsy
- Poor weight gain
- Coughing and choking during mealtimes; long mealtimes
- Recurrent chest infections
- Gastro-oesophageal reflux
- Malnutrition
- Premature death
- Special diets, adjustment of food consistency and child positioning during mealtimes, adaptive equipment to aid feeding, gastrostomy for unsafe swallow or to augment existing oral intake

Drooling

- Impaired social interactions and participation
- Secretions compromising airway
- Behavioural therapies, biofeedback exercises, anticholinergic drugs, intraglandular botulinum toxin type A injections, surgical rerouting of salivary glands

Intellectual impairment, mental health, and behavioural problems

- Affect 60% of children
- Cognitive impairment
- Anxiety and depression
- Exclude pain and seizures as underlying causes; review treatment and stop unnecessary drugs (especially sedatives); encourage participation and independence with all aspects of life (for example, mobility, school, work, independent living) through adaptive equipment or facilitating communication (for example, toys, books, computers, picture communication boards, electronic communication aids); offer counselling for emotional support and psychological challenges particularly at times of transition in the child's life; consider formal psychiatric assessment

Seizures

- Affect 30-40% of children (many are under-recognised as most are focal seizures)
- Head protection orthosis, drugs for control and monitoring

Communication difficulties

- Impaired social interactions and participation
- Speech therapy, use of gestures (sign language) and eye gaze for communication cards and books, electronic communication aids

Impaired vision and hearing (40%)

- Affects 12% of children
- Retinopathy of prematurity
- Visual field defects
- Myopia
- Strabismus, which may lead to amblyopia, and blindness
- Hearing impairments
- Screen for in all children with developmental impairment; retinopathy of prematurity and squint may require surgery

Abnormal pain and touch sensations

- Sensory and physical stimulation programmes and oral drugs

Bladder dysfunction

- Incontinence or retention secondary to impaired motor control of bladder muscles
- Nappies or padding in underwear, biofeedback exercises, drugs, urological procedures

Sleep disturbance

- Commonly secondary to pain from a variety of causes (see table 2)
- Anxiety
- Assessment and treatment of underlying cause (pain, gastro-oesophageal reflux), counselling and emotional support for psychological challenges, which are particularly apparent at transitional times in the child's life (for example, moving from junior to senior school)

Constipation

- See table 2 for advice

of a multifactorial aetiology that includes environmental factors.[17]

In the developed world, data from systematic reviews suggest that in more than 80% of children, cerebral palsy is caused by brain lesions or maldevelopments; magnetic resonance imaging can demonstrate these abnormalities (fig 1).[3][18] The majority of abnormalities occur prenatally and, contrary to popular belief, hypoxia around the time of birth (hypoxic-ischaemic encephalopathy) accounts for only 10% of cases. Evidence from a systematic review suggests that postnatal head cooling can lessen the adverse neurodevelopmental effects of hypoxic-ischaemic encephalopathy.[19] Postnatal causes such as meningitis, near drowning, and intentional injury account for 10%.[13] In many developing countries, the epidemiology and causation of cerebral palsy differ, with a greater proportion of perinatal and postnatal causes (for example, cerebral malaria). Prospective cohort data suggest that the incidence of postnatal cerebral palsy has decreased with improved childhood nutrition, vaccination policies, and public health initiatives that have reduced the number of automobile and drowning incidents.[5] The exact causes of some cerebral palsies are still poorly understood, and for many children will never be formally determined.

How is cerebral palsy diagnosed?

The diagnosis of cerebral palsy is made on clinical grounds after taking a detailed antenatal and family history and carrying out a full examination. Failure of children to achieve expected milestones in motor development (table 1) in the presence of abnormal movement or muscle tone (excessive stiffness or floppiness) is characteristic. An assessment of general movements in the first five months of life is the most reliable way to identify children who may later have a diagnosis of cerebral palsy.[20][21] In normal, awake infants, fidgety spontaneous general movements, defined as an ongoing stream of small, circular, moderate speed, and elegant controlled movements of the neck, trunk, and limbs in all directions, are seen between ages 2 and 5 months.[20] They are continual in the awake infant, except during focused attention, fussing, and crying, and are best seen in the reclined or supine position. Absent or abnormal fidgety movements (exaggerated amplitude, speed, or jerkiness) at age 3 months is 95% sensitive and 96% specific for the development of neurological deficits,[20] and when coupled with findings from magnetic resonance imaging in preterm babies, is almost 100% accurate in predicting cerebral palsy.[21] It can be difficult to identify early subtle changes and if there are any concerns the child should be referred to a specialist. Occasionally, associated features of cerebral palsy (box 2), such as difficulties with feeding, predominate over motor symptoms in the early years.

The diagnosis of cerebral palsy is usually made in the second year of life and confirmed when other diagnoses can be excluded with reasonable certainty.[4] The major cerebral palsy registries of Europe will not classify children as having the condition until age 4 years, to minimise false positive results.[3] The diagnosis of cerebral palsy can be made at younger ages if the clinical signs correlate with the clinical history and neuroimaging. If there are any concerns about a child's physical or cognitive development at any age they should be referred to a general paediatrician or child development pediatrician for more specialised assessment and investigation. Brain injury is static but the clinical signs and difficulties that children face evolve with time, so

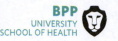

Table 1 Expected milestones in motor development that may be abnormal in neurodevelopmental conditions

Expected timing of milestone	Features of neurodevelopmental abnormality	Additional features/comments
6 to 20 weeks post-term:		
"Fidgety" movements on assessment of spontaneous general movements	Fidgety general movements are absent or abnormal at 3 months. Abnormal movements look like fidgety movements but their amplitude, speed, and jerkiness are greatly exaggerated	Young infants have a repertoire of distinct spontaneous movement patterns. One set of these patterns is known as general movements. Fidgety general movements are defined as an ongoing stream of small, circular, moderate speed, and elegant controlled movements of neck, trunk, and limbs in all directions. They are continual in awake infants, except during focused attention, fussing, and crying and are best observed when infants are in a reclined position or lying supine. Absent or abnormal fidgety general movements at 3 months are highly predictive for cerebral palsy
3 months:		
Head control	Head control not present by 6 months	Infant should be able to lift head off floor. Not specific
6 months:		
Sitting unsupported (little or no trunk support)	Infant cannot sit unsupported by 9 months	Posture abnormalities (excessive stiffness, floppiness, or involuntary movements) are common in cerebral palsy
12 months:		
Walking	Child not walking by 18 months	The time children start to walk varies widely. Gait abnormalities are common in cerebral palsy and include limp, persistent toe walking, scissor walking (knees come in and cross), ataxia, and weakness
After 15 months:		
Development of hand preference	Hand preference develops before 15 months	Hand preference before 15 months suggests a contralateral hemiparesis

repeated assessments are essential. Large cohort studies suggest that most motor impairments become apparent by 18 months. Early clues include persistent fisting, drooling, and feeding difficulties, asymmetrical movements, delayed motor development, and toe walking.[3] It is essential to differentiate a static from a progressive clinical course: loss of previously acquired motor milestones (regression) is characteristic of neurodegenerative and metabolic disorders.[22]

Once the diagnosis is considered, magnetic resonance imaging (often under general anaesthesia) is usually performed. Evidence from a systematic review of observational studies suggests that findings on magnetic resonance imaging are abnormal in 86% of cases.[23] The type of lesion seen may help determine the cause and timing of injury and predict clinical outcome in terms of motor and cognitive impairment, bulbar involvement, seizures,

and visual or perceptual difficulties.[24] A normal magnetic resonance imaging scan with non-classic history requires investigation for an alternative diagnosis.

How and why is cerebral palsy classified?

Many classification systems are used in cerebral palsy, and these fall broadly into two groups: those that describe physical motor abnormalities and those that describe function.[25 26 27 28 29] The Surveillance of Cerebral Palsy in Europe collaboration[25] recommends describing distribution as unilateral or bilateral and classifies the main motor tone types into one of four groups: spastic, dyskinetic, ataxic, and mixed (box 3). Physical classification systems do not provide information on children's activity status or level of participation, defined as involvement in life situations.[30] Functional classification systems[26 27 28] are now the ideal method for classifying children with cerebral palsy, as

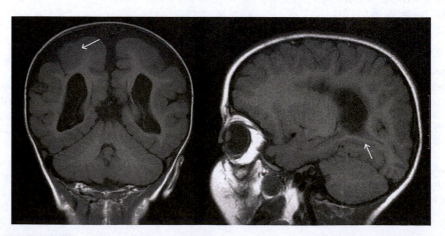

Fig 1 Examples of developmental brain abnormalities in cerebral palsy: (left) lissencephaly (smooth brain), shown on coronal T1 weighted magnetic resonance imaging, is a non-progressive brain maldevelopment resulting from failure of brain folds (gyri) and grooves (sulci) to develop (arrow). (Right) Periventicular leukomalacia (arrow) typically results from preterm (24-32 weeks) insults causing a spastic motor picture worse in the legs

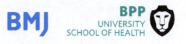

they focus on what children can actually do and how they participate in society. They aid in answering two common questions parents ask: will my child walk, will my child live independently? The age dependent Gross Motor Function Classification System (GMFCS) groups children into one of five levels based on their ability to mobilise and reflects overall gross motor skills and severity of motor impairment (box 4).[26] The system helps predict walking function, the need and type of orthotic and equipment support required to optimise mobility, and the likelihood for orthopaedic surgery.[31] [32]

The World Health Organization's international classification of functioning, disability, and health has redefined the way clinicians understand cerebral palsy.[33] Cerebral palsy impacts on body structure and function (limb movement), activities (walking), and participation (for example, playing sport). There is a move from a focus on body structure and function in the treatment of cerebral palsy, and instead towards optimising quality of life, activity, and participation.

What are the aims of management of cerebral palsy?

Cerebral palsy has no cure. Management strategies should be viewed in a life course context, focused on increasing activity and facilitating participation. Children with cerebral palsy experience a range of impairments, ranging from isolated disturbances in gait and balance that may not be apparent until later childhood (GMFCS level 1) to

profound cognitive and physical disability evident from birth (GMFCS level 4 or 5). Management programmes should be individualised to tackle all impairments, with the involvement of multiple health and social care professionals and families. Family centred services allow parents and children to share and discuss anxieties, which are particularly apparent at transitional times in the child's life (for example, moving schools).[34]

Facilitating communication is important. Home programmes should be tailored to the child's cognitive ability and use toys, communication boards, and technology aids where appropriate. Adaptive equipment is essential to maximise the developmental potential of affected children and allow them to participate more effectively in social activities. Commonly used adaptive devices include mobility aids (k-walkers and wheelchairs to participate in outdoor events, fig 2) and postural support seating (for table activities and feeding at mealtimes).

One of the limitations of evidence based care in cerebral palsy is that most of the research evidence comes from clinically based cohort studies. Information is often skewed by the sources (for example, specialty programmes), age, and case definitions, and thus outcome data (for example, rates of intellectual impairment) may be inaccurate even if they are the best available. Evidence on the impact of many interventions is lacking; this does not mean that the intervention is unhelpful but more likely that the right outcome has failed to be measured.[35]

How are motor tone abnormalities in cerebral palsy assessed and managed?

Tone abnormalities are the primary pathology in cerebral palsy, and effective management of tone can considerably improve quality of life and participation. A cross sectional study of 1174 children with cerebral palsy reported that impaired self mobility and pain were major determinants of quality of life[36]; both can be improved by good tone management.

Registry data suggest that 88% of children have the spastic form of cerebral palsy.[2] [3] [13] Spasticity is one part of the upper motor neurone syndrome in cerebral palsy, which includes hypertonicity, hyperreflexia, clonus, and important "negative signs" such as weakness, poor coordination, and poor selective muscle control. Spasticity is associated with loss of muscle excursion, reduced joint movement, secondary contractures, bony deformity, joint dislocations, and chronic pain.

Dystonia is commonly mistaken for spasticity as both involve hypertonic movements, but treatment and prognosis differ. Dystonia results in muscle co-contracture, a resistance to joint movement, and stiff, slow movements. In contrast with spasticity, tone normalises during sleep and fluctuates considerably with emotional state. Joint contractures and dislocations are less common, but pain can be a considerable problem. Figure 3 outlines the assessment of motor type.

The management of spasticity requires a multidisciplinary approach.[37] Treatment should be goal directed with a view to improving general health (for example, nutrition), alleviating pain (for example, controlling spasms), and facilitating participation (for example, help with walking to attend social events). The National Institute for Health and Care Excellence recently developed guidelines on the management of spasticity in the United Kingdom (summarised below).[38]

Physiotherapy

Physiotherapy should have specific goals, either facilitating participation or preventing the consequences of spasticity, such as pain and joint contractures. Physiotherapists also teach parents how to handle and position their child at home for feeding, bathing, dressing, and other activities of daily living. Referral is indicated for children with weak muscles and those with impaired joint movement. Physiotherapy is used widely and recommended by NICE[38]; however, evidence for its effectiveness is conflicting. Three systematic reviews suggested that strength training physiotherapy programmes can lead to improvements in strength, function, and participation without adverse effects.[39] [40] [41] These reviews were not restricted to randomised controlled trials. A recent systematic review of 22 randomised controlled trials concluded that the evidence for effectiveness of physiotherapy in the arms is moderate and of most physiotherapy interventions is limited overall and that well designed trials are needed.[42] Parents should understand the important but limited role that formal physiotherapy has in the overall management of affected children and that all programmes require input at home as well as at school.

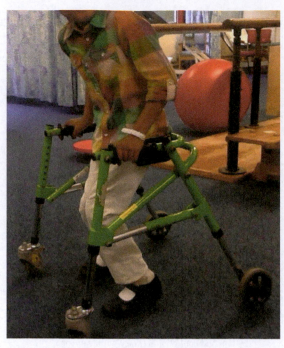

Fig 2 A k-walker frame is commonly used in children with GMFCS level 3 cerebral palsy, to aid mobility

Orthoses

The most commonly used orthoses (ankle-foot orthoses, AFOs) aim to maintain a plantigrade foot and facilitate an upright standing posture and walking. Referral is indicated for ambulant children (GMFCS levels 1-3) with deteriorating walking function as a result of weakness of the legs or joint contractures, or at an earlier stage to improve standing posture and balance so that children have the prerequisites to develop their gait. In non-walkers (GMFCS level 4 or 5), AFOs may improve foot position for comfort during sitting and transfers and may have a role in preventing progression of joint contractures and limb or spinal deformity. Although AFOs are widely prescribed, a systematic review found only weak evidence for their effectiveness.[43] For children with poor postural control, seating supports are helpful at mealtimes and for using a wheelchair, although evidence for their use is lacking. Carers and doctors should be vigilant for pressure sores.

Medical treatment

Oral baclofen or diazepam is indicated to reduce spasticity in children of any GMFCS level when spasticity contributes to pain, muscle spasm, or functional disability.[38] Diazepam is particularly useful when a rapid effect is desirable (for example, painful night spasms), and baclofen for a sustained long term effect (for example, to relieve continuous discomfort or improve motor function). Baclofen works at the spinal level and produces a systemic effect. Large oral doses are often required for treatment effect owing to poor penetration of the blood-brain barrier. Start oral baclofen with a low dose and increase the dose stepwise over four weeks to achieve optimum therapeutic effect. Diazepam may be started at bedtime, and a daytime dose added if initial response is unsatisfactory. As all muscle groups are affected, treatment may produce side effects: muscle weakness manifesting as a loss of head or neck control, or sedation and feeding difficulties, which may limit a child's participation in school. Continue using these treatments if they have benefit and are well tolerated, but consider dose reduction or stopping these drugs whenever the child's management programme is reviewed and at least every

six months. When stopping, ensure the dose is reduced in stages to avoid withdrawal. One small randomised controlled trial of 15 children reported improved scores for goal attainment (for example, in transfers, ease of walking frame use, and improved sleep) in children treated with baclofen compared with placebo.[44] Most relevant studies are observational, small series and provide limited evidence of effectiveness.[38]

Intrathecal baclofen pumps are inserted under the skin of the abdomen and deliver a continuous infusion to the subarachnoid space at a fraction of the oral dose (1%). Pumps are used for the management of both spasticity and severe dystonia when children are refractory to oral treatment or systemic side effects are excessive. Children who benefit typically have moderate to severe functional problems (GMFCS levels 3-5) and bilateral spasticity/dystonia.[38] Prospective observational studies support its effectiveness in managing hypertonia in terms of hypertonia rating scales, functional goals, patient satisfaction, and cost effectiveness, but infection rates are high (18%).[45] Well conducted research with a focus on activity and participation status is needed to critically analyse the indications and outcomes of antispasticity drugs in cerebral palsy.

Botulinum neurotoxin type A (BoNT-A) injections

Botulinum neurotoxin type A (BoNT-A) blocks the release of acetylcholine at the neuromuscular junction, thus providing a focal treatment for spasticity in one muscle group where there is a correctable muscle imbalance. It can also be used for dystonia. It is indicated in children of any GMFCS level when localised spasticity impedes motor control, compromises care or hygiene, causes pain, impedes the use of other treatments (for example, AFOs or postural support equipment), or causes cosmetic concern, such as abnormal posture.[38] The chemical effect lasts for three or four months, whereas the clinical benefits often last longer. BoNT-A can be administered by any qualified practitioner (surgeon, paediatrician, physiotherapist, or nurse specialist) under sedation or general anaesthesia, using ultrasound or a

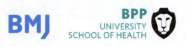

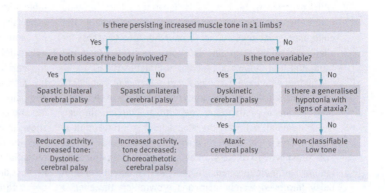

Fig 3 Algorithm for assessing abnormality in tone in cerebral palsy. Adapted from Surveillance of Cerebral Palsy in Europe[5]

nerve stimulator to aid localisation. BoNT-A may be used as a first line treatment and repeated as necessary.

Systematic review evidence has shown that BoNT-A is effective in the management of focal leg spasticity in children, and that when combined with physiotherapy and orthoses, may improve gait and goal attainment.[46] There is moderate evidence that BoNT-A reduces tone in the arms but inconclusive evidence that it improves activity and function.[47] Adverse events (localised weakness, continence issues, breathing and swallowing difficulties) after the use of BoNT-A may occur in up to 23% of children, but these effects are temporary and usually mild.[48] Although BoNT-A is considered a safe treatment for spasticity, there are still many unanswered questions about its use (for example, long term efficacy and chronic changes to muscle structure).

Surgical treatment for abnormal muscle tone

Neurosurgery
Selective dorsal rhizotomy involves the cutting of selected sensory (afferent) nerve roots between L2 and S1. Spasticity is reduced as a result of decreased afferent input to the reflex arc. The procedure is indicated to improve walking ability in children with spasticity at GMFCS level 2 or 3. Assessment of indications and outcome is currently being evaluated. Careful preoperative multidisciplinary assessment is essential as the rehabilitation period is long and demanding. Systematic reviews of small prospective case series have shown improvement in spasticity and gait parameters, but evidence that selective dorsal rhizotomy improves quality of life or participation is lacking and further studies are needed.[49]

Orthopaedic surgery
In general the treatment for localised spasticity tends to move from BoNT-A to surgery as children age and as the abnormal muscle tone leads to soft tissue contractures and secondary bone deformity (as these are not amenable to medical treatments).[50] It is still unclear whether BoNT-A or selective dorsal rhizotomy lessens the long term need for orthopaedic surgery.[51]

How are other symptoms in cerebral palsy managed?
In addition to treating altered muscle tone, management programmes should be proactive in identifying and treating feeding difficulties, pain, dental problems, visual and hearing impairment, bladder and bowel dysfunction, seizures, behavioural and communication problems as

these have a considerable impact on quality of life and activity (see box 2).

Feeding difficulties
Poor feeding is one of the major risk factors for early death and is related to GMFCS level.[52] Limited data exist about the true prevalence of feeding difficulties, with rates often skewed by ascertainment sources and age.[53] Cross sectional studies suggest that problems with sucking (57%), chewing (69%), and swallowing (38%) are common.[54] Children with more severe motor impairment (GMFCS level 4 or 5) have the greatest risk,[53] with 91- 99% having clinically important oromotor dysfunction.[53 55] This can lead to major impairment in feeding ability, lengthy distressing mealtimes, growth disturbance, and malnutrition. Multicentre cross sectional studies estimate that malnutrition affects 50% of children with cerebral palsy and is more common in those at GMFCS levels 3-5.[56 57 58] Feeding difficulties can also result in aspiration of food and fluid into the lungs.

Cross sectional studies show that difficulties with feeding are often severely underestimated by parents[59]; a detailed eating and drinking history must be elicited, with particular reference to weight gain; coughing and choking during mealtimes; fluid intake; time spent feeding each day; and recurrent chest infections and associated problems of gastro-oesophageal reflux.

Useful feeding interventions that family doctors may recommend include adjustment of food consistency or child positioning during mealtimes and adaptive equipment. A well conducted systematic review on the role of feeding interventions in cerebral palsy found potential benefits for growth, nutrition, and participation; however, the current level of evidence was considered poor.[60] Although the exact prevalence is unknown, gastro-oesophageal reflux is common and causes painful muscle spasms. These can be difficult to detect; subtle clues include an irritable child, night waking, and "dystonic" movements with posture changes.[61] Modification of diet, good management of tone, and antacids help. Gastrostomy and oesophageal dilatation for strictures are occasionally required and, after orthopaedic surgery, are the second commonest surgical procedures for children with cerebral palsy.[61 62]

Children at GMFCS level 4 or 5 are at the highest risk of aspiration and premature death.[55] Aspiration can be silent, with no history of coughing or choking during mealtimes; it is often overlooked as a reason for poor weight gain or recurrent chest infections. If there are concerns with feeding, early involvement of a speech and language therapist with experience in dysphagia is essential to provide comprehensive individualised advice on swallowing. The child may undergo videofluoroscopy; indicated to assess for silent aspiration, determine safe consistencies for food and fluid, and trial therapeutic feeding techniques (fig 4).

Children who have dysphagia with evidence of inability to eat and drink sufficiently or safely for a minimum of six weeks may require a gastrostomy "peg" to be inserted through the abdominal wall into the stomach. This intervention is being increasingly used to augment existing oral intake. Two prospective cohort studies showed that gastrostomy feeding of malnourished children with bilateral cerebral palsy improved weight gain and growth.[62] [63] However, a recent Cochrane review found insufficient evidence to report on efficacy.[64] A well conducted prospective study reported improved quality of life in the carers of disabled children who had undergone gastrostomy.[65]

Drooling
Drooling may have an effect on children's quality of life and social interactions. Anticholinergic drugs such as glycopyrrolate and scopolamine used as skin patches can reduce saliva flow but may thicken secretions, making them difficult to clear. Surgical rerouting of salivary gland ducts or intraglandular BoNT-A injections may also reduce secretions and result in an improved appearance; however, long term data on effectiveness and safety are lacking.[66]

Hip dislocation and scoliosis
Large cohort studies have shown an overall incidence of hip displacement and scoliosis in children with cerebral palsy of 35% and 28%, respectively, which increases to 90% and 50% in children at GMFCS level 4 or 5.[67] [68] There is a linear relation between risk and GMFCS level; children at GMFCS level 1 or 2 have a low risk, at level 3 an intermediate, and at level 4 or 5 a high risk.[67] [68] Several countries are screening children with cerebral palsy annually for hip dislocation using pelvic radiography and range of movement data.[69] [70] Early detection of a laterally displacing hip may enable simple treatments (for example, baclofen or BoNT-A, or soft tissue surgery) to prevent progression of subluxation to dislocation, when major orthopaedic surgery would be required. Swedish registry data have shown that screening in combination with appropriate medical and surgical treatment has abolished hip dislocation and reduced scoliosis.[69]

Quality of life and pain management
Pain is a common experience for children with cerebral palsy. Multicentre cross sectional studies estimate that pain affects approximately 70% of affected children on a regular basis.[71] [72] Pain is related to mobility and other demanding motor activities. It interferes with sleep and results in less participation and reduced quality of life.[72] Self report by children is the ideal way to determine the degree of pain but is often not possible because of impaired communication.[71] Better management can start by increasing clinicians' awareness and asking children and their parents about pain, as children with cerebral palsy may always have had pain and assume it to be normal. Discussion about pain itself by family doctors is helpful,[73] and pain diaries may identify the cause, which is often related to motor problems. Pain scoring tools are available for children who cannot communicate, but identifying the cause of pain in children with cerebral palsy can be difficult;

table 2 lists the common causes and treatment. Analgesics, especially non-steroidal anti-inflammatory drugs, are good for bone pain and muscle aches and antispasticity drugs help painful neurological spasms, including those secondary to gastro-oesophageal reflux and constipation. Scoliosis and hip dislocation are common causes of chronic discomfort and pain. Despite a common misconception about quality of life and cerebral palsy, multinational cross sectional studies show that provided pain is controlled, parents can be reassured that most children with cerebral palsy have the potential to gain a similar quality of life to their peer group in most domains.[36] This should guide social and educational policy to ensure that disabled children participate fully in society.

Epilepsy
Epilepsy is present in 30-40% of children with cerebral palsy and is often under-recognised because many seizures are focal (partial) with or without secondary generalisation.[74] Epilepsy may be a reversible cause of learning impairment and behavioural disturbance.

Speech and language difficulties
Poor hearing and vision interfere with development and should be screened for in all children with cerebral palsy who have developmental delay. Efforts should be made to facilitate communication in these children, as difficulties with speech are one of the causes of impaired quality of life.[36] The communication aids need to be matched to the child's learning level and may range from simple pictures to electronic devices. Speech and language therapists aim to maximise communication skills in children with cerebral palsy. A well conducted Cochrane systematic review found positive trends but weak evidence for the beneficial effect of using a speech and language therapist in children with cerebral palsy: more research is needed.[75]

Bowel and bladder dysfunction
Constipation is common and may result from many factors, including primary tone abnormality, poor feeding, and immobility. It is important to recognise constipation as a cause of painful muscle spasms. Regular water and

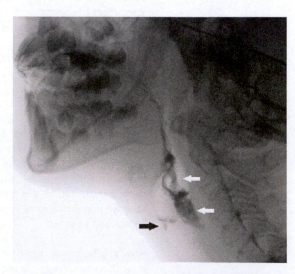

Fig 4 Videofluoroscopy showing normal contrast in oesophagus (white arrows) and silent aspiration into trachea (black arrow) in a 4 year old with GMFCS level 3 cerebral palsy. This child had a classic history of recurrent chest infections requiring antibiotics but no history of coughing or choking while eating and drinking

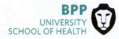

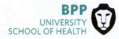

ADDITIONAL EDUCATIONAL RESOURCES

Resources for healthcare professionals
- CanChild (www.canchild.ca/en/#)—research and educational centre that provides evidence based information to improve the lives of children and young people with disabilities and their families
- NHS newborn and infant physical examination programme (NIPE) (http://newbornphysical.screening.nhs.uk/)—new National Health Service screening programme guidelines aimed at improving health outcomes for all children through early detection of disability and disease
- NICE (www.nice.org.uk/CG145)—guidelines on spasticity management in children and young people with non-progressive brain disorders
- Rosenbaum P, Rosenbloom L. Cerebral palsy: from diagnosis to adult life. MacKeith Press, 2012—book describing cerebral palsy from childhood to adulthood, offering perspectives on the lives of parents of children with cerebral palsy and discussing the condition in adulthood

Resources for patients
- SCOPE (www.scope.org.uk/)—charity providing support for people with disability and their families
- Pathways Awareness Foundation (www.pathwaysawareness.org/)—useful resource for families and professionals in the early detection of motor delay
- HemiHelp (www.hemihelp.org.uk/)—UK based charity for people with disability and their families

fibre intake is usually effective, and oral bowel softening laxatives such as lactulose and glycerine suppositories are occasionally necessary. Most children can achieve regular bowel movements with appropriate management. Urinary incontinence due to impaired control of bladder muscles can be treated with biofeedback exercises, drugs, and occasionally surgery, although the evidence for these treatments is lacking. Constipation often has an adverse effect on the bladder and urinary continence, and treatment of one may help the other.

Intellectual impairment

Registry data from multicentre collaborative studies suggest that 30% of children with cerebral palsy have severe intellectual impairment.[5] The highest incidence was shown in those with bilateral involvement.[76] Well conducted, multinational cross sectional studies found that intellectual impairment negatively impacted on quality of life regarding moods and emotions and autonomy.[36]

Cerebral palsy is a condition that affects individuals and their families for life. Child services have become better at promoting participation for growing children and meeting their developmental needs. However, large cohort studies show that young people with disability during transition from paediatric to adult services still face many challenges, have a lower quality of life, and are restricted in participation in work, housing, and intimate relationships.[77] To protect the gains these children make during their developing years, there is an international challenge to incorporate a lifespan perspective in paediatric, transition, and adult healthcare services for those with childhood onset disability.[77]

Contributors: MDS wrote the first draft. NW and DME were involved in all areas of manuscript production and finalised the manuscript. They are the guarantors.

Competing interests: We have read and understood the BMJ policy on declaration of interests and declare the following interests: none.

Provenance and peer review: Commissioned; externally peer reviewed.

1 Rosenbaum P, Paneth N, Leviton A, Goldstein M, Bax M. A report: the definition and classification of cerebral palsy April 2006. Dev Med Child Neurol 2007;49(s2):8-14.
2 Surman G, Bonellie S, Chalmers J, Colver A, Dolk H, Hemming K, et al. UKCP: a collaborative network of cerebral palsy registers in the United Kingdom. J Public Health 2006;28:148-56.
3 Johnson A. Prevalence and characteristics of children with cerebral palsy in Europe. Dev Med Child Neurol 2002;44:633-40.
4 Andersen GL, Irgens LM, Haagaas I, Skranes JS, Meberg AE, Vik T. Cerebral palsy in Norway: prevalence, subtypes and severity. Eur J Paed Neurol 2008;12:4-13.
5 Surveillance of Cerebral Palsy in Europe. A collaboration of cerebral palsy surveys and registers. Surveillance of cerebral palsy in Europe (SCPE). Dev Med Child Neurol 2000;42:816-24.
6 Surveillance of Cerebral Palsy in Europe. Prevalence and characteristics of children with cerebral palsy in Europe. Dev Med Child Neurol 2002;44:633-40.
7 Jarvis S, Glinianaia SV, Torrioli MG, Platt MJ, Miceli M, Jouk PS, et al. Cerebral palsy and intrauterine growth in single births: European collaborative study. Lancet 2003;362:1106-11.
8 Report of the Australian Cerebral Palsy Register, birth years 1993-2006, Feb 2013.
9 Vohr BR, Wright LL, Poole WK, McDonald SA. Neurodevelopmental outcomes of extremely low birth weight infants <32 weeks gestation between 1993 and 1998. Pediatrics 2005;116:635-43.
10 Platt MJ, Cans C, Johnson A, Surman G, Topp M, Torrioli MG, et al. Trends in cerebral palsy among infants of very low birthweight (<1500g) or born prematurely (<32 weeks) in 16 European centres: a database study. Lancet 2007;369:43-50.
11 Hetzel BS. Iodine and neuropsychological development. J Nutr 2000;130 (S2):S493-5.
12 Escobar GJ, Littenberg B, Petitti DB. Outcome among surviving very low birthweight infants: a meta-analysis. Arch Dis Child 1991;66:204-11.
13 Krageloh-Mann I, Cans C. Cerebral palsy update. Brain Dev 2009;31:537-44.
14 Wu YW, Croen LA, Shah SJ, Newman TB, Najjar DV. Cerebral palsy in a term population: risk factors and neuroimaging findings. Pediatrics 2006;118:690-7.
15 Bundey S, Griffiths MA. Recurrence risks in families of children with symmetrical spasticity. Dev Med Child Neurol 1977;19:179-91.
16 Hughes I, Newton R. Genetic aspects of cerebral palsy. Dev Med Child Neurol 1992;43:80-6.
17 Tollanes MC, Wilcox AJ, Lie RT, Moster D. Familial risk of cerebral palsy: population based cohort study. BMJ 2014;349:g4294.
18 Krageloh-Mann I, Horber V. The role of magnetic resonance imaging in elucidating the pathogenesis of cerebral palsy: a systematic review. Dev Med Child Neurol 2007;49:144-51.
19 Jacobs SE, Berg M, Hunt R, Tarnow-Mordi WO, Inder TE, Davis PG. Cooling for newborns with hypoxic ischaemic encephalopathy. Cochrane Database Syst Rev 2013;1:CD003311.
20 Prechtl HF, Einspieler C, Cioni G, Bos AF, Ferrari F, Sontheimer D. An early marker for neurological deficits after perinatal brain lesions. Lancet 1997;349:1361-3.
21 Spittle AJ, Boyd RN, Inder TE, Doyle LW. Predicting motor development in very preterm infants at 12 months corrected age: the role of qualitative magnetic resonance imaging and general movements assessments. Pediatrics 2009;123:512-7.
22 Leonard JM, Cozens AL, Reid SM, Fahey MC, Ditchfield MR, Reddihough DS. Should children with cerebral palsy and normal imaging undergo testing for inherited metabolic disorders? Dev Med Child Neurol 2011;53:226-32.
23 Ashwal S, Russman BS, Blasco PA, Miller G, Sandler A, Shevell M, et al. Practice parameter: diagnostic assessment of the child with cerebral palsy: report of the Quality Standards Subcommittee of the American Academy of Neurology and the Practise Committee of the child neurology society. Neurology 2004;62:851-63.
24 Martinez-Biarge M, Diez-Sebastian J, Rutherford MA, Cowan FM. Outcomes after central grey matter injury in term perinatal hypoxic-ischaemic encephalopathy. Early Hum Dev 2010;86:675-82.
25 Cans C. Surveillance of cerebral palsy in Europe: a collaboration of cerebral palsy surveys and registers. Dev Med Child Neurol 2000;42:816-24.
26 Palisano R, Rosenbaum P, Walter S, Russell D, Wood E, Galuppi B. Development and reliability of a system to classify gross motor function in children with cerebral palsy. Dev Med Child Neurol 1997;39:214-23.
27 Eliasson AC, Krumlinde-Sundholm L, Rosblad B, Beckung E, Arner M, Ohrvall AM, et al. The Manual Ability Classification System (MACS) for children with cerebral palsy: scale development and evidence for validity and reliability. Dev Med Child Neurol 2006;48:549-54.
28 Hidecker MJ, Paneth N, Rosenbaum PL, Kent RD, Lillie J, Eulenberg JB, et al. Developing and validating the communication function classification system for individuals with cerebral palsy. Dev Med Child Neurol 2011;53:704-10.
29 Fauconnier J, Dickinson HO, Beckung E, Marcelli M, McManus V, Michelsen SI, et al. Participation in life situations of 8-12 year old children with cerebral palsy: cross sectional European study. BMJ 2009;338:b1458.
30 Gorter JW, Rosenbaum PL, Hanna SE, Palisano RJ, Bartlett DJ, Russell DJ, et al. Limb distribution, motor impairment, and functional classification of cerebral palsy. Dev Med Child Neurol 2004;46:461-7.
31 Dobson F, Boyd RN, Parrott J, Nattrass GR, Graham HK. Hip surveillance in children with cerebral palsy. Impact on the surgical management of spastic hip disease. J Bone Joint Surg Br 2002;84:720-6.
32 Rosenbaum P. Cerebral palsy: what parents and doctors want to know. BMJ 2003;326:970-4.
33 World Health Organization. International classification of functioning, disability and health. WHO, 2001.

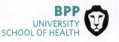

Table 2 Common causes of pain and treatment in children with cerebral palsy[61]

Causes	Symptoms/signs	Treatment
Spasticity	Muscle tone abnormality (see box 3)	Protect joints and head during abnormal spasms; physiotherapy and orthoses (for example, ankle-foot orthoses for weak muscles or shoe raise for discrepancy in leg length); diazepam for acute spasms (for example, at night or postoperatively, but consider what other drugs are being taken); baclofen for persistent increased tone; consider appropriateness of botulinum neurotoxin type A or selective dorsal rhizotomy; orthopaedic surgery
Gastro-oesphageal reflux	Poor feeding, irritability, night waking, malnourished, dystonic movements with posture changes (Sandifer syndrome), anaemia and weight loss	Upright posture (with orthoses/seating adaption), regular small meals; review anti-spasticity drugs ; omeprazole; ranitidine; surgery for strictures or reflux
Hip subluxation	Pain on transfers, sitting, walking, or activities involving hip movement; usually not before late childhood	Request hip radiography and monitor changes; orthotic changes to seat to assist with sitting; paracetamol; non-steroidal anti-inflammatory drugs; codeine; tricyclic antidepressants; oral morphine; orthopaedic surgery
Scoliosis and back pain	Pain on sitting or changes in shape of back, or uneven shoulders when sitting or standing; associated often with hip subluxation and pelvic obliquity	Request whole spine radiography; orthotic changes to seat to assist with sitting or positioning; physiotherapy; paracetamol; non-steroidal anti-inflammatory drugs; codeine; tricyclic antidepressants; oral morphine; orthopaedic spine or hip surgery
Constipation	Solid, infrequent motions; overflow diarrhea; irritability	Good tone management; regular water, fruit, and fibre intake; oral bowel softening laxatives (for example, lactulose); glycerine suppositories
Period pain	Associated with menstruation	Oral contraceptives
Tooth decay	Poor oral hygiene; irritability	Regular teeth cleaning; dental review
Physiotherapy sessions	Associated with physiotherapy	Paracetamol or non-steroidal anti-inflammatory drugs given one hour before sessions

34 Rosenbaum P, King S, Law M, King G, Evans J. Family-centred service: a conceptual framework and research review. *Phys Occup Ther Pediatr*1998;18:1-20.

35 Novak I, McIntyre S, Morgan C, Campbell L, Dark L, Morton N, et al. A systematic review of interventions for children with cerebral palsy: state of the evidence. *Dev Med Child Neurol*2013;55:885-910.

36 Dickinson HO, Parkinson KN, Ravens-Sieberer U, Schirripa G, Thyen U, Arnaud C, et al. Self-reported quality of life of 8-12-year-old children with cerebral palsy: a cross-sectional European study. *Lancet* 2007:369:2171-8.

37 Mugglestone M, Eunson P, Murphy MS. Spasticity in children and young people with non-progressive brain disorders: summary of NICE guidance. *BMJ*2012;345:e4845.

38 National Institute for Health and Care Excellence. Spasticity in children and young people with non-progressive brain disorders. (Clinical guideline 145.) 2012. www.nice.org.uk/CG145.

39 Darrah J, Fan JSW, Chen LC, Nunweiler J, Watkins B. Review of effects of progressive resisted muscle strengthening in children with cerebral palsy: a clinical consensus exercise. *Pediatr Phys Ther*1997;9:12-7.

40 Dodd KJ, Taylor NF, Damiano DL. A systematic review of the effectiveness of strength-training programs for people with cerebral palsy. *Arch Phys Med Rehabil* 2002;83:1157-64.

41 Verschuren O, Ketelaar M, Takken T, Helders PJ, Gorter JW. Exercise programs for children with cerebral palsy: a systematic review of the literature. *Am J of Phys Med Rehabil*2008;87:404-17.

42 Anttila H, Autti-Ramo I, Suoranta J, Makela M, Malmivaara A. Effectiveness of physical therapy interventions for children with cerebral palsy: a systematic review. *BMC Pediatr*2008;8:14.

43 Morris C. A review of the efficacy of lower-limb orthoses used for cerebral palsy. *Dev Med Child Neurol*2002;44:205-11.

44 Scheinberg A, Hall K, Lam LT, O'Flaherty S. Oral baclofen in children with cerebral palsy: a double-blind cross-over pilot study. *J Paediatr Child Health* 2006;42:715-20.

45 Ward A, Hayden S, Dexter M, Scheinberg A. Continuous intrathecal baclofen for children with spasticity and/or dystonia: goal attainment and complications associated with treatment. *J Paed Child Health*2009;45:720-6.

46 Love SC, Novak I, Kentish M, Desloovere K, Heinen F, Molenaers G, et al. Botulinum toxin assessment, intervention and after-care for lower limb spasticity in children with cerebral palsy: international consensus statement. *Eur J Neurol*2010;17(Supp 2):9-37.

47 Fehlings D, Novak I, Berweck S, Hoare B, Stott NS, Russo RN, Cerebral Palsy Institute. Botulinum toxin assessment, intervention and follow-up for paediatric upper limb hypertonicity: international consensus statement. *Eur J Neurol*2010;17(Supp 2):38-56.

48 O'Flaherty SJ, Janakan V, Morrow AM, Scheinberg AM, Waugh MC. Adverse events and health status following botulinum toxin type A injections in children with cerebral palsy. *Dev Med Child Neurol*2011;53:101-2.

49 Grunt S, Becher JG, Vermeulen RJ. Long-term outcome and adverse effects of selective dorsal rhizotomy in children with cerebral palsy: a systematic review. *Dev Med Child Neurol*2011;53:490-8.

50 Bache CE, Selber P, Graham HK. The management of spastic diplegia. *Curr Orthop*2003;17:88-104.

51 Tedroff K, Lowing K, Jacobson DN, Astrom E. Does loss of spasticity matter? A 10-year follow-up after selective dorsal rhizotomy in cerebral palsy. *Dev Med Child Neurol*2011;53:724-9.

52 Strauss D, Brooks J, Rosenbloom L, Shavelle R. Life expectancy in cerebral palsy: an update. *Dev Med Child Neurol*2008;50:487-93.

53 Weir KA, Bell KL, Caristo F, Ware RS, Davies PS, Fahey M, et al. Reported eating ability of young children with cerebral palsy: is there an association with gross motor function? *Arch Phys Med Rehabil* 2013;94:495-502.

54 Reilly S, Skuse D, Poblete X. Prevalence of feeding problems and oral motor dysfunction in children with cerebral palsy: a community survey. *J Pediatr*1996;129:877-82.

55 Calis EA, Veugelers R, Sheppard JJ, Tibboel D, Evenhuis HM, Penning C. Dysphagia in children with severe generalised cerebral palsy and intellectual disability. *Dev Med Child Neurol*2008;50:625-30.

56 Benigni I, Devos P, Rofidal T, Seguy D. The CP-MST, a malnutrition screening tool for institutionalized adult cerebral palsy patients. *Clin Nutr*2011;30:769-73.

57 Odding E, Roebroeck ME, Stam HJ. The epidemiology of cerebral palsy: incidence, impairments and risk factors. *Disabil Rehabil*2006;28:183-91.

58 Fung EB, Samson-Fang L, Stallings VA, Conaway M, Liptak G, Henderson RC, et al. Feeding dysfunction is associated with poor growth and health status in children with cerebral palsy. *J Am Diet Assoc* 2002;102:361-73.

59 Eckstein KC, Mikhail LM, Ariza AJ, Thomson JS, Millard SC, Binns HJ, Pediatric Practice Research Group. Parents' perceptions of their child's weight and health. *Pediatrics*2006;117:681-90.

60 Sidner L, Majnemer A, Darsaklis V. Feeding interventions for children with cerebral palsy: a review of the evidence. *Phys Occup Ther Pediatr*2011;31:58-77.

61 Nolan J, Chalkiadis GA, Low J, Olesch CA, Brown TC. Anaesthesia and pain management in cerebral palsy. *Anaesthesia*2000;55:32-41.

62 Vernon-Roberts A, Wells J, Grant H, Alder N, Vadamalayan B, Eltumi M, et al. Gastrostomy feeding in cerebral palsy: enough and no more. *Dev Med Child Neurol*2010;52:1099-105.

63 Arrowsmith F, Allen J, Gaskin K, Somerville H, Clarke S, O'Loughlin E . The effect of gastrostomy tube feeding on body protein and bone mineralization in children with quadriplegic cerebral palsy. *Dev Med Child Neurol*2010;52:1043-7.

64 Sleigh G, Sullivan PB, Thomas AG. Gastrostomy feeding versus feeding alone for children with cerebral palsy. *Cochrane Database Syst Rev*2004;2:CD003943.

65 Sullivan PB, Juszczak E, Bachlet AM, Thomas AG, Lambert B, Vernon-Roberts A, et al. Impact of gastrostomy tube feeding on the quality of life of carers of children with cerebral palsy. *Dev Med Child Neurol*2004;46:796-800.

66 Reddihough D, Erasmus CE, Johnson H, McKellar GM, Jongerius PH, Cerebral Palsy Institute. Botulinum toxin assessment, intervention and aftercare for paediatric and adult drooling: international consensus statement. *Eur J Neurol*2010;17(Supp 2):109-21.

67 Soo B, Howard JJ, Boyd RN, Reid SM, Lanigan A, Wolfe R, et al. Hip displacement in cerebral palsy. *J Bone J Surg Am*2006;88:121-9.

68 Persson-Bunke M, Hagglund G, Lauge-Pedersen H, et al. Scoliosis in a total population of children with cerebral palsy. *Spine*2012;37:E708-13.

69 Hagglund G, Andersson S, Duppe H, Lauge-Pedersen H, Nordmark E, Westbom L. Prevention of dislocation of the hip in children with cerebral palsy. The first ten years of a population-based prevention programme. *J Bone J Surg Br*2005;87:95-101.

70 Wynter M, Gibson N, Kentish M, Love S, Thomason P, Graham HK. The consensus statement on hip surveillance for children with cerebral palsy: Australian standards of care. *J Ped Rehab Med* 2011;4:183-95.

71 Parkinson K, Gibson L, Dickinson H, Colver A. Pain in children with cerebral palsy: a cross-sectional multicentre European study. *Acta Paediatr*2010;99:446-51.

72 Parkinson KN, Dickinson HO, Arnaud C, Lyons A, Colver A. Pain in young people aged 13-17 years with cerebral palsy: cross-sectional, multicentre European study. *Arch Dis Child*2013;98:434-40.

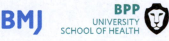

73 Castle K, Imms C, Howie L. Being in pain: a phenomenological study of young people with cerebral palsy. *Dev Med Child Neurol* 2007;49:445-9.

74 Zafeiriou DI, Kontopoulos EE, Tsikoulas I. Characteristics and prognosis of epilepsy in children with cerebral palsy. *J Child Neurol* 1999;14:289-94.

75 Pennington L, Goldbart J, Marshall J. Speech and language therapy to improve the communication skills of children with cerebral palsy. *Cochrane Database Syst Rev* 2004;2:CD003466.

76 Russman BS, Ashwal S. Evaluation of the child with cerebral palsy. *Semin Pediatr Neurol* 2004;11:47-57.

77 Roebroeck ME, Jahnsen R, Carona C, Kent RM, Chamberlain MA. Adult outcomes and lifespan issues for people with childhood-onset physical disability. *Dev Med Child Neurol* 2009;51:670-8.

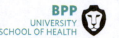

Diagnosis and management of autism in childhood

Stephanie Blenner assistant professor of pediatrics[1], Arathi Reddy developmental behavioral pediatrician[2], Marilyn Augustyn associate professor of pediatrics, division director[1]

[1]Division of Developmental Behavioral Pediatrics, Boston University School of Medicine, Boston, MA 02118, USA

[2]Boston Medical Center, Boston, MA, USA

Correspondence to: S Blenner stephanie.blenner@bmc.org

Cite this as: *BMJ* 2011;343:d6238

‹DOI› 10.1136/bmj.d6238
http://www.bmj.com/content/343/bmj.d6238

Autism spectrum disorder is a commonly used umbrella term for a class of neurodevelopmental disorders characterised by a triad of deficits in social reciprocity, impaired communication, and repetitive restricted patterns of behaviour or interests. Symptoms are evident in early childhood, often before age 3 years, and result in functional impairment. Autism was first described in the 1940s; it was originally thought to be relatively rare because only the most severely affected people were identified. However, epidemiological studies have documented an increasing prevalence over the past 15 years, with one UK cohort study from 2006 reporting a prevalence rate of about one in 110 children compared with four to five cases per 10 000 before the 1990s.[1] This reflects, in part, recognition of a broader phenotype of affected individuals who share impairments within the three core areas.[2]

It is crucial that general clinicians are familiar with the diagnosis and management of autism because the importance of early identification and intervention, and the benefit of supporting families in navigating the myriad of decisions once a diagnosis is made, are well recognised. We review the current nosology, identification, and evaluation of autism spectrum disorders, along with up to date research into their causes and medical management on the basis of recent studies, systematic reviews, and consensus statements.

How are autism spectrum disorders classified?

Currently, autism spectrum disorders comprise three medical diagnoses, as outlined in the *Diagnostic and Statistical Manual of Mental Disorders*, fourth edition, text revision (DSM-IV TR) under pervasive developmental disorders, with corresponding diagnoses in ICD-10 (international classification of diseases, 10th revision). These are autistic disorder; pervasive developmental disorder, not otherwise specified (PDD-NOS); and Asperger's disorder.

Autistic disorder is diagnosed when an individual exhibits six or more symptoms across the three core areas. PDD-NOS is not as clearly defined but is diagnosed when there are five or fewer symptoms or an atypical presentation. Children diagnosed with Asperger's disorder do not have clinically significant delays in language development before age 3 and their greatest difficulties are in the areas of social interaction and restricted interests. Children with all three diagnoses have marked impairment in social reciprocity, which is considered the defining feature of all autism spectrum disorders. Importantly, there has been much debate in the field over recent years about terminology and construct validity, and it is anticipated that DSM-V—planned for release in 2013—will replace the three current diagnoses with the single diagnosis "autism spectrum disorder" accompanied by dimensional descriptors.[3]

What causes autism spectrum disorder?

Genetic vulnerability

Autism is a complex heterogeneous disorder that has an established genetic basis. Twin studies have identified high heritability, with median concordance rates across studies of 88% for monozygotic twins.[4] Siblings of children with autism are at higher risk of being diagnosed with autism, or other developmental disorder.[5] The reported risk of recurrence is at least 4-7% for an autism spectrum disorder, with one recent study making the risk as high as 18%, although this has not yet been replicated. Although single gene disorders, such as fragile X syndrome (*FMR1* gene) and tuberous sclerosis (*TSC1* and *TSC2* genes), account for a small proportion of cases,[6] the proportion of individuals who have an abnormality on genetic evaluation is increasing as more sophisticated testing becomes available. A larger proportion of people with autism are thought to have "idiopathic autism"—with no identifiable genetic abnormality. Although this partly reflects the limitations of available testing, it also suggests that autism is a final manifestation of multiple aetiological pathways. Autism probably develops when an array of possible genetic vulnerabilities, possibly in concert with epigenetic factors or gene-environment interaction, affect neural connectivity and neurodevelopment.[7][8]

SOURCES AND SELECTION CRITERIA

We searched PubMed, PsychInfo, the Cochrane database of systematic reviews, and citation lists of relevant publications using the subject headings and key words "autism," "autism spectrum disorder," "(a)etiology," "screening," "diagnosis," and "treatment." We also searched guidelines from the National Research Council, the American Academy of Pediatrics, and the National Institute for Health and Clinical Excellence.

SUMMARY POINTS

- Autism spectrum disorders are neurodevelopmental conditions that share core impairments in social reciprocity, communication, and behaviour but have a range of presentations
- The prevalence of autism has increased over the past 15 years, partly because the definition now includes milder forms of the disorder
- Genetic factors and potential environmental causes are being studied; vaccines have been shown not to be associated with autism in multiple studies
- Surveillance and screening by the general clinician allow affected children to be identified early and to gain access to crucial early interventions
- Most management strategies aim to improve communication, cognitive abilities, and social and daily living skills, while decreasing maladaptive behaviour
- Involvement of general clinicians and paediatricians in ongoing care helps families access services and prioritise and plan for future needs

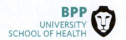

Environmental factors

Environmental factors, as well as prenatal and perinatal factors,[9] that might play a role in the development of autism are being investigated. Childhood immunisations have been a highly publicised area of focus, and clinicians are often confronted with questions about vaccine safety. Theories about how vaccines could contribute to the development of autism include the thimerosal hypothesis; the role of measles, mumps, and rubella vaccine; and exposure to multiple vaccine antigenic components. These theories have been intensely studied in a range of countries and no association or aetiological link to childhood immunisations has been identified.[10]

Another controversial area has been the role of gastrointestinal atypicality and diet in the development of autism. Inadequate metabolism of gluten—a wheat protein—and casein—a milk protein—have been hypothesised to result in peptides that cross the blood-brain barrier, bind to endogenous opioid receptors, and negatively affect behaviour, cognition, and interaction. To date, however, no large well designed study has identified significant changes in core symptoms after the elimination of gluten and casein from the diet of children with autism.[11]

How do children with autism present?

Typical presentation

About half of parents of children with an autism spectrum disorder report having concerns before 12 months of age, with many more reporting recognition of abnormalities between 12 and 24 months in retrospective studies.[12] [13] A recent prospective study of the emergence of early behavioural signs of autism in children found differences in social communication evident by the second year of life.[14] Despite behavioural markers being identified within the first 2 years of life, the current average age of diagnosis remains around 3 years or more.[15]

The most common presenting parental concern in young children subsequently diagnosed with autism is delayed language development. Other common behavioural concerns include lack of or inconsistent use of eye contact, social smile, imitation, response to name, interest in others, emotional expression, directed vocalisations, joint attention skills (pointing to "show," following a point, monitoring others' gaze, and referencing objects or events), requesting behaviours, and gestures (such as waving, clapping, nodding, and shaking head). Pretend play is also deficient in toddlerhood in many children with autism.[16]

Regression is seen in about 25% of children according to several studies using structured parent interviews or parent report coupled with medical record review.[17] [18] This usually occurs between 15 and 24 months of age and can present with loss of previously attained language abilities or social and play skills. Regression can occur in apparently typically developing children or be superimposed on existing developmental delay.

Presenting concerns in older children

Although the average age of diagnosis for autism is 3.1 years, it is 3.9 years for PDD-NOS, and 7.2 years for Asperger's disorder. This delay may occur because the child meets early language milestones but presents with other concerns such as difficulty with transitions, extremes of behaviour, and perseverative interests; these symptoms may be difficult to identify until the child is older. In one study of children in community mental health settings, school aged children with autism spectrum disorder were more likely to be referred for social interaction difficulties and strange behaviour but were less likely to be referred for behaviours like drug use, truancy, or running away.[19]

Associated medical problems

Seizures are seen in 20-35% of children with autism and are more common in those with dysmorphic findings or cognitive delay.[20] Pica or mouthing of objects in the environment is also common. Studies have reported varying rates of gastrointestinal problems. A cohort study in 2009 found that constipation and feeding problems were higher in children with autism, but not reflux or diarrhoea, suggesting that the increased incidence has behavioural, rather than organic, causes.[21] Sleep disorders are common and usually more severe in children with autism. Reported problems include difficulties with sleep onset, maintenance, and duration.

How should non-specialists assess children with suspected autism?

Developmental surveillance—which includes flexible questioning about a child's development (box) accompanied by observation of the child in the surgery—conducted as part of comprehensive medical care at each visit will help the clinician identify concerns.[22] Clinicians can also use autism specific screening to assess symptoms. Recommendations and practices around screening for autism vary by country; the American Academy of Pediatrics recommends using an autism specific screening tool at 18 and 24 months,[23] whereas several other countries, including the United Kingdom, do not currently endorse routine population screening.

Multiple screening tools have been devised to try to standardise screening for potential autism spectrum disorder prospectively (table 1). The most common tools designed for use with children as young as 18 months are the checklist for autism in toddlers (CHAT), pervasive developmental disorders screening test (PDDST), screening tool for autism in two year olds (STAT), checklist for autism

---

QUESTIONS GENERAL CLINICIANS MIGHT ASK PARENTS

Children age 4 years or under

- How does your child communicate with you?
- Does your child point using an index finger?
- Does your child look you in the eyes when communicating?
- What does your child do if he or she sees something interesting, such as a plane or a dog?
- Does your child turn to look to you when you call his or her name?
- What does your child like to play with? Describe what he or she does while playing
- Has your child ever stopped doing something he or she could previously do (such as talking, using eye contact)?

Children over 4 years

- Does your child have friends? Tell me about your child's friendships
- What does your child like to do with his or her time?
- Can you give an example of a recent conversation you had with your child?
- How does your child handle change? Describe how your child reacted to a recent change or new situation

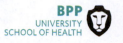

in toddlers-23 (CHAT-23), and the modified checklist for autism in toddlers (M-CHAT).[24][25] All use questions that assess core symptoms such as joint attention, non-verbal communication, and play. The infant toddler checklist (ITC) is used for even younger children, and it focuses on social and communication skills specific to the younger child. It has been evaluated recently in a large sample and shown to have potential for identifying 12 month olds at risk of autism spectrum disorder, but this has yet to be replicated in other samples.[26] When concerns present in school aged children, instruments such as the social communication questionnaire (SCQ)—designed for children aged 4 years or more—can be used.[27][28]

A positive score on a screening test can support referral to a specialist team for comprehensive evaluation, but a negative score does not rule out autism.

Physical examination

Unless there is an associated genetic or neurological condition, children with autism often have no distinct physical findings on examination. Some studies had identified acceleration of head size between 6 and 12 months, with macrocephaly in toddler years,[29] although a recent population study did not find a higher rate of macrocephaly in children with autism at 24 or 36 months.[30]

When to refer to a specialist

If the clinician or family is persistently worried about communication or developmental problems or a screening test identifies that a child is at "high risk" of autism, referral to a specialist team for a comprehensive evaluation is indicated.

Initial investigations

Before evaluation by a specialist, the primary care clinician should order a hearing assessment to rule out hearing loss as a contributory factor. If the child has pica with frequent mouthing of items, measurement of haemoglobin and lead will identify anaemia or a raised lead concentration. A detailed history will uncover chronic sleep difficulties; similarly, history and abdominal radiography if necessary can diagnose common gastrointestinal problems, such as constipation. Any other presenting medical symptoms are evaluated appropriately—for example, consider electroencephalography or magnetic resonance imaging in children with seizures.

How does the specialist team perform a diagnostic assessment?

Because there is currently no specific diagnostic "test" for autism spectrum disorders, the diagnosis is established through a comprehensive evaluation that includes lifetime and family history, review of medical and educational records, behavioural observation, physical examination, administration of standardised instruments such as the autism diagnostic observation schedule, cognitive and adaptive assessment, and review of established DSM or ICD diagnostic criteria. Given the complexity and range of presentation, diagnostic evaluation is best done by paediatric neurologists, developmental and behavioural paediatricians, child psychiatrists or psychologists, or ideally, a multidisciplinary team, with specific training and experience in evaluating children with autism. Involving other professionals—such as speech and language and occupational therapists, special educators, and social workers when available—allows for more detailed assessment of specific domains, such as communication skills, sensory and motor problems, and family stressors and coping abilities. Multidisciplinary input also helps tailor interventions to a specific child's strengths and weaknesses.

Which additional investigations will specialists perform?

An important role of the specialist evaluation is to look for causes and co-occurring conditions. Identification of genetic or metabolic diagnoses allows the family to be given more accurate information on prognosis and risk of recurrence. When a child is diagnosed with autism, the specialist will complete a detailed physical examination to look for dysmorphic and neurological findings and Wood's lamp examination of the skin to assess for hypopigmented macules seen in tuberous sclerosis. High resolution karyotyping, DNA for fragile X syndrome, and chromosomal microarray testing have been recommended as standard laboratory tests, although the replacement of karyotyping with microarray analysis as first tier testing is being advocated by some consortium groups.[31] Additional genetic testing is done in the context of specific findings—for example, MECP2 (methyl-CpG binding protein 2; Rett syndrome) testing in young girls and PTEN (phosphatase and tensin homologue) testing in children with macrocephaly greater than 2.5 standard deviations above mean values for age and sex. Metabolic testing may be indicated in children with serious neurological abnormalities, particularly those born in countries where newborn metabolic screening

Table 1 Developmental screening tools for use in children with suspected autism spectrum disorder

Screening tool	Age range	Administration	Accessibility*
Communication and symbolic behavior scales-developmental profile (CSBS-DP), infant toddler checklist (ITC)	6-24 months	1 page, parent completed; 5-10 min to complete	Public domain (http://firstwords.fsu.edu/toddlerChecklist.html); available in English, Spanish, Slovenian, Chinese, and German
Modified checklist for autism in toddlers (M-CHAT)	16-48 months	23 item parent questionnaire; 5-10 min to complete	English version, public domain (www.firstsigns.org/screening/tools/rec.htm); also available in more than 20 languages, validations currently under way
Screening tool for autism in two year olds (STAT)	24-35 months	Directly administered by clinician and requires training workshop; 20 min to complete	Wendy Stone, PhD (author's email: triad@vanderbilt.edu); available in English
Pervasive developmental disorders screening test-II (PDDST), stage 1-primary care screener	12-48 months	Parent completed questionnaire; 10-15 min to complete and 5 min to score	Psychological Corporation (www.pearsonsassessment.com); available in English
Social communication questionnaire (SCQ)	≥4 years (for children with mental age of at least 2 years)	40 item parent completed questionnaire; 5-10 min to complete	Western Psychological Corporation (www.wpspublish.com); available in English
Social responsiveness scale	≥4 years	65 item parent teacher questionnaire; measures severity of autistic symptoms; 5-10 min to complete	Western Psychological Corporation (www.wpspublish.com); available in English

Screening tools that are not in the public domain can be purchased through the links provided.

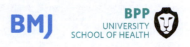

is not routine. Mitochondrial disorders are rare but will be considered if a child with symptoms of autism shows excessive fatigability, abnormities on neurological examination, marked delay in early gross motor milestones, or unusual patterns of regression (repeated regression or regression after age 3 years).[32]

The specialist will also look for medical and psychiatric comorbidities not identified during the general practitioner's initial history and investigations. The specialist will make a detailed review of symptoms and previous laboratory results; order tests that have not been done; and use screening tools to identify clinically relevant behaviours, such as hyperactivity or aggression, or emotional concerns, such as anxiety or depression, and to assess family functioning and level of support. Cognitive tests to determine the degree of intellectual impairment—seen in about 50% of children—can be useful for making a long term prognosis.[33] However, traditional cognitive testing is not always accurate in children with autism, and adaptive deficits often disproportionately affect functioning, even when cognition is within or above the average range.

What kinds of treatment are available for autism?

Although autism is a medical diagnosis, intervention is typically delivered in the educational setting. This requires the paediatric clinician to be familiar with community and educational resources and laws on educating children with disabilities. Clinicians need to be able to counsel families about appropriate treatments, in consultation with specialists involved in the child's care.

Much recent research has focused on the development of intervention programmes for young children with autism. Multiple intervention approaches (table 2) are currently used, such as applied behavior analysis (ABA), the Denver model, and TEACCH. The underlying principles of these approaches vary (for example, behaviour analytical, developmental, and structured teaching) but target common goals. In a recent systematic review, studies of ABA approaches, early intensive behavioural intervention variants, and the early start Denver model improved cognitive performance, language skills, and adaptive behaviour skills in some young children with autism, although the literature is limited by methodological concerns.[34] Educational programmes may use one or more approach (see table 2).

Although approaches vary, there is growing consensus about the crucial components of an educational programme for children with autism.[35] Intensive intervention should start as soon as the diagnosis is seriously considered. The Institute of Medicine's National Research Council recommends year round, systematically planned intervention of at least 25 hours a week. Appropriate educational settings consist of classrooms with a high degree of structure and a low student to teacher ratio. The curriculum promotes academic skills as appropriate for the child's developmental level. Therapists and special educators involved in the child's care help parents incorporate the techniques being used at home and provide opportunities for interaction with typically developing peers. Disruptive behaviours are best targeted with functional behavioural assessment, which identifies potentially modifiable factors (things that happen before and after a challenging behaviour that when changed can decrease the problem behaviour). Appropriate treatment targets include the development of functional communication, as well as social and adaptive skills to maximise independence. Establishing time specific

measureable goals helps to assess achievement and allows the intervention programme to be adjusted if a child is not progressing.

Many children, particularly those who have progressed with intensive intervention or who have milder symptoms, will benefit from consistent interaction with typically developing peers. Integrated classroom programmes, which include a mix of typical students and children with autism, may be appropriate for these children. For high functioning children with autism who have strong verbal skills and are achieving academically, a regular education classroom with supportive services may be an option. Support can include speech and language services to deal with pragmatic language and communication problems and social skills groups to teach appropriate social interaction.

Are drugs indicated in the management of children with autism?

Children with autism often have psychiatric comorbidities or exhibit difficult behaviours, such as aggression, self injurious behaviour, hyperactivity, impulsivity, sleep disorder, and anxiety.[36] When a new difficult behaviour emerges, a thorough search must be undertaken for underlying treatable medical causes (such as otitis media, dental pain, constipation, gastero-oesophogeal reflux). If a medical condition is ruled out, implement a functional behavioural assessment and behavioural plan supporting positive alternative behaviours as first line intervention. This is best done in consultation with a behavioural specialist or psychologist. If the behaviour does not respond to this intervention and functioning is seriously impaired, consider drug treatment to deal with target symptoms such as aggression, anxiety, or emotional lability.[37] Table 3 summarises available drug options, target symptoms, and evidence of efficacy.

Drugs—mainly risperidone and aripiprazole to deal with challenging behaviours—are currently viewed as adjuncts in the treatment of autism.[38] Some studies have associated older age at diagnosis, low adaptive skills and social competence, and higher levels of challenging behaviours with increased use of psychopharmacology.[39] It is important that families are aware that currently used drugs do not treat the core symptoms of autism and should be used only as part of a comprehensive treatment programme.

What about complementary and alternative treatments?

Parents of children with autism are often interested in complementary and alternative treatments.[40] Many of these treatments claim to improve symptoms, but few have been fully evaluated and even fewer shown to be effective by rigorous scientific study. Melatonin is efficacious in the management of sleep disorders associated with autism, particularly in improving sleep onset.[41] However, other treatments, such as chelation therapy, can be directly harmful, with case reports of deaths in children with autism receiving chelation. Clinicians should be open to discussing these treatments with parents, so they can counsel them appropriately and encourage them to seek additional information when necessary.

What is the prognosis for a child diagnosed with autism?

One of the challenging aspects of treating children with autism spectrum disorders is the great variability in long term outcomes. Several small longitudinal studies have found that children who have absence of language by age

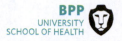

Table 2 Educational approaches for children with autism spectrum disorder

Approach	Details
Early start Denver model	Integrates applied behaviour analysis with developmental and relationship based approaches; aimed at toddlers and uses a developmental curriculum; principles include bringing the child into interactive social relationships, using positive emotional exchanges, and developing joint play activities to target deficits
TEACCH method	This structured teaching approach emphasises organisation of the physical environment, predictable sequence of activities, visual schedules, routines with flexibility, structured work/activity systems, and visually structured activities
Applied behaviour analysis	Uses behavioural principles to systematically change behaviour; the methods are used to teach new skills, increase and maintain desirable adaptive behaviours, reduce maladaptive behaviours, and generalise behaviours to new environments
Speech and language therapy	Communication therapy that is most effective when therapists train and work in collaboration with teachers, families, and peers to promote functional communication in natural settings; to enhance communication, augmentative and alternative communication modalities, such as the picture exchange communication system, may also be taught as part of the treatment
Social skills instruction	Training in the social skills that are typically impaired in autism, such as joint attention, interactive play, responding to social overtures, and initiating and maintaining social behaviour; in verbal, school aged children with autism, social skills groups and approaches like video modelling (using videos) and social stories (using formatted brief stories) can help teach specific social skills
Occupational therapy	Focuses on development and maintenance of fine motor and adaptive skills, but can also tackle deficits in processing and integration of sensory input; the efficacy of sensory integration therapy has not been shown through rigorous scientific study

Table 3 Drugs for treating challenging behaviours in children with autism

Drug	Target symptoms	Strength of evidence
Risperidone	Hyperactivity; irritability; maladaptive behaviours; sleep problems	Effective; side effects include weight gain (with increased risk of metabolic complications), prolactinaemia, and sedation; low risk of extrapyramidal symptoms
Aripiprazole	Maladaptive behaviours	Effective; similar side effect profile to risperidone, but can be used as an alternative when weight gain is prominent
Methylphenidate	Inattention; hyperactivity; restricted repetitive behaviours; irritability	Effective, although response rate may be lower in children with autism than in typical children with attention deficit hyperactivity disorder; lack of research on benefits and tolerability of extended release formulas
Noradrenalin reuptake inhibitor antidepressants and atypical antipsychotics (beyond risperidone)	Behavioural symptoms; hyperactivity	Marginal evidence
SSRIs (especially fluoxetine and escitalopram)	Restricted repetitive behaviour	Marginal evidence

SSRIs=selective serotonin reuptake inhibitors.

QUESTIONS FOR FUTURE RESEARCH

- What is contributing to the prevalence of autism?
- Do particular environmental factors play a role in autism and how do they interact with genetic factors?
- Is there a biomarker for autism spectrum disorder?
- Can we identify which educational approaches and techniques would be most beneficial on the basis of each child's presentation?
- What drugs are effective in treating the core symptoms of autism?
- What are the long term adult outcomes in children who receive specialised intensive early intervention from the time of diagnosis?

TIPS FOR NON-SPECIALISTS

- Assess for developmental delay at every well child visit
- The use of an autism specific screening tool will increase the detection of autism, particularly if you are concerned about developmental delay or if parents report concerns about delayed language development or impaired social interaction
- A negative screen does not rule out autism
- Refer children for whom there are persistent concerns or who score positive on a screening tool to a specialist or multidisciplinary team, if available, for a diagnostic assessment
- Initial investigations before referral should include a hearing evaluation and a detailed history to identify comorbidities such as seizures or constipation

ADDITIONAL EDUCATIONAL RESOURCES

Resources for healthcare professionals

- First Signs Video Glossary (www.firstsigns.org/asd_video_glossary/asdvg_about.htm)—free video clip examples of symptoms of autism
- American Academy of Pediatrics Toolkit (www.aap.org/publiced/autismtoolkit.cfm)—Useful resource for clinicians caring for children with autism; available for purchase
- OCALI Autism Internet Modules (www.autisminternetmodules.org/)—A series of online learning modules about autism related topics and interventions

Resources for families

- First Signs (www.firstsigns.org/)—Free parental education about autism
- First Signs Video Glossary (www.firstsigns.org/asd_video_glossary/asdvg_about.htm)—Free video clip examples of symptoms of autism
- Autism Speaks First 100 Days Kit (www.autismspeaks.org/docs/family_services_docs/100_day_kit.pdf) and OCALI Autism Internet Modules (www.autisminternetmodules.org/)—Free online learning modules about autism related topics and interventions

---

5 and low cognitive functioning have poorer outcomes in adolescence and adulthood on measures of self sufficiency and adaptive functioning,[42] and one noted that higher cumulative early intervention hours were associated with better outcome.[43] Many people with autism require supportive living arrangements into adulthood and relatively few are independently employed without support as young adults.[44]

When counselling families, stress that recent outcome studies looking at adolescents or adults diagnosed with autism in childhood reflect identification and intervention practices in place 10-20 years ago. Children who are less severely affected or benefiting from current intensive interventions may have a better prognosis. The clinician can emphasise that—although many people with autism may experience challenges with independent living, employment, social relationships, and mental health over their life course—the expectation is for developmental progress over time and that all children with autism can be supported in maximising their potential.

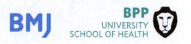

Contributors: SB, AR, and MA all helped write this article and are all guarantors.

Competing interests: All authors have completed the ICMJE uniform disclosure form at www.icmje.org/coi_disclosure.pdf (available on request from the corresponding author) and declare: SB, AR, and MA had support from Boston University School of Medicine and Boston Medical Center for the submitted work; no financial relationships with any organisations that might have an interest in the submitted work in the previous three years; no other relationships or activities that could appear to have influenced the submitted work.

Provenance and peer review: Commissioned; externally peer reviewed.

1   Baird G, Simonoff E, Pickles A, Chandler S, Loucas T, Meldrum D, et al. Prevalence of disorders of the autism spectrum in a population cohort of children in South Thames: the Special Needs and Autism Project (SNAP). Lancet2006;368:210-5.

2   Hertz-Picciotto I, Delwiche L. The rise in autism and the role of age at diagnosis. Epidemiology2009;20:84-90.

3   Marja-Leena M, Kielinen M, Linna SL, Jussila K, Ebeling H, Bloigu R, et al. Autism spectrum disorders according to DSM-IV-TR and comparison with DSM-5 draft criteria: an epidemiological study. J Am Acad Child Adolesc Psychiatry 2011;50:583-92.e11.

4   Ronald A, Hoekstra RA. Autism spectrum disorders and autistic traits: a decade of new twin studies. Am J Med Genet 2011;156B:255-74.

5   Schaefer GB, Mendelsohn NJ; Professional Practice and Guidelines Committee. Clinical genetics evaluation in identifying the etiology of autism spectrum disorders [published correction in: Genet Med 2008;10:464]. Genet Med2008;10:301-5.

6   Freitag CM, Staal W, Klauck SM, Duketis E, Waltes R. Genetics of autistic disorders: review and clinical implications. Eur Child Adolesc Psychiatry2010;19:169-78.

7   Betancur C. Etiological heterogeneity in autism spectrum disorders: more than 100 genetic and genomic disorders and still counting. Brain Res2011;1380:42-77.

8   Wass S. Distortions and disconnections: disrupted brain connectivity in autism. Brain Cogn2011;75:18-28.

9   Gardener H, Spiegelman D, Buka SL. Perinatal and neonatal risk factors for autism: a comprehensive meta-analysis. Pediatrics2011;128:344-55.

10   Immunization Safety Review Committee. Immunization Safety Review: Vaccines and Autism. Institute of Medicine. National Academies Press, 2004.

11   Millward C, Ferriter M, Calver SJ, Connell-Jones GG. Gluten- and casein-free diets for autistic spectrum disorder. Cochrane Database Syst Rev2 008;2:CD0034982009.

12   Werner E, Dawson G, Osterling J, Dinno N. Brief report: recognition of autism spectrum disorder before one year of age: a retrospective study based on home videotapes. J Autism Dev Disord2000;30:157-62.

13   Young R, Brewer N, Pattison C. Parental identification of early behavioural abnormalities in children with Autistic Disorder. Autism 2003;41:332-40.

14   Ozonoff SJ. A prospective study of the emergence of early behavioral signs in autism. Am Acad Child Adolesc Psychiatry2010;49:256-66.e1-2.

15   Mandell DS, Novak MM, Zubritsky CD. Factors associated with age of diagnosis among children with autism spectrum disorders. Pediatrics 2005;116:1480-6.

16   Barbaro J, Dissanayake C. Autism spectrum disorders in infancy and toddlerhood: a review of the evidence on early signs, early identification tools, and early diagnosis. J Dev Behav Pediatr2009;30:447-59.

17   Parr JR, Couteur AL, Baird G, Rutter M, Pickles A, Fombonne E, Bailey A. Developmental regression in autism spectrum disorder. Evidence from an international multiplex sample. J Autism Dev Disord 2011;30:157-62.

18   Baird G, Carman T, Pickles A, Chandler S, Loucas T, Meldrum D. Regression, developmental trajectory and problems in disorders in the autism spectrum: the SNAP Study. J Autism Dev Disord. 2008;38:1827-36.

19   Mandell DS, Walrath CM, Manteuffel B, Sgro G, Pinto-Martin J. Characteristics of children with autistic spectrum disorders served in comprehensive community-based mental health settings. J Autism Dev Disord2005;35:313-21.

20   Angkustsiri K, Krakowiak P, Moghaddam B, Wardinsky T, Gardner J, Kalamkarian N, et al. Minor physical anomalies in children with autism spectrum disorders. Autism2011; published online 24 May.

21   Ibrahim S, Voight R. Incidence of gastrointestinal symptoms in children with autism: a population-based study. Pediatrics2009;124:680-6.

22   American Academy of Pediatrics, Council on Children With Disabilities, Section on Developmental Behavioral Pediatrics, Bright Futures Steering Committee, and Medical Home Initiatives for Children With Special Needs. Identifying infants and young children with developmental disorders in the medical home: an algorithm for developmental surveillance and screening [published correction Pediatrics 2006;118:1808-9]. Pediatrics2006;118:405-20.

23   Johnson CP, Myers SM; American Academy of Pediatrics Council on Children with Disabilities. Identification and evaluation of children with autism spectrum disorders. Pediatrics 2007;120:1183-215.

24   Dumont-Mathieu T, Fein D. Screening for autism in young children: the modified checklist for autism in toddlers (M-CHAT) and other measures. Ment Retard Dev Disabil Res Rev2005;11:253-62.

25   Kleinman JM, Robins DL, Ventola PE, Pandev J, Boorstein HC, Esser EL, et al. The modified checklist for autism in toddlers: a follow-up study investigating the early detection of autism spectrum disorders J Autism Dev Disord2008;38:827-39.

26   Pierce K, Carter C, Weinfeld M, Desmond J, Hazin R, Bjork R, et al. Detecting, studying, and treating autism early: the one-year well-baby check-up approach. J Pediatr2011;159:458-65.e1-6.

27   Chandler S, Charman T, Baird G, Simonff E, Loucas T, Meldrum D, et al. Validation of the social communication questionnaire in a population cohort of children with autism spectrum disorders J Am Acad Child Adolesc Psychiatry2007;46:10.

28   Johnson S, Hollis C, Hennessy E, Kochhar P, Wolke D, Marlow N. Screening for autism in preterm children: diagnostic utility of the social communication questionnaire. Arch Dis Child2011;96:73-7.

29   Lainhart J, Piven J, Wzorek M, Landa R, Santangelo SL, Coon H, et al. Macrocephaly in children and adults with autism J Am Acad Child Adolesc Psychiatry1997;36:282-90.

30   Barnard-Brak L, Sulak T, Hatz JK. Macrocephaly in children with autism spectrum disorders. Pediatric Neurol2011;44:97-100.

31   Miller D, Adam MP, Aradhya S, Biesecker LG, Brothman AR, Carter NP et al. Consensus statement: chromosomal microarray is a first-tier clinical diagnostic test for individuals with developmental disabilities or congenital anomalies. Am J Hum Genet 2010;86:749-64.

32   Weissman JR, Kelley RI, Bauman ML, Cohen BH, Murray KF, Mitchell RL, et al. Mitochondrial disease in autism spectrum disorder patients: a cohort analysis. PLoS One2008;3:e3815.

33   Charman T, Pickles A, Simonoff E, Chandler S, Loucas T, Baird G. IQ in children with autism spectrum disorders: data from the Special Needs and Autism Project (SNAP). Psychol Med2011;41:619-27.

34   Warren Z, McPheeters ML, Sathe N, Foss-Feig JH, Glasser A, Veenstra-Vanderweele J. A systematic review of early intensive intervention for autism spectrum disorders. Pediatrics2011;127:e1303-11.

35   National Research Council, Committee on Educational Interventions for Children with Autism. Educating children with autism. Lord C, McGee JP, eds. National Academies Press, 2001.

36   Simonoff E, Pickles A. Psychiatric disorders in children with autism spectrum disorders: prevalence, comorbidity, and associated factors in a population-derived sample. J Am Acad Child Adolesc Psychiatry2008;47:921-9.

37   Huffman L, Sutcliffe TL, Tanner IS, Feldman HM. Management of symptoms in children with autism spectrum disorders: a comprehensive review of pharmacologic and complementary-alternative medicine treatments. J Dev Behav Pediatr2011;32:56-68.

38   McPheeters ML, Warren Z, Sathe N, Bruzek JL, Krishnaswami S, Jerome RN, et al. A systematic review of medical treatments for children with autism spectrum disorders. Pediatrics2011;127:e1312-21.

39   Myers SM, Johnson CP; American Academy of Pediatrics Council on Children with Disabilities. Management of children with autism spectrum disorders. Pediatrics 2007;120:1162-82.

40   Committee on Children with Disabilities. Counseling families who choose complementary and alternative medicine for their child with chronic illness or disability. Pediatrics2001;107:598.

41   Giannotti F, Cortesi F. An open-label study of controlled release melatonin in treatment of sleep disorders in children with autism. J Autism Dev Disord2006;36:741-52.

42   Billstedt E, Gillberg C, Gillberg C. Autism after adolescence: population-based 13-22 year follow-up study of 120 individuals with autism diagnosed in childhood. J Autism Dev Disord2005;35:351-60.

43   Baghdadli A, Assouline B, Sonie S, Pernon E, Darrou C, Michelon C, et al. Developmental trajectories of adaptive behaviors from early childhood to adolescence in a cohort of 152 children with autism spectrum disorders. J Autism Dev Disord2011; published online 18 September.

44   Taylor JK, Seltzer MM. Employment and post-secondary educational activities for young adults with autism spectrum disorders during the transition to adulthood. J Autism Dev Disord2011;41:566-74.

Related links

bmj.com

- How the autism epidemic came to be (2011;342:d852)Summary points

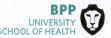

Evaluating the child who presents with an acute limp

Daniel C Perry Monk research fellow and PhD student, orthopaedic surgery[1], Colin Bruce consultant paediatric orthopaedic surgeon and honorary senior lecturer[1]

[1]University of Liverpool and Alder Hey Hospital, Liverpool L12 2AP

Correspondence to: D C Perry
danperry@doctors.org.uk

Cite this as: *BMJ* 2010;341:c4250

‹DOI› 10.1136/bmj.c4250
http://www.bmj.com/content/341/
bmj.c4250

A child may limp after trivial trauma, as a sign of local or systemic disease, or for no apparent reason. When there is a clear history of injury evaluation is usually straightforward. The diagnostic challenge is to distinguish between disease processes that are benign and self limiting (such as transient synovitis), acute or life threatening (such as septic arthritis or acute leukaemia), or chronic and disabling (such as Perthes' disease). In most cases the causes are benign and self limiting, and around two thirds of patients can be managed in the emergency department and do not require referral to hospital.[1 2]

How common is limping in children?

Few studies have outlined the incidence of limping in the children. A hospital based study in Edinburgh identified 243 cases of non-traumatic limps over six months and suggested an annual incidence of 3.6 cases per 1000 children aged 0-14 years.[1] A nationwide community based study from the Netherlands identified an annual incidence of 1.5 cases per 1000 children of non-traumatic hip pathology.[4] The true incidence probably varies by country and region. These figures suggest that family practitioners are likely to meet such a problem several times throughout their career.

What constitutes a limp in a child?

A limp is an abnormal gait pattern usually caused by pain, weakness, or deformity. The term is most commonly used to described a shortened "stance phase" in the gait cycle, in which a person "hurries" off one leg to offload a source of pain; it is better described as an antalgic gait. Parents often use the term "limping" to describe any abnormality of gait. A fundamental difficulty of assessing a limp is that children do not have a mature, reproducible, rhythmic gait cycle until after 7 years of age,[3] so discussion between doctor and parents must elicit specific changes in the child's gait.

Here, we review the epidemiology of acute limp and outline the pitfalls in diagnosis. We provide a framework for early assessment and management of the child who presents with a limp based on evidence from case series, laboratory studies, observational studies, and expert reviews.

How do I assess the limping child?

History

It is most important when trying to establish a working diagnosis to consider the child's age. Children become vulnerable to a variety of diseases that manifest as a limp at different stages in their childhood (box 1).

Listen to the child and observe their interaction with the parents, and be aware that in cases of abuse the history the

---

BOX 1 PRIMARY DIFFERENTIAL DIAGNOSIS OF AN "ATRAUMATIC LIMP" BY AGE*

0-3 years
- Septic arthritis or osteomyelitis
- Developmental hip dysplasia
- Fracture or soft tissue injury (toddler's fractures or non-accidental injury)

3-10 years
- Transient synovitis or irritable hip
- Septic arthritis or osteomyelitis
- Perthes' disease
- Fracture or soft tissue injury (stress fracture)

10-15 years
- Slipped upper femoral epiphysis
- Septic arthritis or osteomyelitis
- Perthes' disease
- Fracture or soft tissue injury (stress fracture)

Other diagnoses
- Haematological disease, such as sickle cell anaemia
- Infective disease, such as pyomyositis or discitis
- Metabolic disease, such as rickets
- Neoplastic disease, such as acute lymphoblastic leukaemia
- Neuromuscular disease, such as cerebral palsy or muscular dystrophy
- Primary anatomical abnormality, such as limb length inequality
- Rheumatological disease, such as juvenile idiopathic arthritis

*Based on studies of the common diagnoses encountered in atraumatic limps[1] and atraumatic hip disease in children.[4 5] Non-accidental injury is included because of the importance of making a prompt diagnosis. We examined age distribution in the more common diagnoses to allow classification of the diagnosis by age (transient synovitis[4 6] Perthes' disease,[7 8] slipped capital femoral epiphysis,[9] late presenting developmental dysplasia of the hip,[10] osteomyelitis,[11 12] toddler's fracture,[13] and orthopaedic injuries in non-accidental injury[14 15])

SOURCES AND SELECTION CRITERIA

We searched Google Scholar and Medline (1965-2010) using the terms "limp", "hip", "Perthes", "developmental dysplasia", "transient synovitis", "irritable hip", and "slipped epiphysis". We also searched bibliographies of retrieved articles for articles not indexed elsewhere and identified references from searches of our files. Only papers published in English were reviewed. No related Cochrane reviews were available. We selected articles if they were the best evidence available or best summary of the evidence. Some articles were included to place the review in historical context.

SUMMARY POINTS

- Atraumatic limps are a source of concern to both the family doctor and emergency practitioner
- Age is the key factor in forming a list of differential diagnoses
- The hip is the most common source of pathology, and pain is often referred to the knee
- A delay in the diagnosis of a slipped upper femoral epiphysis may worsen the outcome
- Transient synovitis and septic arthritis may be difficult to differentiate so any clinical concern warrants urgent investigation

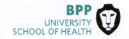

BOX 2 MODIFIED PAEDIATRIC "GAIT, ARMS, LEGS, AND SPINE" EXAMINATION FOR THE LIMPING CHILD

Screening questions

- "Do you have any pain or stiffness in your joints, muscles, or back?"

Gait/general

- Record the child's temperature*
- Observe the child walking. Ask the child to walk on his or her tiptoes and heels

Arms

- Not directly applicable

Legs

- Feel for effusion of the knee
- Ask the child to: "Bend and then straighten your knee" and feel for crepitus
- Apply passive flexion (90°) with internal rotation of hip

Spine

- Observe the spine from behind
- Ask the child: "Can you bend and touch your toes?" Observe the curve of the spine from the side and behind

*Item added to the standard examination

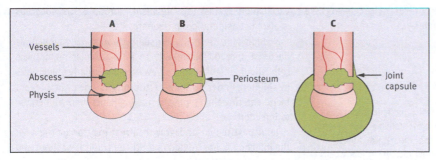

Fig 2 Development of septic arthritis. Infection often begins as a metaphyseal focus of osteomyelitis (A). The thin cortex of the metaphysis is easily breached and the infection spreads to the subperiosteal space forming a periosteal abscess (B). If the metaphysis is intra-articular, inoculation of the joint space may occur, resulting in septic arthritis (C)

BOX 3 AN ORTHOPAEDIC "LOOK, FEEL, MOVE" APPROACH TO THE CHILD WITH A LIMP

Look

- Is the child unwell, feverish, or tachycardic?
- Can the child stand?
- Is the spine straight?
- Is there any evidence of spinal dysraphism (tufts of hair or sacral pit)?
- Is the pelvis level?
- Are the legs of equal length?
- Are the joints swollen or bent?
- Do the muscles look hypotrophic or hypertrophic?

Feel

- Can the patient localise the pain?
- Is focal tenderness present? (Systematically palpate the spine, pelvis, lower limbs, and perhaps the abdomen and testicles)
- Is there increased heat over joints?

Move

- Can the child walk?
- Is there any evidence of a gait abnormality, such as antalgic or trendelenburg gait (downward tilt of the pelvis when standing on one leg on the side of abnormality)?
- Does each joint move fully and without pain?
- Pay special attention to the hips. Do the hips move normally? Do they internally rotate symmetrically and without pain (pain or restricted internal rotation is a sensitive sign of pathology of the hip joint)?

parents give may not accurately reflect the mechanism of injury. A child may commonly associate a symptom with a previous injury, to which it may or may not be related. For example, children presenting with Perthes' disease often describe a traumatic origin to their symptoms.[16]

Elicit the nature of the limp and take the duration of symptoms and presence of pain into account. Like adults children may present with referred pain. Children present with knee pain in a variety of hip disorders,[4] so the clinician must consider hip pathologies when knee pain is reported.

Systemic illness, such as transient synovitis or leukaemia, may present with a limp. The birth and developmental history help to identify risk factors for diseases such as hip dysplasia and cerebral palsy and to gauge global motor development.

Examination

In practice the history may be vague, the patient uncooperative, and clinical signs scant, so a clear idea of how to approach the examination and where to seek pathology is necessary. The musculoskeletal examination in children can be difficult for doctors of all grades and specialties.[17] The "paediatric gait, arms, legs, and spine" examination is a quick to perform, acceptable, and validated musculoskeletal screening examination in school aged children.[18] Box 2 shows a slightly modified version of the examination that is useful when examining a limping child. Box 3 details an orthopaedic "look, feel, move" approach to assessment using questions that we believe are helpful in making a diagnosis.

Meticulous examination of the hips is crucial because this joint is a common source of unexplained limp.[1] Expert opinion generally agrees that restricted internal rotation is the most sensitive marker of hip pathology in children, followed by a lack of abduction. Loss of abduction in a child can be difficult to assess even in experienced hands because children often tilt their pelvis to give a false impression of hip abduction.

Both intra-abdominal pathology[19] and testicular torsion[20] may present simply as a limp, so examination of the abdomen and, in boys, the testicles is important.

What are the potential causes of a limp?

Trauma is the most common cause of limping in children. This is apparent to anyone who has attended a children's fracture clinic or emergency department although evidence to substantiate this statement is lacking. Children have growth plates that are more vulnerable to injury than ligaments, and a "sprain" in a child should raise suspicion of a physeal injury. Children are also more flexible than adults, so seemingly trivial force can cause joint subluxation or dislocation in normal children.[21] The threshold for radiographic assessment in the child is therefore low, especially when the diagnosis is uncertain.

In a prospective series from Edinburgh of 243 children presenting to the emergency department with an acute atraumatic limp, the pathology arose from the hip in more than 60% of cases in which a diagnosis was made.[1] In this series the most common diagnosis was transient synovitis or irritable hip (40%). Chronic muscle sprains or unreported trauma accounted for a further 16% of diagnoses. No diagnosis was made in 30% of cases. Other common diagnoses were Perthes' disease (2%), osteomyelitis (1.5%), toddler's fracture (1%), and slipped capital femoral epiphysis

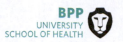

(1%). Less common diseases made up the remainder (see box 1).

What key diagnoses should be considered?

Toddler's fracture
This is a subtle undisplaced spiral fracture of the tibia usually seen in preschool children.[22] It is caused by a sudden twist, often after an unwitnessed fall. The unclear history may prompt the clinician to consider abuse. Examination may be difficult in the child with few clinical signs. Localised tenderness over the tibial shaft may be present or gentle strain on the tibia may provoke symptoms. Diagnosis may be delayed if initial radiographs show little evidence of fracture. In one series of 37 cases, five fractures were not present on initial radiographs, although this result may be biased by poor case ascertainment.[13] If the history and clinical examination suggest a fracture and other differential diagnoses are excluded, the child can be immobilised and managed expectantly. The diagnosis may be confirmed by follow-up radiographs that show evidence of callus at the fracture site (box 4). In the absence of a clear diagnosis a bone scan may identify the pathology.

Transient synovitis
Atraumatic limp is usually caused by transient synovitis.[1 4 5] It is most common in boys aged 4-8.[1 6] It is self limiting and is thought to follow a viral illness, although the evidence is weak. A recent small case-control study confirmed reports of recent viral illness in cases,[23] but information was prone to recall bias. Microbiological investigations have failed to identify a pathogen and the evidence for a viral aetiology comes from old studies that showed activation of the interferon system.[24] Definitive diagnosis is based on a confirmed hip effusion and the exclusion of other potential causes. A link between transient synovitis and the development of Perthes' disease has been suggested, but again the evidence is weak.[25]

Septic arthritis
Septic arthritis is an infection of the synovium and joint space. Pathogens vary by geography and time, and a recent series of 102 Australian cases found that *Staphylococcus aureus* was the most common organism, with no cases of *Haemophilus influenzae* since the introduction of vaccination against this organism.[12] Group B *Streptococcus* is also a consideration in neonates.[26]

Seeding of the infection is usually through haematogenous bacterial spread. Joints with an intra-articular metaphysis (hip, shoulder, ankle, and elbow) are particularly vulnerable. In children under 18 months the physis does not prevent blood entering the epiphysis, making joints more vulnerable to infection.

Joint destruction and growth arrest may occur (fig 2) if the infection is not treated urgently by surgical washout and intravenous antibiotics.

> **BOX 4 A DIFFICULT CASE OF LIMPING**
> An 18 month child attended with limping. Initial examination, blood tests, and radiographs were unremarkable. Ultrasound of the hips was normal. Given the unclear presentation a technetium labelled bone scan was performed. This test showed increased uptake in the right mid-tibial region (fig 1) and the defect was treated as a toddler's fracture. A further radiograph four weeks later showed the periosteal reaction associated with the healing fracture

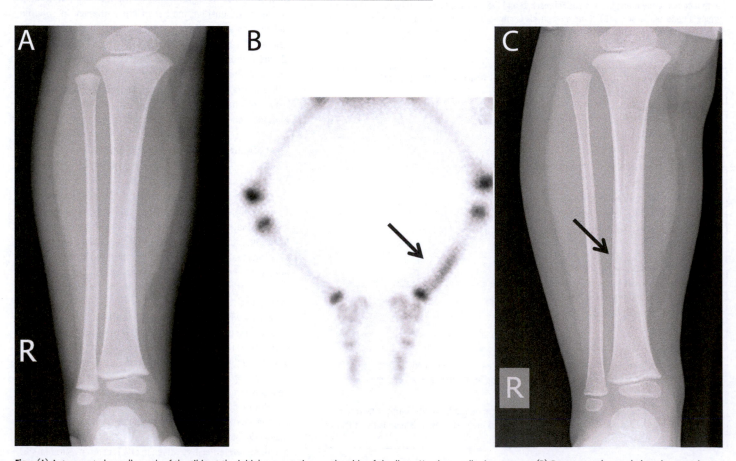

Fig 1 (A) Anteroposterior radiograph of the tibia at the initial presentation on the side of the limp. No abnormality is apparent. (B) Bone scan shows obvious increased uptake in the distribution of the right tibia. (C) After four weeks a florid periosteal reaction can be seen, which supports the diagnosis of toddler's fracture

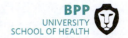
Perthes' disease

Perthes' disease is an idiopathic avascular necrosis of a developing femoral head. It typically presents in boys aged 4-8 years.[7] Affected children are usually shorter than their peers[27] and have a hyperactive tendency.[28] It is diagnosed by plain anteroposterior radiography of the pelvis. Classic radiographic features include sclerosis, fragmentation, and eventual flattening of the proximal femoral epiphysis (fig 3).[29] Radiographic changes may be absent in early disease, and Perthes' disease may initially be mistaken for transient synovitis. Symptoms typically settle within about two weeks in transient synovitis whereas in Perthes' disease they persist. If symptoms persist a technetium bone scan or magnetic resonance imaging can help to identify the pathology, which is seen as an area of reduced perfusion on bone scan or a signal change on magnetic resonance imaging. Both tests are thought to have similar sensitivity and specificity (98% sensitivity, 95% specificity for bone scan[30]), although the evidence for magnetic resonance imaging is weak. Treatment requires "containment" of the hip within the acetabulum by surgical or non-surgical means. Prognosis depends on age, sex, and extent of epiphyseal involvement.[31]

Developmental dysplasia of the hip

Developmental dysplasia of the hip is the term that has replaced congenital dislocation of the hip. Most cases are identified through routine infant clinical screening and selective ultrasound screening of high risk groups. It mostly affects girls and when presentation is delayed typically presents as a limp.[10] Diagnosis is based on a plain radiograph of the pelvis in children of walking age (fig 4). Bilateral developmental dysplasia of the hip may be more difficult to detect than unilateral disease, because the resultant loss of abduction, limb shortening, and altered gait are symmetrical and difficult to identify.

Slipped capital femoral epiphysis

Slipped capital femoral epiphysis, otherwise known as slipped upper femoral epiphysis, usually affects children over 10 years.[9] The proximal femoral epiphysis displaces relative to the metaphysis. It is slightly more common in boys and patients are often overweight.[32] It is associated with endocrinal abnormalities such as hypothyroidism and growth hormone deficiency.[33]

Knee pain is common, and a review of 106 cases of slipped capital femoral epiphysis found this to be the primary feature in 15% of cases.[34] Periadolescents who have pain or discomfort on internal rotation of the hip require further radiographical testing. Plain anteroposterior radiographs of the pelvis may be unremarkable if the slip is subtle. A lateral projection is better at identifying such slips and is therefore essential (fig 5).[35] To minimise radiation exposure many radiology departments do not routinely obtain lateral projections of children's hips, so such views must be specifically requested if this defect is suspected.

This defect must be diagnosed promptly. A recent meta-analysis of five studies assessed the urgency of surgical fixation in unstable slipped capital femoral epiphysis (<24 hours v >24 hours). Although the results were not statistically significant, early fixation seemed to improve outcome.[36] Similarly two retrospective studies of 102 and 65 cases of mainly stable slipped capital femoral epiphysis found a significant tendency to greater deformity in the group with a delayed diagnosis.[34] [37] Delayed diagnosis was most commonly caused in both studies by a presentation with knee pain that was not appropriately investigated.

A pragmatic approach to managing limps not attributable to trauma

Advice on how to manage a childhood limp varies greatly. Orthopaedic and emergency medicine journals generally suggest immediate investigation, yet general practitioners often take a more considered approach, with one Dutch community based study showing that they often opt for close follow-up rather than immediate investigation.[38] A retrospective study of 350 child hospital emergency attendees in New Zealand who underwent radiography for a limp or hip symptoms found that 38% were afebrile and able to bear weight at presentation. All but one of these patients had transient synovitis.[4] The child with an alternative diagnosis had osteomyelitis, which can go undetected even with blood investigations.[39] On the basis of these reviews and our own experience we suggest a considered approach.

Children under 3 years

These children are vulnerable to septic arthritis and non-accidental injury. Transient synovitis is rare, so this diagnosis should be made with extreme caution and only after excluding more serious pathology. Clinical signs may be scant and the child may simply not move the limb—so called pseudoparalysis. Most practitioners lack experience in assessing children of this age and urgent referral is advised (box 5).

Children 3-9 years

Transient synovitis is most likely in this age group. A brief period of observation is permissible if the child is well, afebrile, mobile, but limping and has had symptoms for

---

BOX 5 RED FLAGS (REQUIRING URGENT INVESTIGATION)

- Child <3 years old
- Unable to bear weight
- Fever
- Systemic illness
- Child >9 years old with pain or restricted hip movements

---

under 48 hours. Manage with rest and advice and follow-up within the next 48 hours. Tell parents to attend the emergency department if symptoms worsen or if fever or systemic illness supervenes. If symptoms are resolving at follow-up the working diagnosis is transient synovitis and no investigations are needed. The child should be reviewed a week later to confirm complete resolution of symptoms. If the symptoms worsen or fail to resolve start investigations.

Children over 9 years

Slipped capital femoral epiphysis becomes a consideration in this group. Patients need urgent investigation (box 5), including anteroposterior and lateral radiographs of the hips. Additional investigations are based on the clinical presentation. An 8 year old child with risk factors for a slipped capital femoral epiphysis (obesity, history of endocrinopathy, radiotherapy) would also need urgent investigation.

Investigations

Investigations depend on the suspected diagnosis but should include a full blood count, erythrocyte sedimentation rate, and C reactive protein, along with radiographs of the

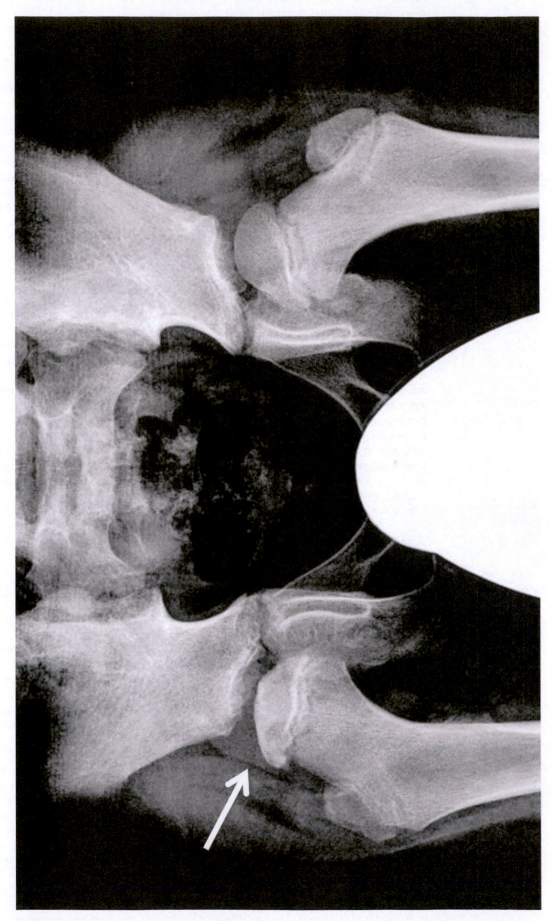

Fig 3 Radiograph showing sclerotic change within right femoral epiphysis in early Perthes' disease

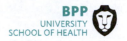

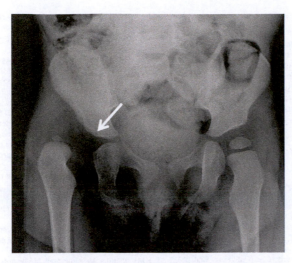

Fig 4 Radiograph of a 16 month old child showing a right dislocated hip

BOX 6 KOCHER'S CRITERIA FOR DIFFERENTIATING SEPTIC ARTHRITIS FROM TRANSIENT SYNOVITIS

Factors for predicting septic arthritis
- Fever >38.5°C
- Cannot bear weight
- Erythrocyte sedimentation rate >40 mm in the first hour
- Serum white blood cell count >12×10⁹/l

Probability of septic arthritis
- No factors: <0.2%
- 1 factor: 3%
- 2 factors: 40%
- 3 factors: 93.1%
- 4 factors: 99.6%

QUESTIONS FOR FUTURE RESEARCH
- What is the true burden of atraumatic limps in primary care?
- What is the best clinical algorithm to distinguish between transient synovitis and septic arthritis?

site of pain and the pelvis if restricted hip movements or knee pain is present.

Ultrasound can identify a hip effusion and help localise the sight of pathology but cannot identify the underlying pathology. A prospective hospital based study found that routine ultrasound of the hips had a low sensitivity (57%) and specificity (59%) for establishing a diagnosis in children

ADDITIONAL EDUCATIONAL RESOURCES

Resources for healthcare professionals
- Sewell MD, Rosendahl J, Eastwood DM. Developmental dysplasia of the hip. *BMJ* 2009;339:b4454
- Clarke NMP, Kendrick T. Slipped capital femoral epiphysis. *BMJ* 2009;339:b4457

Resources for patients
- Patient UK (www.patient.co.uk)—Useful information leaflets for each of the common hip disorders
- STEPS (www.steps-charity.org.uk)—Charity supporting those with lower limb disorders
- Perthes Association (www.perthes.org.uk)—Charity supporting those with Perthes' disease and other osteochondroses

with atraumatic limps. Nevertheless, a negative result was useful in that it prompted further investigation.[40]

In the absence of a working diagnosis, or when symptoms persist, further investigations include technetium labelled bone scans and magnetic resonance imaging. These tests may uncover unexpected diagnoses such as intervertebral discitis, toddler's fractures, or Perthes' disease. Consider additional blood tests, such as creatine kinase (muscular dystrophy), immunogenic markers (rheumatological disease), and a sickle cell screen in high risk groups.

How can transient synovitis and septic arthritis be differentiated?

This is one of the most difficult problems for practitioners faced with a child with an "irritable hip." In 1999 a retrospective series of 168 children with a confirmed hip effusion identified four factors that were useful in differentiating septic arthritis from transient synovitis.[41] When all four variables were positive the probability of septic arthritis was 99.6%. This algorithm (Kocher's algorithm) has since been validated prospectively,[42] although external validation failed to support the strength of the positive predictive value, suggesting only a 59% probability of septic arthritis with all four variables present.[43] Other studies have also tried to identify features that reliably differentiate between these two entities and have suggested that duration of symptoms[44] and previous healthcare visits[43] are independent predictors of pathology. Such additional predictors lack any form of validation. Although the accuracy of Kocher's algorithm is debated, it is currently the most useful tool available (box 6).

Contributors: DCP planned the review, performed literature searches, and is co-author. CB reviewed the literature and is co-author and guarantor.

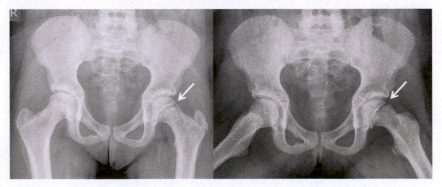

Fig 5 Left sided slipped capital femoral epiphysis. The "frog" lateral radiograph shown on the right is important to detect the abnormality, which is difficult to see on plain anteroposterior radiography

71

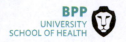

Funding: DCP is funded by John Monk hip research fund.

Competing interests: All authors have completed the Unified Competing Interest form at www.icmje.org/coi_disclosure.pdf (available on request from the corresponding author) and declare: (1) No financial support for the submitted work from anyone other than their employer; (2) No financial relationships with commercial entities that might have an interest in the submitted work; (3) No spouses, partners, or children with relationships with commercial entities that might have an interest in the submitted work; (4) No non-financial interests that may be relevant to the submitted work.

Patient consent obtained.

Provenance and peer review: Commissioned; externally peer reviewed.

1   Fischer SU, Beattie TF. The limping child: epidemiology, assessment and outcome. *J Bone Joint Surg Br*1999;81:1029-34.
2   Mattick A, Turner A, Ferguson J, Beattie T, Sharp J. Seven year follow up of children presenting to the accident and emergency department with irritable hip. *J Accid Emerg Med*1999;16:345-47.
3   Sutherland DH, Olshen R, Cooper L, Woo SL. The development of mature gait. *J Bone Joint Surg Am*1980;62:336-53.
4   Krul M, van der Wouden JC, Schellevis FG, van Suijlekom-Smit LWA, Koes BW. Acute non-traumatic hip pathology in children: incidence and presentation in family practice. *Fam Pract* 2010;27:166-70.
5   Reed L, Baskett A, Watkins N. Managing children with acute non-traumatic limp: the utility of clinical findings, laboratory inflammatory markers and X-rays. *Emerg Med Australas*2009;21:136-42.
6   Landin LA, Danielsson LG, Wattsgård C. Transient synovitis of the hip. Its incidence, epidemiology and relation to Perthes' disease. *J Bone Joint Surg Br*1987;69:238-42.
7   Hall AJ, Barker DJ. The age distribution of Legg-Perthes disease. An analysis using Sartwell's incubation period model. *Am J Epidemiol*1984;120:531-6.
8   Wiig O, Terjesen T, Svenningsen S, Lie SA. The epidemiology and aetiology of Perthes' disease in Norway. A nationwide study of 425 patients. *J Bone Joint Surg Br*2006;88:1217-23.
9   Lehmann CL, Arons RR, Loder RT, Vitale MG. The epidemiology of slipped capital femoral epiphysis: an update. *J Pediatr Orthop*2006;26:286-90.
10 Sharpe P, Mulpuri K, Chan A, Cundy PJ. Differences in risk factors between early and late diagnosed developmental dysplasia of the hip. *Arch Dis Child Fetal Neonatal Ed*2006;91:F158-62.
11 Blyth MJ, Kincaid R, Craigen MA, Bennet GC. The changing epidemiology of acute and subacute haematogenous osteomyelitis in children. *J Bone Joint Surg Br*2001;83:99-102.
12 Goergens ED, McEvoy A, Watson M, Barrett IR. Acute osteomyelitis and septic arthritis in children. *J Paediatr Child Health*2005;41:59-62.
13 Tenenbein M, Reed MH, Black GB. The toddler's fracture revisited. *Am J Emerg Med*1990;8:208-11.
14 Loder RT, Feinberg JR. Orthopaedic injuries in children with nonaccidental trauma: demographics and incidence from the 2000 kids' inpatient database. *J Pediatr Orthop*2007;27:421-6.
15 Kemp AM, Dunstan F, Harrison S, Morris S, Mann M, Rolfe K, et al. Patterns of skeletal fractures in child abuse: systematic review. *BMJ*2008;337:a1518.
16 Wynne-Davies R, Gormley J. The aetiology of Perthes' disease. Genetic, epidemiological and growth factors in 310 Edinburgh and Glasgow patients. *J Bone Joint Surg Br*1978;60:6-14.
17 Jandial S, Myers A, Wise E, Foster HE. Doctors likely to encounter children with musculoskeletal complaints have low confidence in their clinical skills. *J Pediatr*2009;154:267-71.
18 Foster HE, Kay LJ, Friswell M, Coady D, Myers A. Musculoskeletal screening examination (pGALS) for school-age children based on the adult GALS screen. *Arthritis Rheum*2006;55:709-16.
19 Crandall WV, Langer JC. Primary omental torsion presenting as hip pain and limp. *J Pediatr Gastroenterol Nutr*1999;28:95-6.
20 Sheafor DH, Holder LE, Thompson D, Schauwecker DS, Sager GL, McFarland EG. Scrotal pathology as the cause for hip pain. Diagnostic findings on bone scintigraphy. *Clin Nucl Med*1997;22:287-91.
21 Schlonsky J, Miller PR. Traumatic hip dislocations in children. *J Bone Joint Surg Am*1973;55:1057-63.
22 Dunbar JS, Owen HF, Nogrady MB, McLeese R. Obscure tibial fracture of infants—the toddler's fracture. *J Can Assoc Radiol*1964;15:136-44.
23 Kastrissianakis K, Beattie TF. Transient synovitis of the hip: more evidence for a viral aetiology. *Eur J Emerg Med*2010; published online 2 June.
24 Tolat V, Carty H, Klenerman L, Hart CA. Evidence for a viral aetiology of transient synovitis of the hip. *J Bone Joint Surg Br*1993;75:973-4.
25 Mukamel M, Litmanovitch M, Yosipovich Z, Grunebaum M, Varsano I. Legg-Calve-Perthes disease following transient synovitis. How often? *Clin Pediatr (Phila)*1985;24:629-31.
26 Kalliola S, Vuopio-Varkila J, Takala AK, Eskola J. Neonatal group B streptococcal disease in Finland: a ten-year nationwide study. *Pediatr Infect Dis J*1999;18:806-10.
27 Burwell RG, Dangerfield PH, Hall DJ, Vernon CL, Harrison MH. Perthes' disease. An anthropometric study revealing impaired and disproportionate growth. *J Bone Joint Surg Br*1978;60-B:461-77.
28 Loder RT, Schwartz EM, Hensinger RN. Behavioral characteristics of children with Legg-Calvé-Perthes disease. *J Pediatr Orthop*1993;13:598-601.
29 Waldenstrom H. On coxa plana. *Acta Chir Scand*1923;55:577-90.
30 Sutherland AD, Savage JP, Paterson DC, Foster BK. The nuclide bone-scan in the diagnosis and management of Perthes' disease. *J Bone Joint Surg Br*1980;62:300-6.
31 Herring JA, Kim HT, Browne R. Legg-Calve-Perthes disease. Part II: Prospective multicenter study of the effect of treatment on outcome. *J Bone Joint Surg Am*2004;86-A:2121-34.
32 Bhatia NN, Pirpiris M, Otsuka NY. Body mass index in patients with slipped capital femoral epiphysis. *J Pediatr Orthop*2006;26:197-9.
33 Loder RT, Wittenberg B, DeSilva G. Slipped capital femoral epiphysis associated with endocrine disorders. *J Pediatr Orthop*1995;15:349-56.
34 Matava MJ, Patton CM, Luhmann S, Gordon JE, Schoenecker PL. Knee pain as the initial symptom of slipped capital femoral epiphysis: an analysis of initial presentation and treatment. *J Pediatr Orthop*1999;19:455-60.
35 Loder RT. Effect of femur position on the angular measurement of slipped capital femoral epiphysis. *J Pediatr Orthop*2001;21:488-94.
36 Lowndes S, Khanna A, Emery D, Sim J, Maffulli N. Management of unstable slipped upper femoral epiphysis: a meta-analysis. *Br Med Bull*2009;90:133-46.
37 Rahme D, Comley A, Foster B, Cundy P. Consequences of diagnostic delays in slipped capital femoral epiphysis. *J Pediatr Orthop B*2006;15:93-7.
38 Vijlbrief AS, Bruijnzeels MA, van der Wouden JC, van Suijlekom-Smit LW. Incidence and management of transient synovitis of the hip: a study in Dutch general practice. *Br J Gen Pract*1992;42:426-8.
39 Ferguson LP, Beattie TF. Lesson of the week: osteomyelitis in the well looking afebrile child. *BMJ*2002;324:1380-1.
40 Bienvenu-Perrard M, de Suremain N, Wicart P, Moulin F, Benosman A, Kalifa G, et al. [Benefit of hip ultrasound in management of the limping child]. *J Radiol*2007;88:377-83.
41 Kocher MS, Zurakowski D, Kasser JR. Differentiating between septic arthritis and transient synovitis of the hip in children: an evidence-based clinical prediction algorithm. *J Bone Joint Surg Am*1999;81:1662-70.
42 Kocher MS, Mandiga R, Zurakowski D, Barnewolt C, Kasser JR. Validation of a clinical prediction rule for the differentiation between septic arthritis and transient synovitis of the hip in children. *J Bone Joint Surg Am*2004;86-A:1629-35.
43 Luhmann SJ, Jones A, Schootman M, Gordon JE, Schoenecker PL, Luhmann JD. Differentiation between septic arthritis and transient synovitis of the hip in children with clinical prediction algorithms. *J Bone Joint Surg Am*2004;86-A:956-62.
44 Delaney RA, Lenehan B, O'Sullivan L, McGuinness AJ, Street JT. The limping child: an algorithm to outrule musculoskeletal sepsis. *Ir J Med Sci*2007;176:181-7.

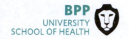

Developmental dysplasia of the hip

M D Sewell specialist registrar trauma and orthopaedics[1], K Rosendahl consultant paediatric radiologist[2], D M Eastwood consultant paediatric orthopaedic surgeon[1][2]

[1]Catterall Unit, Royal National Orthopaedic Hospital, Stanmore HA7 4LP

[2]Department of Radiology, Great Ormond Street Hospital for Children, London, UK

Correspondence to: D M Eastwood
d.m.eastwood@btinternet.com

Cite this as: *BMJ* 2009;339:b4454

‹DOI› 10.1136/bmj.b4454
http://www.bmj.com/content/339/bmj.b4454

Developmental dysplasia of the hip affects 1-3% of newborns.[1][2][w1-w3] A registry based study showed that it was responsible for 29% of primary hip replacements in people up to age 60 years.[3] The effectiveness of screening programmes aimed at early detection varies according to their organisation, methods of ascertainment, and diagnostic criteria.[1][4][5][w4] Delay in diagnosis means that more complex treatments with higher failure rates will be required, so early diagnosis and prompt, appropriate treatment are essential. We describe the diagnosis, management, and screening controversies for hip dysplasia and provide a framework for early assessment, based on the available literature, including studies with level 1 evidence.

What is developmental dysplasia of the hip?

The term refers to a spectrum of pathology, ranging from mild acetabular dysplasia with a stable hip through more severe forms of dysplasia, often associated with neonatal hip instability, to established hip dysplasia with or without later subluxation or dislocation. The condition used to be known as congenital dislocation of the hip (CDH), but the term developmental dysplasia of the hip (DDH) better reflects both the variable presentation and the potentially progressive nature of the condition.[w5] Typically, cases present within the neonatal period, but some cases are recognised later (fig 1).

This review concentrates on "idiopathic" developmental dysplasia of the hip. The management of dislocation secondary to neuromuscular conditions is outside the scope of this article.[w6-w8]

How common is it?

Precise prevalence varies with age and definition of hip dysplasia. A worldwide systematic review of unscreened populations estimated the prevalence of clinically diagnosed, established hip dysplasia to be 1.3 per 1000.[2] In populations screened clinically with Ortolani and Barlow tests, the prevalence is higher (1.6-28.5 per 1000[2]), and it is higher still with ultrasound screening that uses a morphological definition of abnormality.[w9]

What do we know about the causes?

The precise aetiology of developmental hip dysplasia is unknown, but genetic and environmental factors may act as internal or external influences, respectively (box 1). The left

---

BOX 1 FACTORS INFLUENCING DEVELOPMENTAL HIP DYSPLASIA

Internal

- Decreased resistance of the hip to dislocation
- Shallow acetabulum
- Connective tissue laxity

External

- Breech presentation[7]
- Large for gestational age
- Oligohydramnios
- Infant position in utero and in infancy[w11]
- Multiple pregnancy

---

hip is most often affected; 20% of cases are bilateral and 80% are in girls.[w10] Findings from twin and family studies suggest high heritability consistent with a strong genetic susceptibility to onset of disease but not necessarily to progression or severity.[6] Having a sibling with hip dysplasia increases risk by 5%.[6]

Vaginal delivery of babies with breech presentation is associated with a 17-fold increased risk of hip dysplasia, compared with a sevenfold increase for breech babies delivered by elective caesarean section.[7]

Why is early detection important?

The pathology of hip dysplasia changes with time, and so does management. In neonates, soft tissues are lax: a dislocated hip may be reduced by simple manipulation during clinical examination, and stabilisation occurs as the soft tissues tighten. An unstable or dislocatable hip may also stabilise spontaneously. When the femoral head is aligned with the centre of the acetabulum, the dysplastic acetabulum often normalises within the first months of life. If the hip remains dislocated, soft tissue contractures develop rapidly, and surgery is likely to be required to obtain and maintain joint reduction. The longer the hip is left in an abnormal position, the more the anatomy changes, developing abnormalities of both the proximal femur and the acetabulum such that, after the age of 18 months, one or both bones may need surgical correction to provide joint congruity and stability.

Treatment outcomes are difficult to interpret in the absence of a randomised control group, but most observational studies, despite their methodological weaknesses, have

---

SOURCES AND SELECTION CRITERIA

We searched Medline and the Cochrane Library using MeSH terms "DDH", "CDH", "hip dislocation", and "developmental dysplasia of the hip". We included systematic reviews, randomised controlled trials, and good quality prospective observational studies mainly from the past 15 years but did not exclude seminal papers from before this time.

SUMMARY POINTS

- Developmental dysplasia of the hip affects 1-3% of all newborns; it ranges from mild acetabular dysplasia with a stable hip to a frankly dislocated hip with a dysmorphic femoral head and acetabulum

- Delayed diagnosis requires more complex treatment and has a less successful outcome than dysplasia diagnosed early

- Limited hip abduction (<60°) in 90° of hip flexion may be the most sensitive sign for detecting a dislocated hip in neonates; the Barlow and Ortolani tests can be difficult to elicit and must be performed properly

- Ultrasound, assessing both morphology and stability, helps diagnosis in children under 4.5 months; after this, pelvic radiographs are more useful

- Controversy still exists regarding the role of clinical versus ultrasound screening for developmental dysplasia of the hip in the newborn and whether ultrasound screening should be selective (high risk) or universal

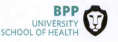

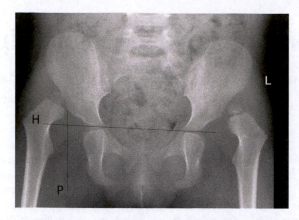

Fig 1 Anteroposterior pelvic radiograph of a 2 year old who presented late with bilateral hip dislocations despite maternal concerns expressed from the first week of life. Hilgenriener's line (H) is drawn through both tri-radiate cartilages; Perkins' line (P) is perpendicular to this and drawn through the most superolateral point of the ossified acetabulum. The ossific nucleus of the femoral head (when present) should be in the inferomedial quadrant formed by the intersection of these two lines; in the dysplastic or dislocated hip the ossific nucleus lies in the superolateral quadrant

shown that early treatment of those most severely affected is important for a good outcome. There is no clear definition of a late diagnosis: we define diagnosis after 6-8 weeks as late since the success rate of simple, conservative treatment falls significantly after age 7 weeks.[8] [9]

How is the diagnosis made?

History

Risk factors are shown in box 2. The prevalence is higher in firstborn children and in girls, but these risk factors are

---

BOX 2 HISTORY AND EXAMINATION FOR DEVELOPMENTAL DYSPLASIA OF THE HIP

History of risk factors

Major
- Positive family history (1 or more first degree relatives or 2 or more second degree relatives)
- Breech presentation
- Birthweight >5 kg
- Congenital calcaneovalgus foot deformity (not "club foot" or equinovarus foot)

Minor
- Oligohydramnios
- Prematurity
- Intrauterine moulding and postnatal positioning or swaddling

Examination

General:
- To exclude a neuromuscular or syndromic problem

Specific:
- Galeazzi test
- Barlow or Ortolani test
- Hip abduction in >90° flexion

Investigation
- <4.5 months—Ultrasound scan for child with clinical hip instability and the high risk child with or without instability
- >4.5 months—Antero-posterior pelvic radiograph (well positioned)

---

not used in screening programmes. Only 15-25% of infants with hip dysplasia are breech births or have a family history of dysplasia, and only 1 in 75 infants with a risk factor has

a dislocated hip.[10] Thus a good clinical examination must supplement a thorough clinical history.

Clinical examination

The 1986 guidelines of the Standing Medical Advisory Committee (SMAC) state that all babies should be screened clinically for congenital hip dislocation within 24 hours of birth; before hospital discharge; at 6 weeks; between 6-9 months; and at walking age.[11] These guidelines were written before the change in nomenclature from congenital to developmental dysplasia and before ultrasound screening was available.

Early period

The Ortolani and Barlow tests, performed as part of the examination at birth and at 6 weeks, are used to detect hip instability. Signs can be difficult to elicit: the baby must be relaxed and lying without its nappy. The Ortolani test aims to relocate a dislocated femoral head; the Barlow test attempts to dislocate an articulated femoral head (fig 2). Both tests will detect an unstable hip, but they will not detect a dislocated, irreducible hip (it is best detected by identifying limited abduction of the flexed hip) or a stable hip with abnormal anatomy, such as acetabular dysplasia (which is best detected by ultrasound examination). Benign "hip clicks" resulting from soft tissues snapping over bony prominences during hip movement should be distinguished from the "clunks" produced during the Ortolani manoeuvre as the dislocated femoral head is reduced and from the subluxation felt during the Barlow test. These tests are useful in neonates (table 1), but they become difficult by 2-3 months of age owing to the development of muscle tone and soft tissue contractures.

Late diagnosis

Limited hip abduction when the hip is flexed to 90° is the single most important sign of a dislocated or dysplastic hip. Most relaxed infants can abduct the flexed hip fully (the examiner's hand, holding the thigh, can touch the examination couch). Asymmetrical movement should alert the examiner to a potential problem, and limited abduction is a useful sign in cases of bilateral hip dysplasia, where asymmetry is absent.

The Galleazzi test identifies a "short" thigh (fig 3). The child is supine with hips and knees flexed to 90° and the height of each knee is compared. Unilateral femoral shortening may signify hip dislocation or rarer abnormalities of the femur. False negative results may occur when bilateral hip dysplasia is present or when the pelvis is not level as when the nappy is left on, for example.

Additional signs, such as a discrepancy in leg length, a widened perineum on the affected side, buttock flattening, and asymmetrical thigh skin folds, may be present. None of these signs is particularly sensitive or specific. Asymmetric skin folds are found in 25% of normal babies: on its own this is not an important clinical finding.[W12]

Making a clinical diagnosis of hip dysplasia in older children is often easier. All subluxed, dysplastic hips will show limited abduction when fully flexed (>90°) (fig 4). The child may walk on its toes on the affected side or may present with a painless limp from weak hip abductor muscles secondary to the unstable hip and unequal leg lengths. Despite this, a delay in walking age is not common.[13]

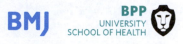

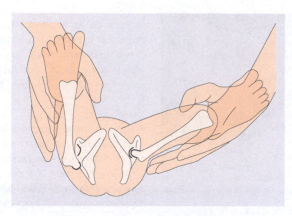

Fig 2 Barlow test (left) and Ortolani test (right). In the Barlow test (baby's right hip), the hip is adducted and flexed to 90°; the examiner holds the distal thigh and pushes posteriorly on the hip joint. The test is positive when the femoral head is felt to slide posteriorly as it dislocates. In the Ortolani test (baby's left hip), the pelvis is stabilised by the examiner and each hip examined separately. In a baby with limited hip abduction in flexion, the hip is flexed to 90° and gently abducted while the examiner's finger lifts the greater trochanter. In a positive test the femoral head is felt to relocate into the acetabulum. The dislocated femoral head (pictured on the opposite hip) has now been reduced back into joint[12]

Imaging

Ultrasonography

Ultrasound scans of the hip are useful from birth until the age of 4-5 months, while the hips are cartilaginous. The Graf technique is based on a standardised coronal section through the mid-acetabulum and assesses hip morphology (static examination). It does not include assessment of stability (dynamic assessment), but a coexisting instability will influence the grading of pathology (fig 5).[14] Modifications allowing hip shape and hip stability to be assessed separately are now commonly used (table 2, fig 6).[15]

Morphologically normal hips have a marginal risk of developing dysplasia in later childhood.[1 16 w13] Immature hips, although dislocatable, develop normally without treatment in 97% of cases.[w14 w15] Reports on the natural course of mild dysplasia are sparse, but two prospective studies suggest that such hips tend to normalise spontaneously.[17 w16]

A second measure of acetabular shape or depth is the percentage of the femoral head covered by the bony rim of the acetabulum (fig 5).[w17 w18] With a centred femoral head, coverage <47% in boys and <44% in girls is pathological, affecting 1-6% of newborns.[1 16 18] When the hip is both unstable and dysplastic, the coverage varies and measurement can be misleading.

It is important to remember that the clinical picture and the ultrasound report should agree—if they don't, presume one is wrong. Ultrasonography and clinical examinations are both operator and situation dependent.

Radiography

In babies older than 4.5 months, as bone develops, anteroposterior pelvic radiographs show hip dysplasia as a delay in acetabular ossification or as dysplasia with or without a subluxed or dislocated femoral head (fig 1, fig 7). As in ultrasonography, a standardised position for the radiograph is crucial for an accurate diagnosis. The acetabular index measures the "shallowness" of the acetabulum: hips with values >2SD[w19] are termed dysplastic and those between 1 and 2 SD indicate delay in acetabular ossification.

Once detected, how is a dysplastic or unstable hip treated?

Abnormal results must be identified and acted on promptly (fig 8), as the window of opportunity for instigating effective treatment of neonatal hip instability is small. In accordance with SMAC guidelines and the National Screening Committee's 2004 report on hip dysplasia,[11 19] and www.library.nhs.uk/specialistlibrarysearch] clinicians need to take responsibility for their assessments and audit the results of their local screening programmes.

Early diagnosis

The primary aim of treatment is to achieve a stable, concentric reduction of the hip to enable normal joint development. Most unstable hips stabilise spontaneously by 2-6 weeks of age. Hips that remain dislocatable or pathologically unstable after this time, most of which also show dysplasia on ultrasound, need prompt treatment. A dynamic flexion-abduction orthosis known as the Pavlik harness, or "splinting," is used to obtain and maintain hip reduction (fig 9).

The harness remains in place at all times, allowing loose capsular soft tissues of the hip to tighten and tight hip adductor muscles to stretch. The harness may be adjusted as the child grows and the hip stabilises. The child is followed up clinically and with ultrasound scans (radiographs after age 4.5 months), the frequency of which will vary with the pathology being treated, until the hip is clinically stable and ultrasonography shows a stable, centred, and normal or only slightly immature hip (Graf type 1 or 2a+). A longitudinal study showed that when harness treatment was started by 90 days of age, only 5.7% of 332 babies required further treatment.[20]

Table 1   Developmental hip dysplasia in neonates

Type of pathology	Clinical finding	Ultrasound finding; morphology and stability (assessed separately)	Treatment
Dislocated irreducible hip	Ortolani negative, limited hip abduction in flexion <60° at birth	Severe dysplasia; dislocated, irreducible	Trial of harness treatment if considered appropriate by the orthopaedic surgeon
Dislocated reducible hip	Ortolani positive	Severe dysplasia; dislocated, reducible	Start harness treatment by 6-8 weeks
Dislocatable hip	Barlow positive	Normal, immature, or dysplastic (of varying severity); dislocatable.	Start harness treatment by 6-8 weeks
Hip subluxation	Barlow negative*	Normal, immature or dysplastic; unstable	Start harness treatment at 6-8 weeks if still unstable
Stable acetabular dysplasia	Barlow negative	Mild dysplasia, stable (50° >α-angle ≥43°)	No treatment required; follow up until anatomically normal

*Some movement of the femoral head may be felt but this head does not dislocate.

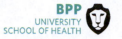

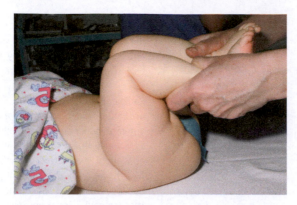

Fig 3 Galeazzi test: the child's hips and knees are flexed to 90° and the relative heights of the knees noted. In this example, viewed from the patient's right side, the right knee is "lower" and represents an apparent shortening of the right thigh because of a dislocated hip. (Child is under general anaesthesia before operative reduction of her hip)

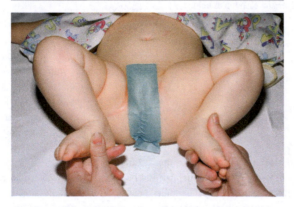

Fig 4 Late presenting dysplasia of the right hip: asymmetry in abduction of the flexed hip (the right hip has reduced abduction in flexion); the right thigh seems short; thigh skin creases are asymmetrical. (The child was under general anaesthetic, so we could show limited abduction without hands obscuring the picture. Hands should be positioned as in fig 2 for this test)

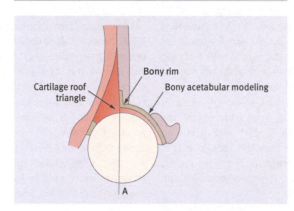

Fig 5 Graf's technique for hip ultrasonography. The diagrams are usually presented in this orientation, but the ultrasound is commonly presented with a 90° change in orientation, as in fig 6. Line A is a continuation of the sonographic iliac wing and helps to define the percentage of the femoral head that is covered by (or contained within) the bony acetabulum, as described by Morin and modified by Terjesen[w17] [w18]

A Pavlik harness is contraindicated with teratological hip dislocation, in children older than 4.5-6 months, when the hip is irreducible (Ortolani negative), and in cases of parental non-compliance. The main risk of splinting is that pressure on the immature, dislocated femoral head may

cause avascular necrosis (reported in up to 2% of those treated) or occasionally a temporary femoral nerve palsy.[5] [9]

Two small randomised trials have shown that stable hips with mild dysplasia on ultrasonography can be observed safely for six weeks before a decision to treat is made.[17] [21]

Late diagnosis
Harness or splint treatment is much less successful if it is started after the age of 6-8 weeks.[8] [9] Firmer abduction braces may be more successful when the major problem is instability, but there is a risk of damaging the vulnerable, developing femoral head, particularly in cases of fixed dislocation. Abduction braces should be used with care.

When is surgery indicated?
Children who require surgery arise from two groups: those who fail early splint or harness treatment, and those who are diagnosed late and are not suitable for such treatment. The most common operation is closed reduction with adductor or psoas tenotomy, followed by 3-4 months in a plaster cast or abduction brace. The older the child, the more likely it is that an extensive procedure will be required: open reduction with soft tissue stabilisation of the joint, followed by a cast. Over the age of 18-24 months, an additional pelvic or femoral osteotomy (or both) is often required to create a more normal anatomical shape and orientation of the hip joint (fig 10).

What is the long term outlook?
Premature degenerative joint disease[3] and low back pain are potential long term sequelae of hip dysplasia, depending on type and duration of the untreated instability, treatment, age at which it was instigated, and the presence of avascular necrosis. Untreated dislocated hips may fare better than treated dislocated or dysplastic hips. Cases must be assessed individually; a unilateral hip dislocation is probably more amenable to surgery than a bilateral dislocation. Most surgeons are reluctant to treat bilateral dislocations after the age of 6-8 years because of the limited remodelling potential as children get older.

Screening
A successful screening programme is defined by several criteria, and international debate continues as to whether hip screening fulfils them. The main aim of screening is to reduce the prevalence of late diagnosis as early detection allows early treatment, reducing the need for surgical treatment and the risk of residual dysplasia.

One controversy is whether screening should be by clinical examination alone or with selective or universal ultrasound assessment. In the United Kingdom, clinical screening with the Ortolani and Barlow tests has failed to reduce the prevalence of late diagnosed developmental hip dysplasia.[22w20] Both clinical tests have a high specificity, but low sensitivity, especially with non-trained examiners.[23] [24w21-w23].

Only two randomised controlled trials have addressed the effect of neonatal ultrasound screening on presentation of hip dysplasia: both compared universal to selective (high risk) screening, and one included a clinically screened control group.[16] [25] Trained examiners performed both the clinical screening and the ultrasound examinations. Although there were more late cases in the selective screening groups than in the universally screened groups, this was not statistically significant (p=0.22).[16] Had non-trained examiners performed

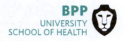

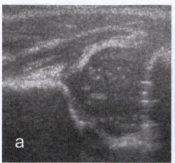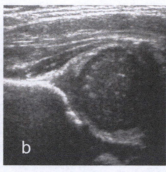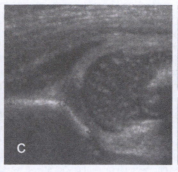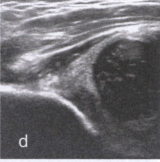

Fig 6 Ultrasound scans performed using a modified (Rosendahl) Graf's technique, based on the coronal standard section and measurements of the α-angle, with the femoral head centred in the acetabulum. The α-angle is a measure of acetabular depth: (a) normal, α.60°; (b) immature, 50°,α<60°; (c) mild dysplasia 43°,α<50°; (d) significant dysplasia (with or without changes of the labrum), α<43°. This technique also includes a separate assessment of hip stability

Table 2 Relation of hip morphology to stability as assessed on ultrasound[23]

Morphological diagnosis	% of cases	Functional diagnosis	% in group
Normal	84.3%	Dislocatable	0.1%
Immature	13.3%	Dislocatable	0.6%
Mild dysplasia	2.4%	Dislocatable	62%
Severe dysplasia	0.7%	Dislocatable *or* dislocated	100%

the clinical screening, the results may have been different. The advantage offered by ultrasound screening becomes evident only in comparison to clinical screening by non-trained examiners.[16] [w24]

In countries where universal ultrasound screening is practised, initial treatment rates (and costs) have been high initially but, with experience, both have fallen.[26] [w25] [w26] Late diagnosis of dysplasia has become less common, and few children require surgical reduction.[27] One German study showed an ascertainment adjusted rate of first operative procedures of 0.26 per 1000 live births (95% CI 0.22 to −0.32) after universal ultrasound screening, compared with a UK equivalent estimate of 0.78 (0.72 to 0.84) after clinical screening.[4] [28]

In the UK and parts of Europe, selective ultrasound screening has become common practice, despite the uncertain evidence base for screening for hip dysplasia, including effectiveness of treatment, as highlighted in two systematic reviews.[5] [29] The US Preventive Services Task Force did not recommend universal ultrasound screening in North America and acknowledged that even when newborn and infant hip examinations are normal, a late presentation occurs in 1 in 5000 infants.[30] In Coventry, three years after the instigation of a universal ultrasound screening programme, there had been no late presentations of hip dysplasia.[1] [26]

Where are we now?

As early harness or splint treatment avoids operative treatment in some cases, early diagnosis is important. Many studies emphasise that if the neonatal clinical examinations are performed by experienced practitioners, be they physicians, surgeons, or physiotherapists, then the late diagnosis rate is low, and in this context universal ultrasound screening may add little more in terms of clinical efficacy than selective ultrasound screening.[23] [24] [31] [w22] [w27] Late diagnosed hip dysplasia is still common in the UK.[w28] This may be related to variable quality or completeness of clinical screening, which is often performed by junior and inexperienced clinicians, or to the selective use of ultrasound screening. Although no system at national level has been shown to eliminate late presenting developmental dysplasia of the hip, improved outcomes have resulted

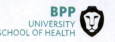

A PATIENT'S STORY

The baby was born at term by head first vaginal delivery after an uncomplicated pregnancy. Her mother had had a delayed diagnosis of hip dysplasia as a child and was consequently having residual problems with her hips. Clinical screening was normal but the GP sent the baby for an ultrasound scan on account of the family history. Ascan at 6 weeks showed bilateral hip dysplasia (Graf 2C in the right hip and 2A in the left). The baby was placed in a Pavlik harness at 8 weeks of age.

The mother was concerned that the baby might develop chronic hip problems. "I received very little information about the Pavlik harness at first. I didn't understand why it had to be on all the time. It looked so restrictive, especially when other babies were kicking and having fun. It got dirty when I changed nappies, and getting clothes to fit was a real problem. I kept wanting to take it off but knew I wasn't meant to." It was only when a follow-up scan after 6 weeks showed normal hips (Graf 1) that the mother began to feel confidence with the harness: "It was a huge relief. I could now see it had helped."The baby remained in the Pavlik harness for a further six weeks and went on to develop normal hips.

from conscientiously applied screening programmes implemented in different regions.[23 24 27 31 W25 W27]

Contributors: MDS wrote the first draft. DME was involved throughout with the review and finalised the manuscript. KR provided figures and contributed to the intellectual content. DME is guarantor.

Competing interests: None declared.

Provenance and peer review: Not commissioned; externally peer reviewed.

Patient consent obtained.

1   Marks DS, Clegg J, Al-Chalabi AN. Routine ultrasound screening for neonatal hip instability. Can it abolish late-presenting congenital dislocation of the hip. *J Bone Joint Surg Br*1994;76-B:534-8.
2   Leck I. Congenital dislocation of the hip. In: Wald N, Leck I, eds. *Antenatal and neonatal screening*. 2nd ed. Oxford: Oxford University Press, 2000:398-424.
3   Furnes O, Lie SA, Espehaug B, Vollset SE, Engesaeter LB, Havelin LI. Hip disease and the prognosis of total hip replacements. A review of 53,698 primary total hip replacements reported to the Norwegian arthroplasty register 1987-99. *J Bone Joint Surg Br*2001;83:579-86.
4   Von Kries R, Ihme N, Oberle D, Lorani A, Stark R, Altenhofen L, et al. Effect of ultrasound screening on the rate of first operative procedure for developmental hip dysplasia in Germany. *Lancet*2003;362:1883-7.
5   Shipman SA, Helfand M, Moyer VA, Yawn BP. Screening for developmental dysplasia of the hip: a systematic literature review for the US Preventive Services Task Force. *Pediatrics* 2006;117:557-76.
6   Wilkinson JA. Etiological factors in congenital displacement of the hip myelodysplasia. *Clin Orthop*1992;281:75-83.
7   Chan A, McCaul KA, Cundy PJ, Haan EA, Byron Scott R. Perinatal risk factors for developmental dysplasia of the hip. *Arch Dis Child*1997;76:94-100.
8   Atalar H, Sayli U, Yavuz OY, Uras I, Dogruel H. Indicators of successful use of the Pavlik harness in infants with developmental dysplasia of the hip. *Int Orthop* 2007;31:145-50.
9   Viere RG, Birch JG, Herring JA, Roach JW, Johnston CE. Use of the Pavlik harness in congenital dislocation of the hip. An analysis of failures of treatment. *J Bone Joint Surg Am*1990;72:238-44.
10 Lewis K, Jones DA, Powell N. Ultrasound and neonatal hip screening: the five-year results of a prospective study in high risk babies. *J Paediatr Orthop* 1999;19:760-2.
11 SMAC guidelines. Special report. Screening for the detection of congenital dislocation of the hip. *Arch Dis Child*1986;61:921-6.
12 Donnan L, Angliss L. *Developmental dysplasia of the hip* [DVD]. Melbourne: Royal Children's Hospital, 2008.
13 Kamath SU, Bennet GC. Does developmental dysplasia of the hip cause a delay in walking? *J Paediatr Orthop*2004;24:265.
14 Graf R. The diagnosis of congenital hip-joint dislocation by the ultrasonic Combound treatment. *Arch Orthop Trauma Surg*1980;97:117-33.
15 Rosendahl K, Markestad T, Lie RT. Developmental dysplasia of the hip. A population-based comparison of ultrasound and clinical findings. *Acta Pediatr* 1996;85:64-9.
16 Holen KH, Tegnander A, Bredland T, Johansen OJ, Saether OD, Eik-Nes SH et al. Universal or selective screening of the neonatal hip using ultrasound? *J Bone Joint Surg Br* 2002;84-B:886-90.
17 Wood MK, Conboy V, Benson MK. Does early treatment by abduction splintage improve the development of dysplastic but stable neonatal hips? *J Paediatr Orthop* 2000;20:302-5.
18 Holen KJ, Tegnander A, Eik-Nes SH, Terjesen T. The use of ultrasound in determining the initiation of treatment in instability of the hip in neonates. *J Bone Joint Surg Br*1999;81:846-51.
19 National Screening Committee. Child Health Sub-Group report: dysplasia of the hip. September 2004. www.library.nhs.uk/CHILDHEALTH/ViewResource.aspx?resID=6102 1&tabID=289.
20 Cashman JP, Round J, Taylor G, Clarke NM. The natural history of developmental dysplasia of the hip after early supervised treatment in the Pavlik harness. A prospective, longitudinal follow-up. *J Bone Joint Surg Br*2002;84:418-25.
21 Rosendahl K, Dezateux C, Fosse K, Aukland SM, Aase H, Reigstad H, et al. Congenital dysplasia of the hip in newborns. A randomised, controlled trial on the effect of abduction treatment. *Paediatrics*2009 (in press).
22 Boere-Boonekamp MM, Kerkhoff TMH, Schuil PB, Zielhuis GA. Early detection of developmental dysplasia of the hip in the Netherlands: the validity of a standardised assessment protocol in infants. *Am J Public Health*1998;88;285-8.
23 Macnicol MF. Results of a 25-year screening programme for neonatal hip instability. *J Bone Joint Surg Br* 1990;72:1057-60.
24 Krikler SJ, Dwyer NS. Comparison of results of two approaches to hip screening in infants. *J Bone Joint Surg Br* 1992;74:701-3.
25 Rosendahl K, Markestad T, Lie RT. Ultrasound screening for developmental dysplasia of the hip in the neonate: the effect on treatment rate and prevalence of late cases. *Pediatrics* 1994;94:47-52.
26 Clegg J, Bache CE, Raut VV. Financial justification for routine ultrasound screening of the neonatal hip. *J Bone Joint Surg Br* 1999;8:852-7.
27 Ihme N, Altenhofen L, von Kries R, Niethard FU. Hip ultrasound screening in Germany. Results and comparison with other screening procedures. *Orthopade*2008;37:541-6, 548-9.
28 Godward S, Dezateux C. Surgery for congenital dislocation of the hip in the UK as a measure of outcome of screening. *Lancet* 1998;351:1149-52.
29 Woolacott N, Puhan MA, Misso K, Steurer J, Kleijnen J. *Systematic review of clinical and cost effectiveness of ultrasound in screening for developmental dysplasia of the hip in newborns.* York: Centre for reviews and dissemination, University of York, 2005.
30 Schwend RM, Schoenecker P, Richards BS, Flynn JM, Vitale M. Screening the newborn for developmental dysplasia of the hip. Now what do we do? *J Paediatr Orthop* 2007;27:607-10.
31 Tredwell SJ, Bell HM. Efficacy of neonatal hip examination. *J Pediatr Orthop*1981;1:61-5.

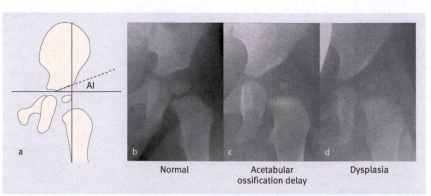

a   AI

b   Normal

c   Acetabular ossification delay

d   Dysplasia

Fig 7 Anteroposterior pelvic radiographs in 6 month old children. (a) The acetabular index (AI) is a measure of the acetabular inclination and dysplasia; (b) normal hip with large ossified femoral head and normal AI; (c) hip with high AI with delayed acetabular ossification (note that the femoral head ossific nucleus is small); (d) hip with dysplasia with greatly abnormal AI and small femoral head ossific nucleus. In both (b) and (c) Shenton's line is disrupted, implying the hip is subluxed

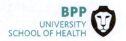

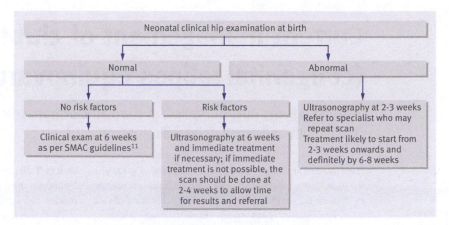

Neonatal clinical hip examination at birth	
Normal	Abnormal

No risk factors	Risk factors	Ultrasonography at 2-3 weeks Refer to specialist who may repeat scan Treatment likely to start from 2-3 weeks onwards and definitely by 6-8 weeks
Clinical exam at 6 weeks as per SMAC guidelines[11]	Ultrasonography at 6 weeks and immediate treatment if necessary; if immediate treatment is not possible, the scan should be done at 2-4 weeks to allow time for results and referral	

Fig 8 Assessing developmental dysplasia of the hip

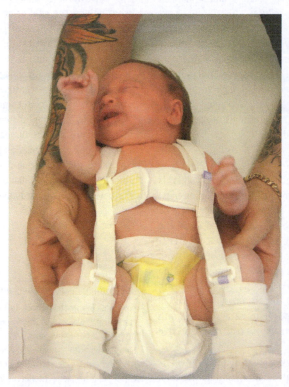

Fig 9 Properly applied Pavlik harness. The hips are in 100° of flexion and considerable abduction. In this position the hip is held reduced, allowing the hip capsule to tighten, which stabilises the hip. The harness is safe, but extreme positions of abduction should be avoided to lessen the risk of femoral head avascular necrosis, which could disturb growth of the proximal femur

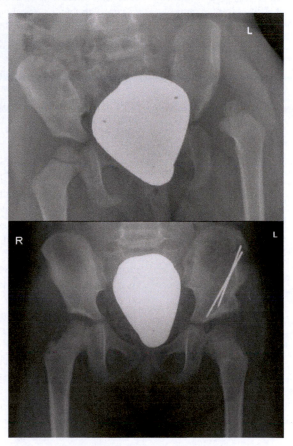

Fig 10 (top) Preoperative anteroposterior pelvic radiograph showing a late presenting (age 2 years) left dislocated hip with considerable acetabular abnormality; (bottom) after open reduction of the joint, the iliac wing of the pelvis was "broken" (a pelvic osteotomy) and the fragments moved into position with better bony coverage of the femoral head. The osteotomy was held with two wires. The improved anatomy helps stabilise a reduced hip joint; movement promotes normal growth

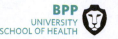

Current management of clubfoot (congenital talipes equinovarus)

Joshua Bridgens post-CCT fellow in paediatric orthopaedic surgery[1], Nigel Kiely consultant paediatric orthopaedic surgeon[1]

[1]Robert Jones and Agnes Hunt Orthopaedic Hospital, Oswestry, Shropshire SY10 7AG

Correspondence to: J Bridgens jpbridgens@doctors.org.uk

Cite this as: BMJ 2010;340:c355

‹DOI› 10.1136/bmj.c355
http://www.bmj.com/content/340/bmj.c355

The standard treatment of clubfoot has changed greatly in the past 10 years. Previously, extensive surgery was common in children born with this condition. The publication of long term evidence of good outcomes with more minimally invasive methods, such as the Ponseti technique, has led surgeons worldwide to change their approach. Ponseti treatment consists of sequential plasters and prolonged bracing, with minor surgical procedures.

This clinical review describes clubfoot and its current management. It is particularly aimed at general readers who are non-specialists but may be involved in the care of patients with this condition. The evidence underpinning this review is largely observational. Although the Ponseti method was first described over 30 years ago, it is only since the publication of long term outcomes of case series that it has been widely adopted.

What is clubfoot and who gets it?

Clubfoot, also known as congenital talipes equinovarus, is a developmental deformity of the foot. It is one of the most common birth deformities with an incidence of 1.2 per 1000 live births each year in the white population.[1] Clubfoot is twice as common in boys and is bilateral in 50% of cases.[1]

It is most often idiopathic but may be associated with other conditions in around 20% of cases. The most common associated conditions are spina bifida (4.4% of children with clubfoot), cerebral palsy (1.9%), and arthrogryposis (0.9%).[2] Although it was previously thought to be associated with developmental dysplasia of the hip a recent prospective study did not support this.[3]

Historical family studies suggest that there is a genetic component but not a recognisable pattern of inheritance. If one child has clubfoot, the risk of clubfoot in a subsequent child is increased 20-fold. The risk to the second of identical twins is one in three.[1] If one parent has clubfoot the risk of having affected offspring is 3-4%, but if both parents are affected the risk is 30%.[4]

How is it diagnosed?

Clubfoot is most commonly diagnosed postnatally during the routine baby check. The foot assumes the position shown in fig 1. The foot points downwards at the ankle (equinus) the heel is turned in (varus), the midfoot is deviated towards the midline (adductus), and the first metatarsal points downwards (plantar flexion). Deep creases may be present behind the heel or on the medial side of the foot. The deformity is not passively correctable by the examiner. The foot and calf muscles are smaller than the unaffected side in unilateral clubfoot. The diagnosis is clinical and is normally straightforward. Imaging, such as radiography, is not needed. It may be confused with other congenital foot deformities that are more common (box 1).

Two grading systems are commonly used for clubfoot—the Pirani score and the Dimeglio grade. The Pirani score is outlined in box 2. A correlation has been shown between the Pirani score and subsequent need for Achilles tenotomy.[5] Clubfoot is increasingly diagnosed on prenatal scans and these have a positive predictive value of around 85%.[6]

SOURCES AND SELECTION CRITERIA

No Cochrane reviews or other systematic reviews are available on the treatment of clubfoot. We searched PubMed for English language peer reviewed articles on clubfoot using search terms that included "clubfoot", "Ponseti", "surgical release clubfoot", and "external fixator clubfoot". We also used standard texts on the management of clubfoot.

BOX 1 OTHER COMMON CONGENITAL FOOT DEFORMITIES

Positional clubfoot: the foot assumes the same position as in congenital clubfoot but the deformity is correctable. This is probably a normal variant.

Metatarsus adductus: medial deviation of the forefoot on the hindfoot creates an adduction deformity. This may be correctable or fixed. The heel is in a neutral position (unlike clubfoot) and there is no equinus. This is more common than clubfoot, although its exact incidence is difficult to determine. Most cases will improve spontaneously, but more severe cases may require serial casting.

Positional calcaneovalgus: dorsiflexion of the whole foot to the extent that it may touch the tibia. This dramatic deformity is unlikely to be confused with clubfoot, but the appearance is concerning and it is important to rule out more serious conditions such as congenital vertical talus. Calcaneovalgus improves spontaneously with time.

Both metatarsus adductus and calcaneovalgus are associated with developmental dysplasia of the hip and if diagnosed should lead to referral for assessment of the hips

---

SUMMARY POINTS

- Clubfoot is a common congenital deformity that affects one in 1000 live births in the United Kingdom
- Most cases are idiopathic and not associated with other conditions
- Babies should be referred early for treatment
- Current best treatment is by casting and bracing according to the Ponseti method
- Results are better with manipulative methods than with surgical release
- Recurrences can occur and are normally caused by non-compliance with bracing

---

BOX 2 GRADING OF CLUBFOOT: THE PIRANI SCORE

In this system, six clinical features of the deformity are graded 0, 0.5, or 1. The six scores are summed giving a total score of 0-6—the higher the score the worse the deformity. The features scored are:

- Hindfoot: heel crease, equinus, and softness of the heel
- Forefoot: lateral border shape, medial border creases, and cover of head of talus

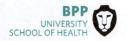

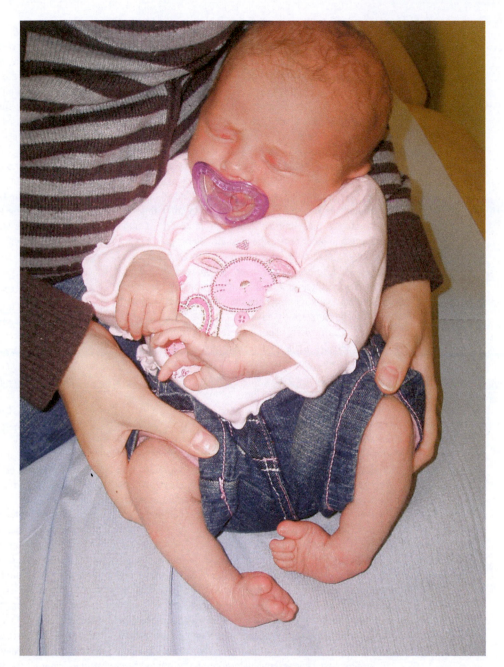

Fig 1 Infant with bilateral clubfoot

Why do I need to know about clubfoot?

If diagnosis and referral to an orthopaedic surgeon do not occur prenatally or in the first few days after birth, the baby must be referred urgently when the deformity is first noticed. This is because the earlier Ponseti treatment is started (ideally around one to two weeks), the easier correction will be.

It is important for non-specialists to have an understanding of the standard treatment because success is largely related to the parents' compliance with the bracing protocol. This is prolonged and can be demanding. Support and encouragement from healthcare professionals can be helpful. It is important for parents to receive a clear message that the long term use of the brace is essential.

What was the standard treatment previously?

Although manipulation and casting were used in the past, this was not performed according to a formal protocol, and extensive surgery was often used. The aim of surgery was to correct the deformity by lengthening or dividing all structures that were tight. Few long term studies on the outcome of surgery are available, and most evidence comes from case series. One case series published in 2006 looked at 73 feet in 45 patients with a minimum follow-up of 25 years. This was a thorough review with the patients completing three independent quality of life questionnaires, including the Laaveg and Ponseti functional score, which is commonly used in clubfoot outcome studies.[7] On this measure, 34 feet (47%) had a poor outcome and most had more than one operation.[8] In a case series looking at staged surgical release, 99 feet in 71 patients with severe clubfoot were studied. The average follow-up was 11.5 years and the relapse rate was 76%.[9] Gait analysis has been used by some investigators to try to quantify the results of treatment. A case-control study using this technique compared the outcomes of surgical and non-surgical treatment. This showed that surgery led to a greater proportion of gait abnormalities.[10]

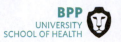

What is the current preferred treatment?

The current preferred treatment for clubfoot is the Ponseti method. This is a detailed method of manipulation and casting without major surgical releases, and it is the treatment of choice of most orthopaedic surgeons worldwide. A review of patients treated by Ponseti published in 1995 showed good long term results.[11] In this study, 45 patients with 71 clubfeet were reviewed after an average of 30 years. Using pain and functional limitation as the outcome criteria, 35 of 45 patients (78%) had an excellent or good outcome compared with 82 of 97 (85%) of age matched patients without foot pathology. Although Ponseti originally published his method in 1963, it was only after this long term review that interest began to increase.[12] Studies performed in other centres have confirmed his good results, although with shorter term follow-up.[13 14 15] Acceptance by orthopaedic surgeons has been encouraged by parents who use the internet to seek out surgeons who use this technique.[16] Parents prefer the more non-surgical approach and can become strong advocates for the technique. This method is particularly useful in developing countries where surgical services are limited. A descriptive study of its use in Malawi showed that it could be successfully carried out by suitably trained non-doctor personnel with similar results to those seen in other studies.[17]

What is the Ponseti method?

Treatment starts as soon after birth as possible. Ponseti defined a precise sequence of manipulations of the clubfoot that lead to correction of the deformity. Exact details of the technique are available free on the internet.[4] Ponseti stressed that the cavus should be corrected by raising the first metatarsal, which initially makes the deformity look "worse," and that correction should occur around the head of the talus without the heel being touched. At weekly intervals the foot is manipulated into the maximum position of correction and then held in a plaster of Paris cast. Several studies have shown that this manipulation and casting can be carried out by doctors and other trained staff.[17 18]

During the time in cast the immature collagen undergoes stress relaxation (stretches); this then allows greater correction at the next manipulation. After about six weeks of weekly cast changes the deformity of the midfoot and forefoot is generally corrected. The foot is often still in the equinus position at this stage (pointing down at the ankle), and in most cases this will not correct further with manipulation. Therefore, around 85% of children have an Achilles tenotomy carried out at this stage. This can be done under local anaesthetic in clinic or under general anaesthesia. The child then goes into a final cast for three weeks.

On removal of this final cast the foot position is reviewed. If correction is complete the child then goes into "boots and bar." This is an orthotic device that holds the feet in an abducted, externally rotated, and dorsiflexed position about a shoulder width apart (fig 2). In a unilateral case the affected side is externally rotated 60-70° and the unaffected side is rotated 30-40°. The child wears this device all the time for three months and then at night time and during naps until 4 years of age. If treatment is successful the child will be left with a supple well corrected foot. It should look similar to the unaffected foot but may be slightly smaller (around one shoe size). The calf may also be smaller than on the unaffected side.

Can clubfoot recur?

Yes, recurrence occurs in around 15% of patients and can be at any stage in the treatment process. It occurs most commonly during the time in the boots and bar device, as a result of poor compliance.[19] At initial signs of recurrence it is important to ensure compliance with the boots and bar. Simple measures and advice may increase compliance and lead to correction of recurrence (box 3). If these measures are not successful, recurrences can be treated with a further period of manipulation and casting. If the recurrent deformity is dynamic supination of the forefoot this can be corrected by a tibialis anterior tendon transfer. This is described by Ponseti and is the only other surgical procedure that is a standard part of the Ponseti method.[4] It is carried out far less often than Achilles tenotomy (around 15% of cases).

BOX 3 IMPROVING COMPLIANCE WITH BRACING

- Parents need to understand why bracing is important and why it must continue for such a long time. Parents should be encouraged to accept responsibility for this phase of the treatment
- For older children, wearing the brace at night must be part of their normal routine. It should not be stopped for reasons such as illness
- Baby sleeping bags may help the boots stay on
- Socks with non-slip areas on the soles may also help the boots stay on
- The boots must fit well and be comfortable, and the bar width should be correct. If concerns exist, the parents should be directed back to the brace provider

---

Are outcomes better with current treatment?

No randomised trials have compared the Ponseti method and surgical management of clubfoot. Long term studies of the Ponseti treatment suggest that the results are much better than with surgical treatment, however.[8 9 10 11 13 14 15 20] In the 30 year review of Ponseti's patients, 35 of 45 (78%) had an excellent or good outcome using the Laaveg-Ponseti functional score. This compares with 24 of 73 feet (33%) in the previously discussed case series, which had a similar follow-up of surgically treated patients.[8] It is unusual to find studies where case series from the same authors can be compared, but in one such paper, with long term follow up, 20 of 47 feet (43%) treated surgically had an excellent or good result compared with 38 of 49 (78%) treated by the Ponseti method.[20]

Can the Ponseti method be used for non-idiopathic clubfoot?

Yes, although syndromic clubfoot is more difficult to treat, may need more plasters, and may not correct fully with Ponseti treatment. However, this treatment will improve the position and make subsequent surgery easier; it also reduced the need for major surgery. The Ponseti method can also be used for late presenting clubfoot.[21]

What risks do less invasive techniques carry?

The Ponseti technique uses serial casts and it is important that these are properly applied to reduce the risk of pressure damage to skin. There is a small risk of neurovascular injury during the percutaneous tenotomy.[22] If parents do not ensure compliance with bracing, the risk of recurrence is high.

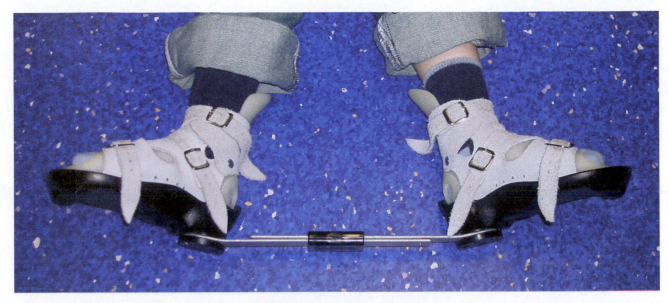

Fig 2 Child wearing the "boots and bar" orthosis

What other forms of treatment are available?

Other specific methods of manipulation have been suggested. One of these is the French method of manipulations (also known as functional or physiotherapy method). This requires daily manipulation of the foot and taping. A non-randomised study in one unit found it to be as effective as the Ponseti method. When given the choice, however, parents were twice as likely to choose the Ponseti method than the French method, probably because of the need for daily attendances with the French method.[23]

Ilizarov frames are external fixators that can be used for gradual correction of deformity. They can be used to stretch soft tissues or to alter the foot shape through osteotomies.

They have been used for recurrences after Ponseti treatment and residual deformity in older patients. Not all studies show good outcomes however.[24]

Surgery still has a part to play in the management of clubfoot. The Ponseti method does not fully correct the defect in a proportion of patients, and these children will need surgery. Patients with syndromic clubfoot are also more likely to need surgery. During surgery, posteromedial structures are released or lengthened to allow the foot position to be corrected. Older patients with residual deformity of the foot may need osteotomies in addition to soft tissue procedures.

QUESTIONS FOR FUTURE RESEARCH

- Which surgical techniques give the best results in feet that do not fully correct after Ponseti treatment?
- How effective is the "reverse Ponseti" technique for congenital vertical talus?
- What surgical technique is the best treatment for the "neglected" clubfoot in older children and adults?

USEFUL RESOURCES FOR NON-SPECIALISTS AND PATIENTS

Resources for healthcare professionals

- Ponseti International Association (www.ponseti.info)—Website of the unit where Dr Ponseti practised. The website promotes the Ponseti method and provides education for healthcare professionals
- Global Help (www.global-help.org)—Clubfoot: Ponseti management. This document contains detailed information on the Ponseti method and practicalities of treating patients with this technique

Resources for parents

- Steps charity (www.steps-charity.org.uk)—A UK charity website that has information on clubfoot as well as other lower limb conditions
- Clubfoot.co.uk (www.clubfoot.co.uk)—Website set up by the parents of a child with clubfoot that contains good basic information and describes their experience
- Ponseti International Association (www.ponseti.info/parents)—Website specifically for parents that is intended to promote the Ponseti method. It has information on the method itself and doctors who offer it

---

A PARENT'S PERSPECTIVE

Erin's clubfeet were first diagnosed when I had my 20 week scan. A week later I had another scan, during which the fetal expert checked for related syndromes and confirmed the diagnosis. My partner and I were asked if we would like to meet an orthopaedic surgeon and discuss the treatment at this stage. This would also give us the opportunity to meet other parents and children with the condition. At about 30 weeks' gestation we met the consultant and other parents at the regular clinic. This was very useful because we then knew what to expect when Erin was born, all of our questions were answered, and the entire procedure was explained. We came away from this very reassured and well informed.

Erin was born full term with moderate bilateral clubfoot. When she was 2 weeks old she was seen by the consultant, who confirmed the diagnosis of clubfoot and started the Ponseti treatment (plasters). She wasn't upset by the application of the plasters, but when we got home the wet plasters seemed to make her feel cold; we overcame this by putting a hot water bottle under her legs. By week three of plastering we noticed a big improvement in her feet. Again, this was very reassuring. As the weeks went by she improved noticeably. Today, at 9 weeks old, Erin has had the bilateral tenotomy, which went well.

On reflection, the only negative aspect was the initial diagnosis at 20 weeks. We think that it could have been handled more sensitively—a lot of emphasis was put on the syndromes that can be associated with clubfoot. We believe that this could have been left until we saw the fetal expert.
Carys Jones, Valley, Anglesey

TIPS FOR NON-SPECIALISTS

- Although patients should be seen as soon after birth as is practical, Ponseti treatment can also be used for late presenting clubfoot
- Recurrence is associated with non-compliance with bracing. Parents must be encouraged to continue using the boots and bar
- Ponseti treatment is successful in around 85% of patients. Parents can be reassured that a good outcome is likely

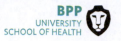

Contributors: JB is the primary author and NK reviewed and amended the article. NK is guarantor

Competing interests: None declared.

Provenance and peer review: Not commissioned; externally peer reviewed.

Parental consent obtained.

1   Wynne-Davis R. Family studies and the causes of congenital clubfoot: talipes equinovarus, talipes calcaneal valgus, and metatarsus varus. *J Bone Joint Surg Br* 1964;46:445-63

2   Chung C, Nemechek R, Larsen I, Ching G. Genetic and epidemiological studies of clubfoot in Hawaii: general and medical considerations. *Hum Hered* 1969;19:321-42

3   Paton RW, Choudry Q. Neonatal foot deformities and their relationship to developmental dysplasia of the hip: an 11-year prospective, longitudinal observational study. *J Bone Joint Surg Br* 2009; 91-B:655-658.

4   Clubfoot: Ponseti management. www.global-help.org.

5   Dyer PJ, Davis N. The role of the Pirani scoring system in the management of club foot by the Ponseti method. *J Bone Joint Surg Br* 2006;88-B:1082-4.

6   Bar-On E, Mashiach R, Inbar O, Weigl D, Katz K, Meizner I. Prenatal ultrasound diagnosis of clubfoot. *J Bone Joint Surg Br* 2005;87:990-3.

7   Laaveg SJ, Ponseti IV. Long-term results of treatment of congenital clubfoot. *J Bone Joint Surg Am* 1980;62:23-31.

8   Dobbs MB, Nunley R, Schoenecker PL. Long term follow up of patients with clubfoot treated with extensive soft tissue releases. *J Bone Joint Surg Am* 2006;88:986-96.

9   Uglow MG, Senbaga N, Pickard R, Clarke NMP. Relapse rates following staged surgery in the treatment of recalcitrant talipes equinovarus: 9- to 16-year outcome study. *J Child Orthop* 2007;1:115-9.

10 Karol LA, O'Brien SE, Wilson H, Johnston CE, Richards BS. Gait analysis in children with severe clubfeet: early results of physiotherapy versus surgical release. *J Pediatr Orthop* 2005;25:236-40.

11 Cooper DM, Deitz FR. Treatment of idiopathic clubfoot: a thirty year follow-up note. *J Bone Joint Surg Am* 1995;77:1477-89.

12 Ponseti IV, Smoley EN. Congenital club foot: the results of treatment. *J Bone Joint Surg Am* 1963;45:261-344.

13 Changulani M, Garg NK, Rajagopal TS, Bass A, Nayagam SN, Sampath J, et al. Treatment of idiopathic clubfoot using the Ponseti method. *J Bone Joint Surg Br* 2006;88:1385-7.

14 Cosma D, Vasilescu D, Vasilescu D, Valeanu M. Comparative results of the conservative treatment in clubfoot by two different protocols. *J Pediatr Orthop B* 2007;16:317-21.

15 Adbelgawad AA, Lehman WB, van Bosse HJ, Scher DM, Sala DA. Treatment of idiopathic clubfoot using the Ponseti method: minimum 2-year follow-up. *J Pediatr Orthop B* 2007;16:98-105.

16 Morcuende JA, Egbert M, Ponseti IV. The effect of the internet in the treatment of congenital idiopathic clubfoot. *Iowa Orthop J* 2003;23:83-6.

17 Tindall AJ, Steinlechner CW, Lavy CB, Mannion S, Mkandawire N. Results of manipulation of idiopathic clubfoot deformity in Malawi by orthopaedic clinical officers using the Ponseti method: a realistic alternative for the developing world? *J Pediatr Orthop* 2005;25:627-9.

18 Janicki JA, Narayanan UG, Harvey BJ, Roy A, Weir S, Wright JG. Comparison of surgeon and physiotherapist-directed Ponseti treatment of idiopathic clubfoot. *J Bone Joint Surg Am* 2009;91:1101-8.

19 Morcuende JA, Dolan LA, Dietz FR, Ponseti IV. Radical reduction in the rate of extensive corrective surgery for clubfoot using the Ponseti method. *Pediatrics* 2004;113:376-80.

20 Ippolito E, Farsetti P, Caterini R, Tudisco C. Long-term comparative results in patients with congenital clubfoot treated with two different protocols. *J Bone Joint Surg Am* 2003;85:1286-94.

21 Lourenço AF, Morcuende JA. Correction of neglected idiopathic clubfoot by the Ponseti method. *J Bone Joint Surg Br* 2007;89:378-81.

22 Dobbs MB, Gordon JE, Walton T, Schoenecker PL. Bleeding complications following percutaneous tendoachilles tenotomy in the treatment of clubfoot deformity. *J Pediatr Orthop* 2004;24:353-7.

23 Richards BS, Faulks S, Rathjen KE, Karol LA, Johnston CE, Jones SA. A comparison of two nonoperative methods of idiopathic clubfoot correction: the Ponseti method and the French functional (physiotherapy) method. *J Bone Joint Surg Am* 2008;90:2313-21.

24 Freedman JA, Watts H, Otsuka NY. The Ilizarov method for the treatment of resistant clubfoot: is it an effective solution? *J Pediatr Orthop* 2006;26:432-7.

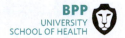

Diagnosis and management of juvenile idiopathic arthritis

Femke H M Prince research fellow (paediatric) rheumatology[12], Marieke H Otten PhD student paediatric rheumatology[1], Lisette W A van Suijlekom-Smit paediatric rheumatologist[1]

[1]Department of Paediatrics/ Paediatric Rheumatology, Erasmus MC Sophia Children's Hospital, Rotterdam, Netherlands

[2]Division of Rheumatology, Immunology and Allergy, Brigham and Women's Hospital, Harvard Medical School, Boston, USA

Correspondence to: F H M Prince
f.prince@erasmusmc.nl

Cite this as: BMJ 2010;341:c6434

<DOI> 10.1136/bmj.c6434
http://www.bmj.com/content/341/
bmj.c6434

Juvenile idiopathic arthritis is the most common cause of chronic arthritis in childhood; a review of 34 epidemiological studies showed that 0.07-4.01 per 1000 children worldwide are affected.[w1] It is characterised by joint inflammation that often leads to joint destruction with physical disability and chronic pain that affects daily life.[1] During the past decade, increased understanding of the disease has improved treatment, particularly through earlier diagnosis and new treatments that help to prevent long term damage to joints. Earlier this year, the British Society for Paediatric and Adolescent Rheumatology published standards of care for children and young people with juvenile idiopathic arthritis, which outlined the importance of involving different disciplines within healthcare.[2] We review recent advances in the diagnosis and management of juvenile idiopathic arthritis, focusing on evidence from randomised controlled trials, cohort studies, systematic reviews, and current guidelines.

What is juvenile idiopathic arthritis and who gets it?

Juvenile idiopathic arthritis (formerly juvenile chronic arthritis in Europe and juvenile rheumatoid arthritis in North America) covers a heterogeneous group of conditions more accurately described as subtypes.[w2-w4] The disease encompasses all forms of arthritis that begin before the age of 16 years, persist for more than six weeks, and are of unknown cause.[3] It is thought to be a multifactorial autoimmune disease with environmental and genetic contributory factors.[4] The heterogeneity of the subtypes and changes in terminology and classification make it difficult to interpret studies on the role of the environment.[5] The most common risk factors are infections in combination with genetic susceptibility. Many other factors, such as stress and maternal smoking, are thought to contribute

to the pathogenesis. Juvenile idiopathic arthritis is a complex genetic disease with multiple genes involved. Individual cohort studies have confirmed and replicated several associations between juvenile idiopathic arthritis and variants in the histocompatibility (HLA) genes but the strength of the associations differ for each disease subtype.[w5] A large number of non-HLA candidate genes have been tested for associations, but only a few such as protein tyrosine phosphatase (PTPN22) and macrophage inhibitory factor (MIF) have been confirmed. A multiethnic Canadian cohort study showed a moderately increased risk for European origin compared with African, Asian, or Indian origin, and that subtypes differ significantly between ethnic groups (table 1).[6] The typical age of onset also depends on subtype.[w6] Table 1 lists the subtypes according to the currently accepted classification. Increased knowledge about the disease will probably refine the classification further. This might provide homogeneous subgroups for research and lead to tailored disease management.

How is the diagnosis made?
No conclusive laboratory tests are available for the diagnosis of juvenile idiopathic arthritis, so a good history and physical examination are important.[7] The diagnosis is made by excluding joint problems with a discernable cause. Box 1 lists causes of joint pain in children.

History
After queries about joint pain and swelling (including previous episodes), ask patients and parents about morning stiffness that lasts for more than 15 minutes but improves during the day.[7 9] Parents, other family members, or teachers may have noticed problems with, for example, walking, running, climbing stairs, standing up, writing, or sleeping. The child might need help with daily activities that were previously performed independently. Also ask about autoimmune disease in relatives, and in suspected psoriatic arthritis and enthesitis related arthritis (table 1) ask about specific family history.[3w7] Lastly, ask about any systemic features such as rash or intermittent pyrexia (see table 1).

Physical examination
Examine all joints for pain or tenderness, swelling, limited movement, decreased strength or muscle atrophy, and bony deformity.[7 9] Observe the child while walking, standing up, sitting down, or climbing on to the examination table. In a general examination look for features such as lymphadenopathy, organ enlargement, systemic rashes, nail abnormalities, psoriatic rash, or enthesitis. Always measure growth parameters. Eyes should be checked by an ophthalmologist for uveitis.

SUMMARY POINTS

- Early recognition and early aggressive treatment of juvenile idiopathic arthritis prevent joint damage and allow for normal development and growth
- The disease is heterogeneous and complex, so patients benefit from regular review and management by experts in a multidisciplinary team
- The disease currently has no cure, but clinical remission is a realistic treatment goal
- Biological disease modifying antirheumatic drugs are a new and effective treatment for severe disease, but they increase the risk of infection; more data on long term adverse events need to be obtained from registries
- Trials need to determine the optimal treatment strategies with synthetic and biological disease modifying antirheumatic drugs

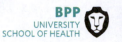

Table 1 Juvenile idiopathic arthritis subtypes[3 6 w6]

Categories	Characteristics	% of total	Onset age	Sex ratio (F:M)	Relative risk (European v non- European)
Systemic juvenile idiopathic arthritis	Arthritis and daily fever .3 days, accompanied by at least one of the following: evanescent (non-fixed) erythematous rash, generalised lymph node enlargement, hepatomegaly or splenomegaly (or both), serositis	4-17	Throughout childhood	1:1	2.5
Oligoarthritis:	Arthritis affecting 1-4 joints during the first 6 months of disease	27-60	Early childhood (peak 2-4 years)	5:1	
Persistent	Arthritis affecting ,4 joints throughout the disease course	40			3.3
Extended	Arthritis affecting >4 joints after the first 6 months of disease	20			6.0
Polyarthritis:	Arthritis affecting .5 joints during the first 6 months of disease				
Rheumatoid factor positive	Two or more positive tests for rheumatoid factor at least 3 months apart	2-7	Late childhood or adolescence	3:1	0.8
Rheumatoid factor negative	Tests for rheumatoid factor negative	11-30	Early peak 2-4 years and late peak 6-12 years	3:1	3.9
Psoriatic arthritis	Arthritis and psoriasis, or arthritis and at least 2 of the following: dactylitis, nail pitting or onycholysis, psoriasis in first degree relative	2-11	Late childhood or adolescence	1:0.95	6.4
Enthesitis related arthritis	Arthritis and enthesitis, or arthritis or enthesitis with at least 2 of the following: sacroiliac joint tenderness or inflammatory lumbosacral pain (or both), HLA-B27 antigen positive, onset in boy over 6 years old, acute anterior uveitis, HLA-B27 associated disease* in first degree relative	1-11	Early peak 2-4 years and late peak 6-12 years	1:7	1.7
Undifferentiated arthritis	Arthritis that fulfils criteria in no specific category or meets criteria for more than one category	11-21			

*Ankylosing spondylitis, enthesitis related arthritis, sacroiilitis with inflammatory bowel disease, Reiter's syndrome, or acute anterior uveitis.

BOX 1 DIFFERENTIAL DIAGNOSIS OF JOINT PROBLEMS IN CHILDREN[8]

Arthritis*

- Infective and reactive: Lyme disease, viral infection, mycoplasma infection, post-streptococcal reactive arthritis
- Juvenile idiopathic arthritis
- Connective tissues disorders: systemic lupus erythematosus, dermatomyositis, systemic sclerosis
- Systemic vasculitis: Henoch-Schönlein purpura, Kawasaki's disease, polyarteritis nodosa
- Other: haemophilia, immunodeficiency (including periodic fever syndromes), sarcoidosis, inflammatory bowel disease

Mechanical and degenerative causes†

- Trauma: accidental and non-accidental
- Hypermobility
- Avascular necrosis including Perthes' disease, Osgood-Schlatter's disease, Scheuermann's disease
- Slipped upper femoral epiphyses
- Anterior knee pain including chondromalacia patallae

Non-organic causes†

- Idiopathic pain syndromes: diffuse or localised (reflex sympathetic dystrophy)
- Benign nocturnal idiopathic limb pains (growing pains)
- Psychogenic causes

Miscellaneous causes‡

- Osteomyelitis
- Tumours: malignant (leukaemia, neuroblastoma) or benign (osteoid osteoma, pigment villonodular synovitis)
- Endocrine and metabolic abnormalities: rickets, diabetes, hypophosphataemic rickets, hypothyroidism or hyperthyroidism
- Genetic disorders: skeletal dysplasias, mucopolysaccharidoses, collagen disorders (Ehlers-Danlos syndrome, Stickler's syndrome)

*Joint(s) show (or mimic) signs of inflammation: redness, swelling, heat, pain, loss of function
†Most likely cause in otherwise well patients with joint pain but no swelling (except for trauma)
‡Most likely cause in patients with overall malaise in addition to joint problems

---

Clinical features

Clinical features strongly depend on the subtype and differ in age at onset of disease, number and location of joints involved, disease course, presence of antinuclear antibodies or rheumatoid factor, presence of chronic or acute uveitis, presence of systemic features, and HLA allelic associations (table 1).[w8] Patients with oligoarthritis (one to four joints affected in first six months of disease) usually present with arthritis in the knees, ankles, or elbows rather than the hips. Chronic anterior uveitis develops in a fifth of these patients and most will be antinuclear antibody positive.[10w8] Most patients with polyarthritis (five or more joints affected in first six months) present with symmetrical arthritis in large and small joints and less commonly with uveitis.[w8] Onset may be acute or insidious. Systemic disease is characterised by fever with one or more daily spikes for at least three days. As well as arthritis, which affects a variable number of joints, there are systemic features (table 1).[3] Arthritis may start weeks or even years after the onset of systemic features and can present as a single episode or become persistent. Patients with enthesitis related arthritis can present with oligoarthritis or polyarthritis of the large or small joints as well as enthesitis (table 1).[3w8] Patients who also have psoriasis, a history of psoriasis in a first degree relative, nail pitting, or dactylitis will probably have psoriatic arthritis unless rheumatoid factor is positive.[3w8]

Further investigations

Other investigations for all subtypes include laboratory tests—a full blood examination, inflammatory markers (erythrocyte sedimentation rate, C reactive protein), and autoimmune markers (rheumatoid factor, HLA B27, and antinuclear antibodies)—and imaging studies.[7 9] Radiography

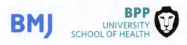

can detect narrowing of the joint spaces or erosions and might show maturation differences or growth abnormalities in bones from an early stage.[w9] Magnetic resonance imaging studies can also show inflamed synovium and increased joint fluid.[w9]

Referral

Refer all children with suspected or confirmed juvenile idiopathic arthritis to a paediatric rheumatologist as soon as possible to prevent delay in treatment. A cohort study of 128 patients with juvenile idiopathic arthritis and a placebo controlled trial showed that time to treatment is an important factor in response to treatment.[11 12]

How does juvenile idiopathic arthritis affect patients?

Patients with active arthritis have pain, fatigue, and limitation in performing daily activities, but the degree to which patients are affected differs. The course of the disease is related to the subtype—persistent oligoarthritis is generally the mildest form and systemic the most severe form. When disease is not completely controlled, long term local or systemic complications can occur, depending on the subtype, severity of the disease, and the treatment given. Case-control studies show that long term localised joint inflammation can lead to flexion deformities, damage of cartilage and bone, and bony overgrowth that results in limb length discrepancies.[13 14] Observational studies show that overall growth can be affected by the disease itself and other factors, such as use of corticosteroids.[w10-w12] Chronic inflammation can cause anaemia.[w13] Uveitis, which occurs in 5-20% of patients, most commonly in the oligoarticular subtype, can be asymptomatic and can lead to cataracts and even blindness.[10] Regular ophthalmology checks are indicated. The systemic subtype is associated with the most serious morbidity and even mortality.[15] Conditions associated with this subtype include amyloidosis and macrophage activation syndrome.[15w14]

Despite improvements in treatment, a review published last year showed that a large proportion of children with juvenile idiopathic arthritis still have active disease throughout childhood and enter adulthood with active disease.[16] Several clinical studies have shown that patients with active disease have low health related quality of life[17] [18]—the disease affects their physical, emotional, and social wellbeing. A review found that affected children have lower self esteem, are more likely to have behavioural problems than their peers, and are limited in their social lives because of mobility problems and pain.[w15] The patient's family is also affected—the disease has an emotional impact on parents and limits family activities. Fortunately, several studies have shown that family cohesion is not affected.[17w15]

How is juvenile idiopathic arthritis treated?

Because there is currently no cure for juvenile idiopathic arthritis, the goal of treatment is clinical remission (complete absence of disease).[2 7w16] Treatment aims to control the inflammatory process by decreasing the number of actively affected joints and to improve the quality of life. A validated set of response variables is used to measure the response to treatment in patients enrolled in clinical trials (box 2).[19] Patients are considered to be in remission if they have had no active arthritis, fever, rash, serositis, or generalised lymphadenopathy attributable to juvenile idiopathic arthritis; no active uveitis; a normal erythrocyte sedimentation rate or C reactive protein; and no disease activity as assessed by a doctor for the past six months.[20]

Old versus new approach to treatment

In the past, juvenile idiopathic arthritis was treated with non-steroidal anti-inflammatory drugs (NSAIDs), with delayed addition of synthetic disease modifying antirheumatic drugs (DMARDs) or systemic corticosteroids (or both), and lastly biological DMARDs. However, accumulating evidence from cohort studies and trials has shown that a more aggressive approach to disease control, with earlier introduction of DMARDs, prevents or minimises long term sequelae of the disease.[11 12 16] Existing guidelines on care have not been revised to include such advice but do advocate "tight" clinical control.[2w16]

Drug treatment

Up to date international guidelines are currently lacking. The British Paediatric Rheumatology Group provided guidelines for the management of childhood arthritis in 2001,[21] but because treatment is changing rapidly, this guideline needs revision. A recent guideline from the Royal Australian College of General Practitioners focuses on NSAID treatment only.[9] New recommendations for the treatment of juvenile idiopathic arthritis were presented at the American College of Rheumatology 2010 November meeting but have not been published yet. They are based on studies also mentioned in this review and on expert opinions when evidence is lacking. The treatment modalities we describe are based on randomised controlled trials, case series, and cohort studies. The figure outlines a simplified approach to treatment.

Non-steroidal anti-inflammatory drugs

During diagnosis, while other causes of arthritis are being excluded, most patients are given NSAIDs. These drugs relieve pain usually within a few days and do not, as more aggressive treatments can, interfere with the disease course in case of misdiagnosis. Several NSAIDs are used, and none has proved to be superior to another.[22] Recent randomised trials found that the newer cyclo-oxygenase-2 inhibitors (rofecoxib, celecoxib, and meloxicam) were no more effective or safer than the most commonly prescribed NSAID, naproxen.[w17-w19] More than half of patients achieved an ACR pediatric 30 response (box 2) after three months of NSAID monotherapy, an NSAID added to a stable dose of a synthetic DMARD, or biological DMARD treatment, although these responses were not compared with placebo.[w17-w19]

Corticosteroids (intra-articular and systemic)

Children with oligoarticular disease are often given NSAID monotherapy, intra-articular corticosteroids alone, or a combination of both. Intra-articular corticosteroids are

---

BOX 2 JUVENILE IDIOPATHIC ARTHRITIS CORE SET OF RESPONSE VARIABLES[19]

- Global assessment of the disease activity by the doctor using a visual analogue scale (VAS) (range 0-100 mm, 0 best score)
- Childhood health assessment questionnaire (CHAQ) (range 0-3, 0 best score) used by the patient or parent (measures functional ability)
- Global assessment of wellbeing by the patient or parent using a visual analogue scale (range 0-100 mm, 0 best score)
- Number of joints with active arthritis
- Number of joints with limited movement
- A laboratory marker of inflammation—erythrocyte sedimentation rate or C reactive protein
- Patients have responded if at least three variables have improved by 30% (50%, 70%, 100%) and no more than one variable has worsened by more than 30% (ACR pediatric 30%, 50%, 70%, or 100% response)[19]

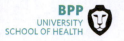

Table 2 Synthetic disease modifying antirheumatic drugs

Agent	Dose*	Contraindication	Common side effects
Methotrexate (Emthexate, Metoject)	10-15 mg/m² once weekly orally or subcutaneously(maximum 25 mg/m²)	Liver dysfunction, kidney dysfunction, immunodeficiency, bone marrow dysfunction, active infection, pregnancy, breast feeding	Gastrointestinal symptoms (nausea, vomiting, anorexia); less commonly transient rises in liver transaminases and haematological disturbances
Sulfasalazine (Salazopyrin)	50 mg/kg orally divided into 2 or 3 doses a day(maximum 2000 mg/day)	Salicylate hypersensitivity, systemic disease	Gastrointestinal symptoms, allergic reactions; less commonly, myelosuppression
Leflunomide (Arava)	<20 kg: 100 mg orally for 1 day and then 10 mg every other day;20-40 kg: 100 mg orally for 2 days and then 10 mg/day;>40 kg: 100 mg orally for 3 days and then 20 mg/day	Severe immunodeficiency, bone marrow dysfunction, serious infection, liver dysfunction, severe hypoproteinaemia, pregnancy, breast feeding	Gastrointestinal symptoms, rash, allergic reactions, headache, reversible alopecia; less commonly, transient rises in liver transaminases, haematological disturbances; can be teratogenetic
Ciclosporin A (Neoral)	3-7 mg/kg daily orally or intravenously	Renal impairment, uncontrolled hypertension, uncontrolled infections, malignancy	Hypertension and nephrotoxicity; depletion of calcium and magnesium can be associated with muscle cramping; hirsuitism and gum hyperplasia often reported at higher doses

*m² refers to body surface; kg refers to body weight.

increasingly being used, and earlier in the disease course. In a retrospective study of 121 injected joints, all joints responded within one week, and after one year 52% were still in remission.[w20] A randomised double blind trial confirmed this rapid and long lasting effect and showed that triamcinolone hexacetonide is superior to triamcinolone acetonide (85% of joints still in remission after one year) and should be the drug of first choice.[23] Skin atrophy at the injection site occurred in 2.3% of the treated joints.[23] The systemic absorption of triamcinolone, which peaks at eight hours after injection, is usually not clinically relevant, although cases of Cushing's syndrome and transient increases in blood glucose in patients with diabetes have been reported after intra-articular injection.[w21 w22]

The long term use of systemic corticosteroids has declined because of side effects, particularly reduced growth and bone health.[w12] These drugs are mainly used while waiting for DMARDs to take effect and in patients with severe systemic or polyarticular juvenile idiopathic arthritis unresponsive to treatment with synthetic and biological DMARDs.[22 w7]

Synthetic disease modifying antirheumatic drugs

Patients with a definite diagnosis of polyarticular disease or oligoarticular disease refractory to intra-articular steroids are candidates for second line agents (DMARDs). Table 2 lists the typical doses, side effects, and contraindications of such drugs used in juvenile idiopathic arthritis.

Methotrexate is the most widely used and first choice synthetic DMARD. A randomised placebo controlled trial (127 patients), a randomised placebo controlled crossover trial (43 patients with extended oligoarticular arthritis), and a dose finding trial (80 patients, mostly unresponsive to low dose methotrexate) found it to be effective—with significant reductions in active and limited joint counts, and high overall improvement—in patients with polyarticular and oligoarticular extended disease.[24 w23 w24] However, it produced no overall improvement in systemic disease—the most difficult subtype to treat.[24] It is unclear how long after remission methotrexate should be withdrawn; a recent randomised clinical withdrawal trial found no differences in relapse rates in patients who continued the drug for six or 12 months (57% v 56%) after induction of remission.[w25]

A randomised placebo controlled trial (69 patients) also found sulfasalazine to be effective in the management of juvenile idiopathic arthritis, with a higher response rate than placebo (69% v 45%) after 24 weeks of treatment.[25] However, the drug was not well tolerated, and nearly a third of patients discontinued treatment.[25] With the development

of newer biological DMARDs, the use of sulfasalazine has decreased. In a relatively small randomised controlled trial, leflunomide was found to be less effective than methotrexate but with similar adverse event rates.[26] There are no controlled studies of ciclosporin A in juvenile idiopathic arthritis, although small case series show a beneficial effect in severe systemic disease.[w26 w27] A large observational study of 329 patients treated with ciclosporin A found a 9% complete response rate; most patients discontinued the drug because of inefficacy.[w28] Case series have shown that ciclosporin A might be effective in macrophage activation syndrome.[w29 w30] The use of leflunomide and ciclosporin A in juvenile idiopathic arthritis is limited. Other synthetic DMARDs (auranofin, penicillamine, and hydroxychloroquine) have not been shown to have a significant therapeutic advantage over placebo, in contrast to findings in adult patients with rheumatoid arthritis.[w31 w32]

Biological disease modifying antirheumatic drugs

With the introduction of biological DMARDs (also know as biologicals or biologics) the goal has shifted from reducing inflammation to "switching off" the autoimmune system by targeting inflammatory cytokines. Table 3 lists the biological DMARDs currently available or under investigation for juvenile idiopathic arthritis.

Tumour necrosis factor is a proinflammatory cytokine that plays a central role in the pathogenesis of juvenile idiopathic arthritis.[w33] In systemic disease, interleukin 1 (a proinflammatory cytokine synthesised by fibroblasts in the synovium and macrophages) and interleukin 6 (concentrations of which correlate with fever, disease activity, and platelet counts) are also thought to be important.[w33-w35] If inhibition of these cytokines is not sufficient, other drugs aimed at T cell blockade and B cell depletion are available.[w36] Only etanercept, adalimumab, and abatacept have been approved by the European Medicines Agency and the Food and Drug Administration for the treatment of juvenile idiopathic arthritis after testing in placebo controlled withdrawal trials.[27 28 29] These trials are designed so that all patients start the drug in an initial open label part of the trial. Those with an ACR pediatric 30 response to treatment (box 2) enter a double blind study and are randomly assigned to receive placebo or the biological DMARD until the disease flares. The response rates (ACR pediatric scores) reported from these trials come from the open label phase and represent the initial responders.[w37] Results from the randomised blinded phase are presented as flare rates. This design is used in paediatric rheumatology trials to minimise the consequences of placebo treatment.

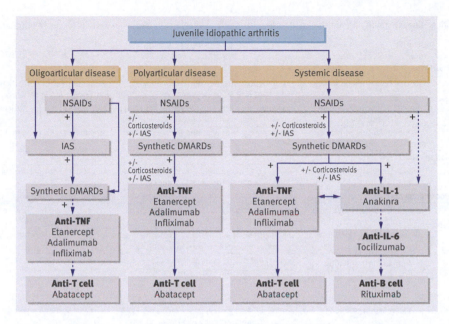

Simplified approach to treatment of patients with juvenile idiopathic arthritis. Steps often rapidly succeed one another or are combined. DMARDs, disease modifying antirheumatic drugs; IAS, intra-articular steroids; IL, interleukin; NSAIDs, non-steroidal anti-inflammatory drugs; TNF, tumour necrosis factor

Other biological DMARDs are prescribed off label, although some (infliximab, anakinra, tocilizumab) have been tested in patients with juvenile idiopathic arthritis in placebo controlled withdrawal trials (table 3).[w38-w40] Choice of biological DMARD is based on effectiveness, safety, route of administration, and arthritis subtype.

Etanercept was the first and for a long time the only registered biological DMARD for the treatment of juvenile idiopathic arthritis; 74% of patients previously resistant to other drugs, including methotrexate, met the ACR pediatric 30 target after three months in the placebo controlled withdrawal trial.[27] Many observational studies have provided data on safety and response; the drug seems to be well tolerated and effective.[w41-w46] It is the most commonly prescribed biological DMARD for patients with this disease, followed by adalimumab. A prospective registry study found that etanercept reduced disease activity and improved quality of life in all aspects affected by the disease.[17] A health related quality of life study of abatacept showed similar results.[w47] A placebo controlled withdrawal trial showed that abatacept was effective in patients for whom anti-tumour necrosis factor was not effective (ACR pediatric 30 response in 39%), thereby providing a valuable alternative treatment.[29]

The treatment of systemic disease is challenging.[15] In a controlled clinical withdrawal trial and case series anakinra seemed to be better than etanercept in reducing systemic symptoms.[15 w38 w48-w50] Other biological DMARDs (table 3) have shown promising results in clinical trials or case series. No head to head trials on choice of biological DMARD exist for these patients. Today, most experts favour anakinra when systemic features are prominent, but the timing of this treatment is debatable.[30] More studies on management of systemic arthritis are needed.

The most commonly encountered adverse events of biological DMARDs are local reactions at injection sites and opportunistic infections.[31 w51] Most injection site reactions resolve as a result of tolerance. Consult a paediatric rheumatologist if the drug has to be discontinued because of a serious infection. Less commonly encountered but important

adverse events are neurological or neuropsychological disorders, new onset autoimmune diseases, and cancer. The most common cancers reported related to anti-tumour necrosis factor treatment are hepatosplenic T cell lymphoma, Hodgkin's lymphoma, non-Hodgkin's lymphoma, and leukaemia, although there is no convincing evidence of an increased risk.[31 w52 w53] Similarly, although safety studies with long term follow-up have shown new onset of the above complications in patients taking biological DMARDs, we have insufficient data to compare incidence rates in patients taking biological DMARDs with those in patients not taking biological DMARDs.[w41-w46] If one of these conditions is suspected in a patient taking a biological DMARD or other immunosuppressive drug, consult the treating paediatric rheumatologist immediately to discuss discontinuing the drug. Box 3 provides recommendations for safety and monitoring of DMARDs.

Other treatments

Depending on the subtype and severity of disease, the British Society for Paediatric and Adolescent Rheumatology standards of care recommends regular checks by a paediatric rheumatologist, ophthalmologist, dermatologist, orthopaedic surgeon, orthodontist, general practitioner, psychologist, and physiotherapist or occupational therapist. The idea is that a well chosen multidisciplinary team will enable the best possible care.[2]

A Cochrane review has shown that physiotherapy is important to maintain normal muscle and joint function.[w63] Rehabilitation—using heat or cold treatment, massage, therapeutic exercise, and splints—is crucial to returning to activities of daily living again once these have been limited by disease.[9] The British Society for Paediatric and Adolescent Rheumatology standards of care guideline also recommends psychological therapy and education.[2]

Supplements may be needed to prevent certain side effects of treatment. During corticosteroid treatment patients are at increased risk of osteoporosis and osteopenia. Several studies, including a randomised clinical trial, found a small but significant beneficial effect of calcium

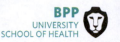

Table 3 Biological disease modifying antirheumatic drugs currently available or under investigation for juvenile idiopathic arthritis

Agent	Action	Dose*	Used in subtypes	Other paediatric indications (approved or off label)
TNF-α blocking agents				
Etanercept (Enbrel)	TNF-α receptor fusion protein	0.4 mg/kg twice weekly SC or 0.8 mg/kg weekly SC (max 50 mg/week)	All patients with polyarticular course and seldom in oligoarticular persistent††	Plaque psoriasis
Adalimumab (Humira)	Human monoclonal anti-TNF antibody	<30 kg: 20 mg every two weeks SC; >30 kg: 40 mg every two weeks SC	All patients with polyarticular course‡	Crohn's disease, ulcerative colitis, uveitis
Infliximab (Remicade)	Chimeric murine-human monoclonal anti-TNF antibody	6-10 mg/kg IV at 0, 2, and 6 weeks, then every 4-8 weeks	All patients with polyarticular course†	Crohn's disease, ulcerative colitis, plaque psoriasis, uveitis
T cell co-stimulation modulator				
Abatacept (Orencia)	T cell co-stimulation modulator	10 mg/kg IV at 0, 2, and 4 weeks (maximum 1000 mg), then every 4 weeks	All patients with polyarticular course¶	
Interleukin 1 blocking agents				
Anakinra (Kineret)	IL-1 receptor anatagonist	1-2 mg/kg daily SC (maximum 100 mg)	Systemic disease†	Cryopyrin associated periodic syndrome
Rilonacept (Arcalyst)	IL-1 receptor-IL1RacP-FC fusion protein	Loading dose of 4.4 mg/kg SC (maximum 160 mg), then weekly doses of 2.2 mg/kg	Systemic disease**	Cryopyrin associated periodic syndrome
Canakinumab (Ilaris)	Human IL-1β antibody	<40 kg: 2-4 mg/kg every 8 weeks SC; >40 kg: 150-300 mg every 8 weeks SC	Systemic disease**	Cryopyrin associated periodic syndrome
Interleukin 6 blocking agent				
Tocilizumab (RoActemra)	IL-6 receptor antibody	<30 kg: 12 mg/kg every 2 weeks SC; >30 kg: 8 mg/kg every 2 weeks SC	Systemic disease††	
B cell depletion agent				
Rituximab (Rituxan)	Chimeric anti-CD20 monoclonal causing B cell depletion	<40 kg: 2 doses of 500 mg IV 2 weeks apart; >40 kg: 2 doses of 1000 mg IV 2 weeks apart	Systemic disease**	Systemic lupus erythematosus, B cell non-Hodgkin's lymphoma

Abbreviations: . IL=interleukin, IV=intravenous, TNF=tumour necrosis factor, SC=subcutaneous.

*kg refers to body weight.

Placebo controlled withdrawal trials published for:

†Subtypes: systemic, oligoarticular extended, and polyarticular (rheumatoid factor positive and negative).

‡Patients with a polyarticular course (any subtype).

¶Subtypes: systemic (without systemic manifestations), oligoarticular extended, and polyarticular (rheumatoid factor positive and negative).

**No randomised trials (yet) published in juvenile idiopathic arthritis.

††Systemic subtype only.

BOX 3 SAFETY AND MONITORING OF SYNTHETIC* AND BIOLOGICAL DISEASE MODIFYING ANTIRHEUMATIC DRUGS

Overall recommendations

- Do not start treatment in patients with an active infection, current or previous tuberculosis, immunodeficiency, cancer, or precancerous state[w54]
- In each infectious episode during treatment, consider the need to discontinue the drug temporarily[w54]
- Perform regular check-ups with full blood counts and liver and kidney function tests[w54]
- Be aware of adverse events, including neurological and neuropsychological disorders, new onset autoimmune diseases, and cancers[w54]
- Avoid live (attenuated) vaccines until more data are available[w55 w56]
- Killed (or inactivated) vaccines are safe, although the immune response may be suboptimal and boosters may be needed[w57-w59]
- Yearly influenza vaccination is recommended[w54]
- Give any susceptible patient exposed to varicella specific immunoglobulin and aciclovir at first sign of infection; consider vaccination before starting disease modifying antirheumatic drugs[w54]

Drug specific recommendations

Methotrexate

- Give folate supplements 24-48 hours after starting methotrexate to reduce the gastrointestinal and hepatic side effects[w60]
- In higher doses parenteral application is recommended because of better bioavailability and tolerability[w61]

Leflunomide and ciclosporin A

- Measure blood pressure regularly[w54]

Infliximab

- Monitor for acute hypersensitivity reactions until two hours after infusion[w54]
- Give methotrexate concomitantly to prevent immunogenicity[w62]

*Applies only to synthetic DMARDs that affect the immune system (methotrexate, leflunomide, ciclosporin A)

---

and vitamin D supplements on bone mineral density.[w64 w65] Children using methotrexate might benefit from folic acid supplements. Although evidence that weekly folic acid reduces methotrexate related adverse effects in children is weak, studies in adults with rheumatoid arthritis have shown significant effects.[w66 w67]

Autologous stem cell transplantation was used in autoimmune diseases before biological agents were available, and several patients with juvenile idiopathic arthritis have been successfully transplanted. [w68 w69] However, because of the risks involved (9% transplant related mortality) and relatively high relapse rates (>30%), this treatment is reserved for patients who are resistant to combinations of synthetic DMARDs, corticosteroids, and biological DMARDs and who have severe, debilitating, and potentially fatal disease.

What will the future hold?

Despite the lack of a cure, biological DMARDs have provided a better quality of life for many patients with juvenile idiopathic arthritis who were previously refractory to treatment. In addition, the current trend of early aggressive treatment has improved long term outcomes. However, a proportion of patients still have ongoing active disease and associated long term sequelae that limit daily life.[w70] Individual children must be managed according to subtype, severity of disease, and prognostic factors. Research into biomarkers and genetic markers of disease subtype, as well as advances in radiographic imaging, may one day provide earlier diagnosis, better monitoring of disease activity, and more tailored treatments. Outcomes improve with earlier disease control, and trials to investigate the efficacy of various treatments (combining different drugs according to different time schedules) are under way.[w71-w73] The new

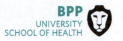

biological DMARDs—targeted at interleukins 1 and 6, T cells, and B cells—have shown promising results and might improve treatment for specific patients groups.

Disease registries are important sources of data from large patient groups. They can be used to compare different outcomes of treatments, while accounting for patient and disease characteristics, disease course, and occurrence of adverse events during (multiple) treatments over long periods. Registry data provide a real life picture of patients as treated by their doctor. Initiatives to combine registries have begun in Europe and the United States and should help us answer questions on the long term safety of biological DMARDs. A worldwide consolidated juvenile idiopathic arthritis registry would be ideal.

Hopefully, these efforts will result in more choice of effective and safe drugs and an optimal treatment strategy for each patient. The ultimate goal is clinical remission off drugs that could be considered as a "cure."[32]

Contributors: FHMP and MHO reviewed the literature and wrote the article. LWAS reviewed and revised the article. FHMP and LWAS are the guarantors.

Funding: FHMP is funded by the Niels Stensen Foundation.

Competing interests: The authors have completed the Unified Competing Interest form at www.icmje.org/coi_disclosure.pdf (available on request from the corresponding author) and declare: FHMP had support from the Niels Stensen Foundation for the submitted work; FHMP received consulting fees from Bristol-Myers Squibb, a travel grant from Wyeth Pharmaceuticals, and financial support for educational purposes from Abbott, Bristol-Myers Squib, Novartis Pharma, Teva Pharma, and Wyeth Pharmaceuticals, MHO received consulting fees from Roche and a travel grant from Wyeth Pharmaceuticals, LWAS received research grants from Abbott, Pfizer, and Wyeth Pharmaceuticals and consulting fees from Bristol-Myers Squibb, Roche and Schering-Plough in the previous three years; no other relationships or activities that could appear to have influenced the submitted work.

Provenance and peer review: Not commissioned; externally peer reviewed.

1   Ostlie IL, Aasland A, Johansson I, Flato B, Moller A. A longitudinal follow-up study of physical and psychosocial health in young adults with chronic childhood arthritis. Clin Exp Rheumatol 2009;27:1039-46.
2   Davies K, Cleary G, Foster H, Hutchinson E, Baildam E. BSPAR standards of care for children and young people with juvenile idiopathic arthritis. Rheumatol (Oxford) 2010;49:1406-8.
3   Petty RE, Southwood TR, Manners P, Baum J, Glass DN, Goldenberg J, et al. International League of Associations for Rheumatology classification of juvenile idiopathic arthritis: second revision, Edmonton, 2001. J Rheumatol 2004;31:390-2.
4   Prakken BJ, Albani S. Using biology of disease to understand and guide therapy of JIA. Best Pract Res Clin Rheumatol 2009;23:599-608.
5   Berkun Y, Padeh S. Environmental factors and the geoepidemiology of juvenile idiopathic arthritis. Autoimmun Rev 2010;9:A319-24.
6   Saurenmann RK, Rose JB, Tyrrell P, Feldman BM, Laxer RM, Schneider R, et al. Epidemiology of juvenile idiopathic arthritis in a multiethnic cohort: ethnicity as a risk factor. Arthritis Rheum 2007;56:1974-84.
7   Wallace CA. Current management of juvenile idiopathic arthritis. Best Pract Res Clin Rheumatol 2006;20:279-300.
8   Davidson J. Juvenile idiopathic arthritis: a clinical overview. Eur J Radiol 2000;33:128-35.
9   Australian Government. Clinical guideline for the diagnosis and management of juvenile idiopathic arthritis. www.racgp.org.au/Content/NavigationMenu/ClinicalResources/RACGPGuidelines/Juvenileidiopathicarthritis/RACGP_JIA_guideline.pdf.
10 Foster CS. Diagnosis and treatment of juvenile idiopathic arthritis-associated uveitis. Curr Opin Ophthalmol 2003;14:395-8.
11 Albers HM, Wessels JA, van der Straaten RJ, Brinkman DM, Suijlekom-Smit LW, Kamphuis SS, et al. Time to treatment as an important factor for the response to methotrexate in juvenile idiopathic arthritis. Arthritis Rheum 2009;61:46-51.
12 Van Rossum MA, van Soesbergen RM, Boers M, Zwinderman AH, Fiselier TJ, Franssen MJ, et al. Long-term outcome of juvenile idiopathic arthritis following a placebo-controlled trial: sustained benefits of early sulfasalazine treatment. Ann Rheum Dis 2007;66:1518-24.
13 Flato B, Lien G, Smerdel A, Vinje O, Dale K, Johnston V, et al. Prognostic factors in juvenile rheumatoid arthritis: a case-control study revealing early predictors and outcome after 14.9 years. J Rheumatol 2003;30:386-93.
14 Sherry DD, Stein LD, Reed AM, Schanberg LE, Kredich DW. Prevention of leg length discrepancy in young children with pauciarticular

juvenile rheumatoid arthritis by treatment with intraarticular steroids. Arthritis Rheum 1999;42:2330-4.
15 Woo P. Systemic juvenile idiopathic arthritis: diagnosis, management, and outcome. Nat Clin Pract Rheumatol 2006;2:28-34.
16 Minden K. Adult outcomes of patients with juvenile idiopathic arthritis. Horm Res 2009;72(suppl 1):20-5.
17 Prince FH, Geerdink LM, Borsboom GJ, Twilt M, Van Rossum MA, Hoppenreijs EP, et al. Major improvements in health-related quality of life during the use of etanercept in patients with previously refractory juvenile idiopathic arthritis. Ann Rheum Dis 2010;69:138-42.
18 Ringold S, Wallace CA, Rivara FP. Health-related quality of life, physical function, fatigue, and disease activity in children with established polyarticular juvenile idiopathic arthritis. J Rheumatol 2009;36:1330-6.
19 Giannini EH, Ruperto N, Ravelli A, Lovell DJ, Felson DT, Martini A. Preliminary definition of improvement in juvenile arthritis. Arthritis Rheum 1997;40:1202-9.
20 Wallace CA, Ruperto N, Giannini E, Childhood Arthritis and Rheumatology Research A, Pediatric Rheumatology International Trials O, Pediatric Rheumatology Collaborative Study G. Preliminary criteria for clinical remission for select categories of juvenile idiopathic arthritis. J Rheumatol 2004;31:2290-4.
21 Hull RG. Management guidelines for arthritis in children. Rheumatol (Oxford) 2001;40:1308.
22 Hashkes PJ, Laxer RM. Medical treatment of juvenile idiopathic arthritis. JAMA 2005;294:1671-84.
23 Zulian F, Martini G, Gobber D, Plebani M, Zacchello F, Manners P. Triamcinolone acetonide and hexacetonide intra-articular treatment of

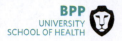

symmetrical joints in juvenile idiopathic arthritis: a double-blind trial. *Rheumatol (Oxford)*2004;43:1288-91.

24 Woo P, Southwood TR, Prieur AM, Dore CJ, Grainger J, David J, et al. Randomized, placebo-controlled, crossover trial of low-dose oral methotrexate in children with extended oligoarticular or systemic arthritis. *Arthritis Rheum*2000;43:1849-57.

25 Van Rossum MA, Fiselier TJ, Franssen MJ, Zwinderman AH, ten Cate R, van Suijlekom-Smit LW, et al. Sulfasalazine in the treatment of juvenile chronic arthritis: a randomized, double-blind, placebo-controlled, multicenter study. Dutch Juvenile Chronic Arthritis Study Group. *Arthritis Rheum*1998;41:808-16.

26 Silverman E, Mouy R, Spiegel L, Jung LK, Saurenmann RK, Lahdenne P, et al. Leflunomide or methotrexate for juvenile rheumatoid arthritis. *N Engl J Med*2005;352:1655-66.

27 Lovell DJ, Giannini EH, Reiff A, Cawkwell GD, Silverman ED, Nocton JJ, et al. Etanercept in children with polyarticular juvenile rheumatoid arthritis. Pediatric Rheumatology Collaborative Study Group. *N Engl J Med*2000;342:763-9.

28 Lovell DJ, Ruperto N, Goodman S, Reiff A, Jung L, Jarosova K, et al. Adalimumab with or without methotrexate in juvenile rheumatoid arthritis. *N Engl J Med*2008;359:810-20.

29 Ruperto N, Lovell DJ, Quartier P, Paz E, Rubio-Perez N, Silva CA, et al. Abatacept in children with juvenile idiopathic arthritis: a randomised, double-blind, placebo-controlled withdrawal trial. *Lancet*2008;372:383-91.

30 Nigrovic PA, Mannion M, Prince FH, Zeft A, Rabinovich CE, van Rossum MA, et al. Anakinra as first-line disease modifying therapy in systemic juvenile idiopathic arthritis. *Arthritis Rheum*2010 online 4 November.

31 Hashkes PJ, Uziel Y, Laxer RM. The safety profile of biologic therapies for juvenile idiopathic arthritis. *Nat Rev Rheumatol*2010;6:561-71.

32 Shenoi S, Wallace CA. Remission in juvenile idiopathic arthritis: current facts. *Curr Rheumatol Rep*2010;12:80-6.

Related links

bmj.com archive

- Diagnosis and management of soft tissue sarcoma (2010;341:c7170)
- Recent advances in the management of rheumatoid arthritis (2010;341:c6942)
- Investigating and managing chronic scrotal pain (2010;341:c6716)
- Commentary: managing oesophageal cancer in a resource poor setting—a Malawian example (2010;341:6723)
- Oesophageal cancer (2010;341:6280)

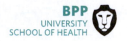

Management of difficult and severe eczema in childhood

M A McAleer specialist registrar[1], C Flohr clinical senior lecturer[2], A D Irvine professor[134]

[1]Department of Paediatric Dermatology, Our Lady's Children's Hospital, Crumlin, Dublin 12, Republic of Ireland

[2]Department of Paediatric Dermatology, St John's Institute of Dermatology, Guy's and St Thomas' Hospitals NHS Foundation Trust and King's College, London, UK

[3]Clinical Medicine, Trinity College, Dublin, Republic of Ireland

[4]National Children's Research Centre, Dublin, Republic of Ireland

Correspondence to: A D Irvine
irvinea@tcd.ie

Cite this as: *BMJ* 2012;345:e4770

‹DOI› 10.1136/bmj.e4770
http://www.bmj.com/content/345/bmj.e4770

Childhood eczema is the most common inflammatory skin disease and affects around 20% of children in the United Kingdom.[w1] The condition is also referred to as atopic dermatitis and atopic eczema. The correct nomenclature is debated by experts. The World Allergy Organisation recommends the term eczema, and this is widely used in the UK literature. Atopic dermatitis is perhaps the more accepted term historically and internationally. In this review we will use the term eczema.

Eczema is associated with several comorbidities, including food and respiratory allergies. It has a serious effect on children's and families' quality of life—for example, through sleep disturbance and a negative impact on schooling.[1][2][3] The resulting impairment in health related quality of life is comparable to that of other chronic diseases of childhood, including diabetes and asthma.[1]

Although mild eczema can often be managed in primary care, around 2% of patients have severe disease that does not respond to topical anti-inflammatory drugs or ultraviolet light treatment alone. These recalcitrant cases require intensive expert management and an individualised approach, especially when systemic immunomodulatory drugs are used. Although these drugs are often life transforming, their side effects require close monitoring. Currently, there is a distinct lack of evidence to help guide the clinician caring for children with severe eczema. This review summarises the management of difficult eczema in primary care, when to refer to secondary care, and treatment options for severe eczema.

How common is childhood eczema?

Eczema is the most common chronic inflammatory disease of early childhood and is often the initial step in the "atopic march," with the subsequent development of food and respiratory allergies (asthma and hay fever).[4]

Eczema affects about 10% of children in the United States and around 20% in the UK.[w2-w4] About two thirds of children with eczema have spontaneous remission before adolescence.[4] The prevalence of eczema has increased in developing countries, especially in urban areas, where populations have adopted a Western lifestyle.[w1][w5]

What causes eczema?

Eczema is a complex disease. Loss of function mutations in the gene that encodes filaggrin (*FLG*), which has a pivotal role in skin barrier function, are strongly linked to the risk of eczema.[w6] Because most cases present in early life and heritability is more strongly linked to the maternal side, environmental influences that operate in utero or in early infancy are probably involved.[w7] For instance, studies have suggested a positive association with water hardness and frequency of washing, as well as exposure to antibiotics in early life.[w7] These influences may be partially due to an effect on the skin microflora, and further research is needed to understand how environmental and genetic factors interact in the development of eczema.[w7] Patients also have well characterised systemic and cutaneous immune abnormalities, including increased total and allergen specific serum IgE; raised cutaneous cytokines, T cells, Langerhans cells, and inflammatory dendritic epidermal cells; and decreased expression of antimicrobial peptides.[w8]

How is eczema diagnosed?

Eczema is diagnosed clinically, usually in primary care. It is characterised by itch, skin inflammation, a skin barrier abnormality, and susceptibility to skin infection.

The disease can be difficult to define because the clinical features vary and presentation depends on age and ethnicity (box 1).[4] It is unclear whether eczema is one disease or whether distinct subphenotypes have different genetic and immunological profiles.

A systematic review concluded that the UK refinement of the Hanifin and Rajka diagnostic criteria is the most extensively validated in hospital based and population based settings as well as a wide range of ethnic groups (box 2).[5][w9] Many healthcare professionals will not need diagnostic criteria in routine clinical practice, however, although such criteria may help diagnose borderline cases.[6]

Approach to management

Severe eczema is a physically and psychologically demanding disease and requires a comprehensive, holistic, medium term or long term strategy (fig 1). Treatment aims to reduce the symptoms, improve quality of life, and decrease the degree and frequency of flares. Furthermore, treatment may modify the overall disease course and possibly reduce atopic comorbidities,[7] although more evidence is needed to determine if this is a robust effect. A personalised

SUMMARY POINTS

- Eczema is associated with serious morbidity for the patient and family
- Patient education is essential for the treatment of this complex chronic disorder
- Topical anti-inflammatory drugs together with regular use of emollients is effective in most children with eczema
- Patients with eczema are susceptible to molluscum contagiosum and infection with *Staphylococcus aureus* and herpes simplex virus; infections can cause disease flares and treatment resistance
- Patients with severe eczema may need systemic immunomodulatory drugs, which require close monitoring by a doctor experienced in their use

SOURCES AND SELECTION CRITERIA

We searched Medline, the Cochrane Collaboration, and the GREAT database (www.greatdatabase.co.uk) using the search terms "eczema", "atopic eczema", "atopic dermatitis", "management", and "treatment". When possible, evidence from randomised controlled trials and systemic reviews was used. Case series were used in the absence of higher level evidence. We also referenced expert review articles and included expert opinion based on clinical experience.

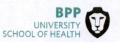

management plan is essential to ensure adherence to treatment recommendations and treatment success. The management of severe eczema in children often requires a multidisciplinary team approach.

Managing eczema in primary care

Mild eczema can be managed in primary care with patient education, regular use of emollients, and topical corticosteroids of mild or moderate potency. The National Institute for Health and Clinical Excellence (NICE) has published guidelines on the treatment of eczema in children.[8]

Patient education

Patient education is an essential and important primary intervention. It has been shown to reduce disease severity and improve quality of life at least over a one year period.[9] [10] A randomised controlled trial (RCT) concluded that nurses may be better placed to offer educational support, but intervention studies are needed to confirm this.[w10]

Bathing and emollients

Daily use of emollients to counteract dry skin is one of the cornerstones of management. Bathing hydrates and cleanses the skin and emollient based soap substitutes moisturise the skin and avoid skin irritation associated with standard soaps. Bathing is usually recommended once a day and emollients once to twice a day, or even more often, depending on the clinical setting.[11] Ointments contain higher concentrations of lipids and are generally more effective moisturisers than creams. Topical preparations should be free of dyes, fragrances, and food derived allergens such as peanut protein.[7] Despite the universal recommendation of the use of emollients and bath additives, no robust evidence from RCTs supports this.[12] [13] Of note, the 2007 NICE guidelines recommended that aqueous cream should not be used because it can cause irritant reactions.[8] More recently, aqueous cream was shown to increase transepidermal water loss in healthy subjects and those with a history of eczema.[w11] [w12] Despite this, aqueous cream is still the most commonly prescribed emollient in England.[w12]

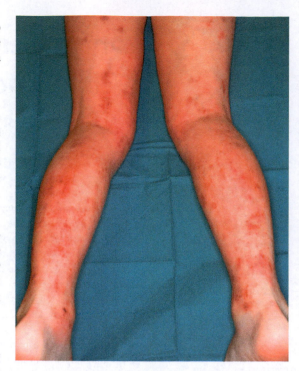

Fig 1 This child had severe eczema despite maximal topical treatment and inpatient management

Topical corticosteroids

Topical corticosteroids are widely used as first and second line agents in the management of eczema. These drugs have anti-inflammatory, antiproliferative, immunosuppressive, and vasoconstrictive actions. Topical corticosteroids are grouped by potency (box 3), and prescribers should tailor them to the severity of the eczema. A proactive rather than reactive approach to treatment is favoured—long term moisturising treatment to maintain remission with short term "step-up" treatment for flares.[11] Corticosteroids of mild to moderate potency are used for maintenance treatment in mild to moderate eczema. Flares are managed with short courses (7-14 days) of such preparations. Do not use long term potent corticosteroids in children without specialist advice. Itch is a key symptom for evaluating response to treatment.[11]

Local adverse effects, such as skin atrophy, striae, and telangiectasia, can occur with inappropriate use of topical corticosteroids, especially on sensitive areas such as the face, neck, or groin. Systemic adverse effects are rare.[7] A systematic review of 10 RCTs found no evidence that

---

BOX 1 CLINICAL FEATURES OF ECZEMA

Clinical manifestations vary with age:

- Typically starts in early infancy with eczematous, erythematous papules and vesicles on the cheeks and scalp; scratching causes crusted erosions (often non-flexural areas)
- After infancy it is often limited to the flexures but may also affect the nape of the neck and extensor surfaces of the limbs; moderate to severe eczema can be much more extensive
- Infections with *Staphylococcus aureus* are common and cause typical honey yellow crusts
- Eczema presents differently in Asian, African, and Afro-Carribean children:
- Skin can appear darkened rather than erythematous
- Extensive lichenification and prurigo lesions can occur
- Follicular and discoid patterns of atopic eczema are more common in children with darker skin

---

BOX 2 UK REFINEMENT OF THE HANIFIN AND RAJKA DIAGNOSTIC CRITERIA[5]

- To qualify as having atopic dermatitis/eczema, the child must have had an itchy skin condition in the past 12 months plus three or more of the following criteria:
- Onset below age 2 years*
- History of flexural involvement
- History of a generally dry skin
- Personal history of other atopic disease**
- Visible flexural dermatitis

*Not used in children under 4 years.
**In children under 4 years, a history of atopic disease in a first degree relative may be included.

BOX 3 TOPICAL CORTICOSTEROID POTENCY CLASSES

- Mild: 1% hydrocortisone
- Moderate: Betamethasone valerate 0.025% (Betnovate-RD) and clobetasone butyrate 0.05% (Eumovate)
- Potent: Betamethasone valerate 0.1% (Betnovate), hydrocortisone butyrate 0.1% (Locoid), mometasone furoate 0.1% (Elocon)
- Suprapotent: Clobetasol propionate 0.05% (Dermovate)
- Combined antimicrobials and corticosteroid: Hydrocortisone acetate 1% (mild) + fusidic acid 2% (Fucidin H); clobetasone butyrate 0.05% (moderate) + oxytetracycline 3% + nystatin (Trimovate); betamethasone valerate 0.1% (potent) + fusidic acid 2% (Fucibet); hydrocortisone butyrate 0.1% (potent) + chlorquinadol 3% (Locoid C)

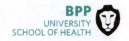

application of topical corticosteroids twice daily is more efficacious than once daily application. Furthermore, once daily application may increase adherence to treatment and reduce side effects and costs.[13] [14] When eczema is not controlled despite potent topical corticosteroids and full adherence to the prescribed emollient and bathing regimen, or when unsafe amounts of potent topical corticosteroids are needed, additional therapeutic approaches are required.

Antimicrobial treatments

Eczema flares are often attributable to infection, most commonly with *Staphylococcus aureus*. These infections can be clinically subtle.[4] Signs of bacterial infection include weeping, crusts, pustules, failure to respond to treatment, and rapidly worsening eczema. However, although skin infection undoubtedly plays a role in eczema flares, two Cochrane reviews of anti-staphylococcal measures (prophylactic and treatment) in routine eczema care found no clear evidence of additional clinical benefit.[15] [16] Nevertheless, it is still accepted clinical practice to use antimicrobial measures in patients with frequent skin infections. Combined corticosteroid and antimicrobial ointments can be used for short periods in infected eczema, but a course of oral antibiotics may be equally effective and bacterial resistance may be less likely to develop. An investigator blinded RCT of 31 patients (aged 6 months to 17 years) with moderate to severe clinically infected eczema reported that bleach baths (0.005% sodium hypochlorite), used together with intermittent nasal mupirocin, decreased the severity of eczema over three months.[17] However, the results could be explained by regression to the mean, and more evidence is needed to determine the exact role of such antiseptic measures in routine clinical practice.

Children with severe eczema are also at increased risk of eczema herpeticum (fig 2), which can be recurrent.[18] Early diagnosis and prompt treatment are essential, and parents should be educated about the clinical signs and the need to seek medical advice. Chickenpox and viral warts can be more severe in children with eczema. Molluscum contagiosum is common in children with eczema and can flare the disease when infected.

Colonisation with the yeast *Malassezia furfur* can also complicate eczema, particularly in the head and neck areas. Clues are a sharp cut-off line between affected and unaffected skin and only partial response to topical anti-inflammatory drugs. In such cases, the addition of a topical antifungal agent can result in great improvement.[w13]

Antihistamines

Systemic antihistamines are widely prescribed in eczema in the belief that they will reduce itch. The role of histamine in the itch of eczema is unclear, and it may play only a small part.[11] There is no good quality evidence for the usefulness of antihistamines in the management of eczema, and they are not routinely recommended. In an acute flare of eczema with serious sleep disturbance, children over 6 months of age can be offered a trial of an appropriate sedating antihistamine.[8]

When should a child with eczema be referred for specialist care?

Comprehensive referral advice is detailed in the recent NICE guidelines.[8] Referral to secondary care is recommended for several clinical scenarios, including if the diagnosis is uncertain, if the disease is not controlled satisfactorily

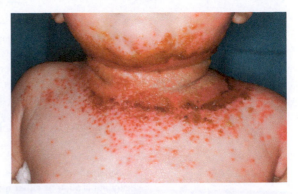

Fig 2 This baby had eczema herpeticum. After an incubation period of 5-12 days, eczema herpeticum presents as multiple, disseminated, vesiculopustular lesions and painful punched out erosions

with appropriate first line treatments, if there are severe or recurrent skin infections, if facial eczema is uncontrolled, if there are serious psychological problems, if the carers need specialist advice on treatment application, or if the child or parent(s) has serious disease associated social or psychological problems. In addition, children with moderate or severe food allergy or growth delay should be referred.[8]

What is severe eczema?

No universally agreed definition of severe eczema exists, but from a clinical point of view, severe disease is eczema that is resistant to first line topical treatments and has a considerable impact on quality of life. The European Taskforce on Atopic Dermatitis defined severe atopic dermatitis as having an eczema severity score (SCORAD) greater than 40 or "persistent" disease, whereas the NICE eczema guidelines refer to "widespread areas of dry skin, incessant itching, and skin redness," but there is no universal consensus on what constitutes a severe case or persistent disease.[11]

The use of validated and reliable severity scores in eczema is important in documenting the treatment response to systemic treatments. It is particularly important to balance safety concerns with efficacious treatment in children, and objective outcome scores can facilitate this. Of 20 severity scales, only three—the scoring atopic dermatitis index (SCORAD), the eczema area and severity index (EASI), and the patient oriented eczema measure (POEM) scores—have been adequately tested.[3] [6] The infant's dermatitis quality of life index (IDQOL) and children's dermatology life quality index (CDLQI) are useful and validated quality of life metrics in children with skin disease.[1]

How common is severe childhood eczema?

Most cases of childhood eczema are mild, but severe eczema is a challenge to manage. A UK study of 1760 children with eczema found that 84% had mild disease, 14% were classified as moderate, and 2% had severe disease.[w14] A Norwegian population survey reported similar findings.[w15]

How is severe eczema managed?

Topical calcineurin inhibitors

Topical calcineurin inhibitors (tacrolimus ointment 0.03% or 0.1% and pimecrolimus ointment 1%) block the production and release of proinflammatory cytokines.[7] They are approved by the Food and Drug Administration and European Medicines Agency as second line agents for the short term and pulsed long term treatment of moderate to severe eczema in immunocompetent patients aged over 2 years.

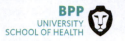

NICE guidelines for childhood eczema recommend their use when first line treatment of moderate to severe eczema with potent topical corticosteroids is contraindicated or has failed in children aged 2 years or more. They are also beneficial in areas of delicate skin, such as around the eyes, the face, the neck, and the nappy area, where the use of potent corticosteroids can cause skin atrophy. NICE recommends that calcineurin inhibitors are used only by physicians (including general practitioners) with a special interest and experience in dermatology.

A systematic review and meta-analysis showed that twice weekly application of either 0.1% tacrolimus ointment or a potent topical corticosteroid (weekend therapy) in patients with stable eczema, compared with vehicle (excipient) alone, significantly increased the time between disease exacerbations and increased the total number of disease-free days.[19] The safety profiles of calcineurin inhibitors are overall reassuring to date, and no causal link with cancer has been shown.[12 20] However, early but unconfirmed epidemiological evidence has emerged of an increased risk of cutaneous lymphoma, but longer term data are needed.[w16]

BOX 4 APPROACH TO NON-RESPONSE TO FIRST LINE TREATMENT

- Assess adherence to treatment recommendations and technique—look at how much of the topical agent is being applied and directly observe application
- Look for the presence of *Staphyloccocus aureus* and herpes simplex infection
- Consider whether allergens might be exacerbating the disease—immediate-type allergy to foods and aeroallergens as well as delayed-type hypersensitivity to a contact allergen, including topically applied drugs

---

BOX 5 POTENTIAL TRIGGERS FOR ECZEMA

- Irritants: Hard soaps, detergents, fragrances
- Infections: Molluscum contagiosum or infection with *Staphyloccocus aureus*, herpes simplex
- Overheating
- Psychological stress
- Aeroallergens: Pollens, grasses, animal dander, house dust mites
- Food allergens: In particular, egg, peanut, and cows' milk

BOX 6 PRETREATMENT SCREENING AND OTHER CONSIDERATIONS FOR SYSTEMIC IMMUNOSUPPRESSANT TREATMENT IN ECZEMA

- Pretreatment screening for infections includes testing for viral hepatitis, tuberculosis, and HIV, in addition to varicella zoster virus antibody (immune status), depending on the population being treated
- Pregnancy prevention should be considered when appropriate. Food and Drug Administration pregnancy categories are: ciclosporin: C, azathioprine: D, mycophenolate mofetil: D, and methotrexate: X
- Live vaccines (such as measles, mumps, and rubella; yellow fever; typhoid) are contraindicated while taking ciclosporin, methotrexate, and azathioprine
- Killed vaccines (such as influenza, hepatitis A, polio, rabies) are less likely to induce immunity in immunosuppressed patients
- Immunosuppressed patients may have more severe forms of infections such as influenza, and vaccination is therefore advised in patients taking systemic immunosuppressants; annual pneumococcal and influenza vaccination is recommended
- Patients and parents should be told about avoiding direct sun while on immunosuppressants because of the increased risk of skin cancer
- Check vitamin D values before and during treatment and supplement as needed (Sun avoidance is recommended in immunosuppressed patients, and this will increase the likelihood of vitamin D deficiency, which is common in northern regions.)
- Each treatment has individual screening protocols for renal, hepatic, and bone marrow impairment, and prescribers need to be familiar with these
- A full and frank discussion with children and parents about the risk-benefit balance is needed before treatment is started

Occlusive treatments (wet wraps)

Occlusion of the skin is widely used in severe eczema. Occlusive dressings increase skin hydration, act as a barrier to scratching, and promote restful sleep. The occlusion also promotes penetration of topical corticosteroids. However, wet wraps can exacerbate infections and increase dryness if not used appropriately, and patients and parents need to be educated in their use.[7] The wraps consist of a bottom (wet) and top (dry) layer. They are generally left in place overnight and applied for five to seven days in a row. In a critical review of 11 studies, only two of which were RCTs, wet wraps were reported as a useful short term treatment to induce disease remission.[20]

Ultraviolet light treatment

A systematic review of nine RCTs of ultraviolet light treatment found it to be effective compared with placebo.[21] It can help to delay or prevent the need for systemic immunomodulatory drugs, especially in children with dark (type V and VI) skin. The inability to comply with safe treatment may, however, preclude its use in younger children, and the practical aspect of treatment three times a week for several months may be difficult for some families. In addition, the long term risk of skin cancer is unknown and of particular concern in white children. When considering such treatment for severe eczema, the doctor should also be aware of the possible need for systemic immunomodulatory drugs later on because such treatment would further increase the risk of skin cancer.

Systemic immunomodulatory treatments

Children with severe eczema may require systemic immunosuppression to achieve disease control. Before considering such therapies, explore the possible reasons for the failure of first and second line treatments (boxes 4 and 5). Topical treatments require some expertise and can be labour intensive for families. Patients with disease refractory to standard treatments can be admitted to hospital or day care for observation of treatment application and response, before treatment is deemed a failure.

Systemic immunomodulatory drugs in severe eczema are not licensed for use in children and adolescents, apart from ciclosporin A, which is licensed in Germany for the management of eczema in patients over 16 years of age. The evidence base for usage and safety of these drugs in childhood eczema is not well established; practice has to be guided by experience in adult patients and the use of these drugs in other severe childhood inflammatory disorders, neither of which is ideal. Differences in prescribing across geographical regions are largely the result of established custom and practice and the familiarity of individual prescribers with the different agents, rather than being based on best evidence, and this is an area that urgently requires more intervention studies. All immunomodulatory drugs need pretreatment screening investigations, as well as close monitoring for side effects throughout the duration of treatment (box 6).

Ciclosporin A

Ciclosporin is a potent inhibitor of T cell dependent immune responses and interleukin 2 production. It is fast acting, allowing prompt induction of remission in severe eczema. The most notable side effects of nephrotoxicity and hypertension limit long term treatment. Ciclosporin A

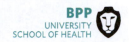

is therefore used as a short term treatment or as a bridge between treatments.

A systematic review of 10 RCTs investigating ciclosporin found that it is more effective in eczema than placebo but that relapse is rapid once treatment is stopped, with clinical scores often returning to baseline values within eight weeks.[13] A systematic review of 11 prospective clinical studies of ciclosporin A found that all showed decreased disease activity.[22] The effectiveness of ciclosporin A was similar in children and adults,[22] with younger patients showing greater tolerance.[23]

Azathioprine

Azathioprine is an inhibitor of purine synthesis that reduces the proliferation of leucocytes. The target cells and mechanism of action in eczema are not fully elucidated.[24] Azathioprine has a complex metabolism with several immunosupressant metabolites. The balance between thiopurine metabolites is governed by thiopurine methyltransferase (TPMT) activity.[24] The pre-treatment determination of TPMT genotype or activity level allows informed drug dosing to minimise myelotoxicity. Other side effects include headache and gastrointestinal upset, hepatotoxicity, and drug hypersensitivity. Azathioprine has a slow onset of action, with a notable clinical improvement at two to eight weeks into treatment.[w17] A double blind placebo controlled crossover RCT of eczema in adults reported that azathioprine significantly improved quality of life measures. There was a mean reduction in disease activity of 27% after 12 weeks of treatment.[25] In a series of 28 children with severe eczema treated with azathioprine, 17 reported significant improvement, six some improvement, and five no improvement. Laboratory abnormalities were seen in seven patients and the dose had to be adjusted.[26] Personal experience is that patients treated with azathioprine take longer to respond and do not rebound as often or as rapidly as those treated with ciclosporin when treatment is stopped.

Methotrexate

Methotrexate is commonly used for other chronic inflammatory diseases including adult psoriasis and childhood arthritis. Its mode of action is not fully understood, but it has anti-inflammatory effects and reduces allergen specific T cell activity.[w18] It is thought to augment concentrations of adenosine, which acts as an endogenous anti-inflammatory agent by mediating cytokine release and adhesion molecule expression, as well as by binding to adenosine cell surface receptors.[27] Gastrointestinal disturbance, liver function abnormalities, and bone marrow suppression are potential side effects, although the drug is generally well tolerated.[27] Evidence for the use of methotrexate in eczema is limited, with a single RCT of methotrexate use in adults.[28] This was a single blind parallel group RCT in 42 patients with severe eczema. Patients were randomly assigned to receive methotrexate or azathioprine for 12 weeks. This study suggests that methotrexate and azathioprine are equally effective in treating eczema in the short term, but larger adequately powered studies with longer follow-up are needed.[w19] A case series of 25 children with refractory discoid eczema treated with methotrexate reported that eczema had cleared in 16 and almost cleared in three. The drug was well tolerated and no adverse events were seen.[29]

Mycophenolate mofetil

Mycophenolate mofetil selectively and reversibly inhibits inosine monophosphate dehydrogenase, which suppresses the de novo pathway of purine synthesis, resulting in selective suppression of lymphocyte function. Unwanted effects on other cell types are minimised. The most common side effect is gastrointestinal disturbance. Mild increases in serum concentrations of liver enzymes are also reported. Severe bone marrow suppression is uncommon.[30] This drug is used in recalcitrant eczema, although no controlled studies have investigated its efficacy. A retrospective case series of 14 children with severe eczema treated with mycophenolate mofetil reported that eczema cleared completely in four and that four children had an excellent response, five a good response, and one an inadequate response. The drug was well tolerated in all patients.[30] In a case series of 12 children who moved from azathioprine to mycophenolate for management of their eczema, eight were reported to have significant improvement and four no improvement.[26]

Are there any new treatment targets for severe eczema?

It is hoped that new insights into the complex pathophysiology of eczema will allow more targeted treatments aimed at dysregulated structural or immune functions, and that a better understanding of eczema endophenotypes will facilitate a more individualised approach to treatment. Furthermore, insights into filaggrin synthesis and function will facilitate strategies aimed at increasing its expression.[w20] Agents that induce antimicrobial peptides might reduce the risk of skin infection,[w20] and biological agents that influence the early development of specific B cell and T cell clones may help reduce the inflammatory cascade.[w21] All this requires more basic research and, eventually, well designed RCTs with clearly defined diagnostic criteria and outcome domains related to disease severity, long term control of flares, and patients' quality of life.[w22]

Thanks to Rosemarie Watson for providing fig 2.

QUESTIONS AND AREAS FOR FUTURE RESEARCH

- Does the regular use of emollients directly after birth in high risk children reduce the risk of developing eczema?
- How effective are nurse led educational interventions?
- Does treating eczema early prevent severe disease?
- Does early intervention prevent respiratory allergies in later life?
- Do robust eczema endophenotypes exist? If so, could personalised treatment be developed?
- Which are the safest and most effective systemic immunosuppressive strategies for severe disease?
- A recent priority setting exercise by the James Lind Alliance involving patients and professionals identified 14 priority areas[w23]

TIPS FOR NON-SPECIALISTS

- Explore the effect of the condition on the child's sleep, schooling, sports, social activities, and family life. Acknowledging and, if possible, dealing with these stressors can improve management
- Ensure that topical treatments, including emollients and topical corticosteroids, are being applied correctly. Education of patients and parents is vital. Directly observed treatment is useful in determining the adherence of patients and parents to treatment
- Phobia about using topical corticosteroids is a common cause of non-adherence and needs to be dealt with
- Consider skin infection, which can be clinically subtle, in patients who do not respond to first line treatment
- Patients on systemic drugs need frequent expert assessments for treatment response, changes in disease status, and potential side effects

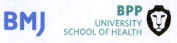

ADDITIONAL EDUCATIONAL RESOURCES

Resources for healthcare professionals

- Centre of Evidence Based Dermatology (www.nottingham.ac.uk/scs/divisions/evidencebaseddermatology/index.aspx)—Evidence based dermatology website including information from the Cochrane Skin Group, the UK Clinical Trials Dermatology Network, and the NHS Evidence website
- Cochrane Skin Group (http://skin.cochrane.org)—Evidence based dermatology website with systematic reviews
- Hoare C, Li Wan Po A, Williams H. Systematic review of treatments for atopic dermatitis. *Health Technol Assess* 2000;4:37. www.hta.ac.uk/fullmono/mon437.pdf
- National Institute for Health and Clinical Excellence. Atopic eczema in children. CG57. 2007. http://guidance.nice.org.uk/CG57

Information resources for patients

- National Eczema Association (www.eczema.org)—UK website with information for parents on eczema and general management principles
- National Eczema Association (www.nationaleczema.org)—US website on eczema for patients and parents, which includes information for schools and teachers
- Under My Skin (www.undermyskin.com)—Online books for children with eczema
- DermNet NZ (www.dermnetnz.org/dermatitis/treatment.html)—Information for patients and parents on treatments for eczema

A PATIENT'S PERSPECTIVE (A, AGED 8 YEARS)

When I had eczema it was hard for me not to scratch. I hated getting blood on my clothes. I felt sad not being able to do stuff like everybody else—not being able to swim and not being able to walk properly. I hated people saying things about my skin and getting in trouble for scratching. When I thought about my skin, scary questions came into my head. Would the eczema go away? Would I ever look normal? Would people laugh at me?

After treatment I feel so much happier. I can do stuff like everybody else. Life is so much easier now. Now my skin is better I don't have to worry about people laughing at me. I don't have to wear gloves at night to stop me scratching. Now I feel just like everybody else.

The mother's story

One of the hardest things was the sleep deprivation. One night seemed to roll into another. As parents we felt out of our depth. Our other children felt neglected as all of our time was consumed by A's skin and creams, baths, and bandages, as well as washing clothes and sheets because they were soiled with blood. It was stressful watching her scratch herself to pieces and nothing we did or said could stop her. The condition can get out of control, not only medically but in the way it affects your mind. It was the worst thing we have been through as a family. I feel blessed to have come out the other side. It may not be a terminal illness but it was very hard to cope with. We now feel we have control of her condition with the help of her medications. We have learnt so much along the way and now just look ahead to good times.

Contributors: MMcA and AI planned the article; MMcA did the background reading, prepared the first draft, and amended subsequent drafts after input from CF and ADI. ADI is guarantor.

Funding: None received.

Competing interests: All authors have completed the ICMJE uniform disclosure form at www.icmje.org/coi_disclosure.pdf (available on request from the corresponding author) and declare: no support from any organisation for the submitted work; no financial relationships with any organisations that might have an interest in the submitted work in the previous three years; no other relationships or activities that could appear to have influenced the submitted work.

Provenance and peer review: Not commissioned; externally peer reviewed.

Patient and parental consent obtained.

1 Lewis-Jones S. Quality of life and childhood atopic dermatitis: the misery of living with childhood eczema. *Int J Clin Pract* 2006;60:984-92.
2 Carroll CL, Balkrishnan R, Feldman SR, Fleischer AB Jr, Manuel JC. The burden of atopic dermatitis: impact on the patient, family, and society. *Pediatr Dermatol* 2005;22:192-9.
3 Schmitt J, Langan S, Williams HC. What are the best outcome measurements for atopic eczema? A systematic review. *J Allergy Clin Immunol* 2007;120:1389-98.
4 Bieber T. Atopic dermatitis. *N Engl J Med* 2008;358:1483-94.
5 Williams HC, Burney PG, Hay RJ, Archer CB, Shipley MJ, Hunter JJ, et al. The UK working party's diagnostic criteria for atopic dermatitis. I. Derivation of a minimum set of discriminators for atopic dermatitis. *Br J Dermatol* 1994;131:383-96.
6 Williams HC, Grindlay DJ. What's new in atopic eczema? An analysis of systematic reviews published in 2007 and 2008. Part 1. Definitions, causes and consequences of eczema. *Clin Exp Dermatol* 2009;35:12-5.
7 Krakowski AC, Eichenfield LF, Dohil MA. Management of atopic dermatitis in the pediatric population. *Pediatrics* 2008;122:812-24.
8 National Institute for Clinical Excellence Lewis-Jones S CM, Clark C et al. Atopic eczema in children. 2007. www.nice.org.uk/nicemedia/live/11901/38597/38597.pdf.
9 Ersser SJ, Latter S, Sibley A, Satherley PA, Welbourne S. Psychological and educational interventions for atopic eczema in children. *Cochrane Database Syst Rev* 2007;3:CD004054.
10 Staab D, Diepgen TL, Fartasch M, Kupfer J, Lob-Corzilius T, Ring J, et al. Age related, structured educational programmes for the management of atopic dermatitis in children and adolescents: multicentre, randomised controlled trial. *BMJ* 2006;332:933-8.
11 Darsow U, Wollenberg A, Simon D, Taieb A, Werfel T, Oranje A, et al. ETFAD/EADV eczema task force 2009 position paper on diagnosis and treatment of atopic dermatitis. *J Eur Acad Dermatol Venereol* 2010;24:317-28.
12 Shams K, Grindlay DJ, Williams HC. What's new in atopic eczema? An analysis of systematic reviews published in 2009-2010. *Clin Exp Dermatol* 2011;36:573-7; quiz 7-8.
13 Hoare C, Li Wan Po A, Williams H. Systematic review of treatments for atopic eczema. *Health Technol Assess* 2000;4:1-191.
14 Williams HC. Established corticosteroid creams should be applied only once daily in patients with atopic eczema. *BMJ* 2007;334:1272.
15 Birnie AJ, Bath-Hextall FJ, Ravenscroft JC, Williams HC. Interventions to reduce Staphylococcus aureus in the management of atopic eczema. *Cochrane Database Syst Rev* 2008;3:CD003871.
16 Bath-Hextall FJ, Birnie AJ, Ravenscroft JC, Williams HC. Interventions to reduce Staphylococcus aureus in the management of atopic eczema: an updated Cochrane review. *Br J Dermatol* 2010;163:12-26.
17 Huang JT, Abrams M, Tlougan B, Rademaker A, Paller AS. Treatment of Staphylococcus aureus colonization in atopic dermatitis decreases disease severity. *Pediatrics* 2009;123:e808-14.
18 Irvine AD, McLean WH, Leung DY. Filaggrin mutations associated with skin and allergic diseases. *N Engl J Med* 2011;365:1315-27.
19 Schmitt J, von Kobyletzki L, Svensson A, Apfelbacher C. Efficacy and tolerability of proactive treatment with topical corticosteroids and calcineurin inhibitors for atopic eczema: systematic review and meta-analysis of randomized controlled trials. *Br J Dermatol* 2011;164:415-28.
20 Williams HC, Grindlay DJ. What's new in atopic eczema? An analysis of the clinical significance of systematic reviews on atopic eczema published in 2006 and 2007. *Clin Exp Dermatol* 2008;33:685-8.
21 Meduri NB, Vandergriff T, Rasmussen H, Jacobe H. Phototherapy in the management of atopic dermatitis: a systematic review. *Photodermatol Photoimmunol Photomed* 2007;23:106-12.
22 Schmitt J, Schakel K, Schmitt N, Meurer M. Systemic treatment of severe atopic eczema: a systematic review. *Acta Dermatovenereol* 2007;87:100-11.
23 Schmitt J, Schmitt N, Meurer M. Cyclosporin in the treatment of patients with atopic eczema - a systematic review and meta-analysis. *J Eur Acad Dermatol Venereol* 2007;21:606-19.
24 Meggitt SJ, Gray JC, Reynolds NJ. Azathioprine dosed by thiopurine methyltransferase activity for moderate-to-severe atopic eczema: a double-blind, randomised controlled trial. *Lancet* 2006;367:839-46.
25 Berth-Jones J, Takwale A, Tan E, Barclay G, Agarwal S, Ahmed I, et al. Azathioprine in severe adult atopic dermatitis: a double-blind, placebo-controlled, crossover trial. *Br J Dermatol* 2002;147:324-30.
26 Waxweiler WT, Agans R, Morrell DS. Systemic treatment of pediatric atopic dermatitis with azathioprine and mycophenolate mofetil. *Pediatr Dermatol* 2011;28:689-94.
27 Weatherhead SC, Wahie S, Reynolds NJ, Meggitt SJ. An open-label, dose-ranging study of methotrexate for moderate-to-severe adult atopic eczema. *Br J Dermatol* 2007;156:346-51.
28 Schram ME, Roekevisch E, Leeflang MM, Bos JD, Schmitt J, Spuls PI. A randomized trial of methotrexate versus azathioprine for severe atopic eczema. *J Allergy Clin Immunol* 2011;128:353-9.
29 Roberts H, Orchard D. Methotrexate is a safe and effective treatment for paediatric discoid (nummular) eczema: a case series of 25 children. *Australas J Dermatol* 2010;51:128-30.
30 Heller M, Shin HT, Orlow SJ, Schaffer JV. Mycophenolate mofetil for severe childhood atopic dermatitis: experience in 14 patients. *Br J Dermatol* 2007;157:127-32.

Related links

bmj.com
- Get Cleveland clinic CME points for this article

bmj.com/archive
Previous clinical reviews
- Management of chronic epilepsy (2012;345:e4576)
- The diagnosis and management of tinea (2012;345:e4380)
- Perioperative management of patients taking treatment for chronic pain (2012;345:e4148)
- Manifestation, diagnosis, and management of foodborne trematodiasis (2012;344:e4093)
- Communicating risk (2012;344:e3996)

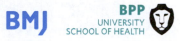

Allergic rhinitis in children

James G Barr core surgical trainee, Hiba Al-Reefy locum consultant rhinologist, Adam T Fox consultant paediatric allergist, Claire Hopkins consultant rhinologist

¹Department of ENT surgery, Guy's and St Thomas' Hospitals NHS Foundation Trust, London SE1 9RT, UK

Correspondence to: J G Barr
jgbarr85@gmail.com

Cite this as: BMJ 2014;349:g4153

‹DOI› 10.1136/bmj.g4153
http://www.bmj.com/content/349/bmj.g4153

Allergic rhinitis is a common paediatric condition. In a worldwide study of over one million adolescents aged 13 and 14 years the prevalence was 14.6%.[1] Allergic rhinitis is characterised by rhinorrhoea, nasal obstruction, epiphora, and nasal itching. Many patients and parents think of seasonal, pollen induced "hay fever"; however, numerous aeroallergens may produce perennial symptoms, and these have an important impact on children's quality of life.[2][3] Evidence based guidelines, advances in drug treatments, and novel specific immunotherapy have all improved the management of allergic rhinitis. We review the current literature, with particular respect to the Allergic Rhinitis and its Impact on Asthma guidelines, produced by the World Health Organization.[2]

What is allergic rhinitis and why is it important?

Allergic rhinitis is an IgE mediated disorder triggered by exposure of nasal mucosa to allergens. This results in rhinorrhoea, itching, and sneezing as well as sleep disturbance, which are easily observed and reported by parents or guardians. However, nasal congestion, the most common symptom of allergic rhinitis, may be more difficult to elicit from young children.[2][4]

Allergic rhinitis is a common form of non-infectious rhinitis, but it is often confused with non-allergic conditions that can cause similar symptoms, including infections, endocrine disorders, and anatomical abnormalities (box 1).[2] Allergic rhinitis is the most common cause of nasal congestion in children.[5]

People with allergic rhinitis predominantly present to primary care. The Allergic Rhinitis in Schoolchildren Consensus Group found that the condition impaired school performance.[6] It can also cause dysfunction in the family and difficulty integrating with peers.[3] A study of 23 children with allergic rhinitis and 69 controls found significantly lower health related quality of life (assessed using the

child health questionnaire) in children with allergic rhinitis compared with healthy controls.[7] Quality of life can, however, be improved with treatment.[3]

How common is it?

The prevalence of allergic rhinitis in children is increasing.[2] In England, 10% of 6 and 7 year olds and 15-19% of 13 and 14 year olds have allergic rhinitis.[8] The International Study of Asthma and Allergies in Childhood surveyed 1.2 million children in 98 countries.[1] In western Europe 8.3% of 6 and 7 year olds had allergic rhinitis, compared with 8.8% in North America and 13.1% in South America.[1] Overall, 80% of patients presenting with symptoms are diagnosed as having allergic rhinitis before 20 years of age.[9] For 80-90% of children with allergic rhinitis symptoms continue into adulthood.[10]

How is allergic rhinitis classified?

In both adults and children allergic rhinitis is subdivided into intermittent or persistent depending on the frequency of symptoms.[2] Intermittent allergic rhinitis is related to infrequently encountered allergens such as animal danders, whereas persistent allergic rhinitis is related to commonly encountered allergens such as house dust mites.[2] Intermittent allergic rhinitis is diagnosed if symptoms occur for less than four days a week or for less than four consecutive weeks.[2] Persistent allergic rhinitis is diagnosed when symptoms occur for more than four days a week and for more than four consecutive weeks.[2]

This classification replaced the previous one, which distinguished between seasonal and perennial allergic rhinitis, because symptoms may be triggered by many different allergens and patients may be exposed to allergens throughout the year.[2] In an observational study of 2347 people with allergic rhinitis, 72% were sensitised to both seasonal allergens (pollens) and perennial allergens (house

---

BOX 1 DIFFERENTIAL DIAGNOSES FOR RHINITIS[2]

Common causes
- Rhinosinusitis
- Deviated nasal septum
- Hypertrophied turbinates
- Adenoid hypertrophy
- Foreign bodies
- Vasomotor rhinitis
- Rhinitis medicamentosa

Rarer causes
- Ostiomeatal complex variants
- Choanal atresia
- Benign and malignant tumour
- Sarcoid
- Wegener's granulomatosis
- Ciliary defects
- Cerebrospinal rhinorrhoea

SOURCES AND SELECTION CRITERIA

We searched Medline for randomised controlled trails, systematic reviews, and meta-analyses using the terms "allergic rhinitis" and "paediatrics". We also reviewed the references used in the Allergic Rhinitis and its Impact on Asthma guidelines and consulted the Cochrane database of systematic reviews. Articles were included if all authors agreed on their relevance.

SUMMARY POINTS

- Allergic rhinitis is an important and common condition that causes major morbidity in children and is a risk factor for the development of asthma
- Nasal irrigation with saline is effective in children, improving symptoms, and reducing the need for drug treatment
- Second generation H1 antihistamines are effective and safe for the treatment of allergic rhinitis and ocular symptoms in rhinoconjunctivitis
- Modern intranasal glucocorticoids such as mometasone furoate and fluticasone propionate have not been found to impair growth; they can be used in children aged 6 and 4 years respectively
- Immunotherapy is the only treatment that can modify disease progress; it also has the potential to reduce the risk of asthma in patients with allergic rhinitis

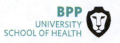

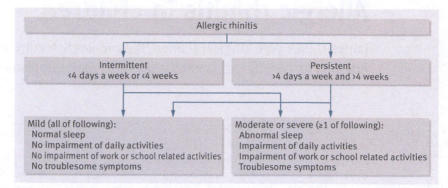

Fig 1 Classification of allergic rhinitis. From Allergic Rhinitis and its Impact on Asthma guidelines, World Health Organization[2]

dust mite, cat and dog dander).[11] In a cross sectional study of 6533 patients assessing the new classification of allergic rhinitis, more than 50% of people sensitised to seasonal allergens had persistent allergic rhinitis.[12]

The classification of severity is based on the impact of symptoms on quality of life. If sleep and daily activities are not affected and symptoms are not too troublesome, then the allergic rhinitis is considered to be mild (fig 1).[2]

What causes it?
The development of allergic rhinitis is mediated by genetic and environmental factors.[2] In a longitudinal cohort study of 8176 families the likelihood of allergic rhinitis developing increased with a personal or parental history of allergy.[13] The odds ratio of having allergic rhinitis at age 4.5 years was 10.21 if the child had a positive food allergy test result at age 4.5 years and 2.21 if the parents had a history of rhinitis.[13]

Common allergens include house dust mites, animal danders, moulds, and tree and grass pollens. In a European study of 3034 adults and children from 14 countries, 33.4% of patients had a clinically relevant allergy to grasses, 26.5% to house dust mites, and 19.4% to cat dander.[14] These allergens stimulate the release of mast cell mediators, which leads to initial symptoms after about 10 minutes.[15] [16] Histamine is one of the key mediators of the early phase response, causing rhinorrhoea, nasal itch, and sneezing.[16] [17] Subsequent recruitment of other inflammatory cells leads to a late phase response characterised clinically by nasal obstruction.[16] [17]

Is allergic rhinitis linked to asthma?
The epidemiological link between asthma and allergic rhinitis is well established.[18] Both conditions are diseases of respiratory tract mucosa, linked by common immunological processes, and they respond to similar treatments.[19] In children with coexisting allergic rhinitis and asthma, exacerbation of allergic rhinitis leads to acute episodes of asthma, whereas treatment of rhinitis improves asthma control.[20] Children with allergic rhinitis are at a greater risk of asthma.[18] [21] In a cohort study of 7383 children, allergic rhinitis in childhood was associated with a sevenfold increased risk of asthma in the preadolescent period.[22] In a smaller cohort study of 1314 children the relative risk for developing wheeze in the preadolescent period was 3.82 in 5 year olds with allergic rhinitis.[23]

How is it diagnosed?
Allergic rhinitis is a clinical diagnosis made according to diagnostic criteria, with allergy testing where necessary. A detailed patient and parental history will provide information about the severity and frequency of the symptoms, triggers, and response to treatment.

Anterior rhinoscopy should be performed in primary care (this may be easily done using a standard auroscope). Young children are best examined while sitting on their parent's or guardian's lap with the caregiver placing one arm around the child's head and one around the arms. The auroscope is inserted into the nose in a posterior superior direction. Whereas normal mucosa is pink, the nasal mucosa in allergic rhinitis is typically swollen and greyish. Examination can identify hypertrophy of the nasal turbinates (fig 2), nasal polyps (rare in children, except in those with cystic fibrosis) (fig 3), foreign bodies, or purulence in the nasal cavity suggestive of adenoiditis or rhinosinusitis.[9] Differentiation between polyps and hypertrophied turbinates can be difficult, and when uncertainty exists about the diagnosis then referral to an ear, nose, and throat specialist is necessary. Nasal swabs for culture are not diagnostically useful.[2] Red flag symptoms in children with allergic rhinitis include unilateral symptoms, recurrent bloody nasal discharge, pain, or visual disturbance. A cranial nerve examination should be performed to assess the eye for visual disturbance and diplopia and the face for paraesthesia and weakness that could indicate a rare sinonasal tumour. Children with any of these symptoms should be referred urgently to an ear, nose, and throat specialist for further assessment.

Children should be routinely referred to secondary care if symptoms remain poorly controlled despite medical treatment (fig 4), treatment causes troublesome side effects, or the diagnosis remains uncertain (box 2). Referral can be made either to an ear, nose, and throat specialist or to an allergy clinic depending on local availability, although if coexistent asthma is poorly controlled an allergist may be preferable.

Investigations in secondary care include nasendoscopy, which allows visualisation of the posterior nasal cavity and middle meatus.[2] Radiology is not routinely required in primary or secondary care.

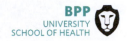

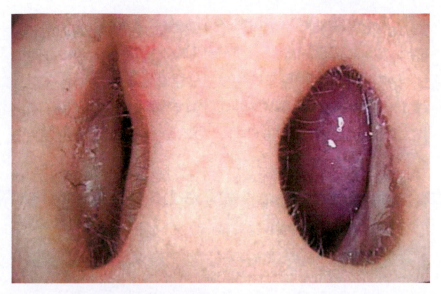

Fig 2 Nasal cavity with hypertrophied inferior turbinate on right

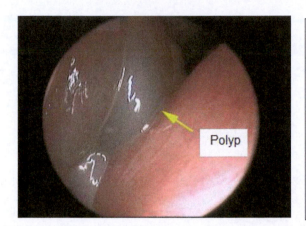

Polyp

Fig 3 Large nasal polyp viewed using a nasendoscope

BOX 2 WHEN TO REFER PATIENTS

- If symptoms are poorly controlled despite medical treatment (see fig 4) or the patient experiences troublesome side effects from treatment
- If there is concern about other diagnoses such as chronic rhinosinusitis and nasal polyps
- If symptoms are atypical—recurrent bloody nasal discharge, pain, disturbance in vision, or neurological signs, warrant consideration for urgent referral
- If nasal obstruction predominates, refer to an ear, nose, and throat specialist
- If itching and rhinorrhoea predominant, particularly in the presence of asthma, refer to an allergy specialist

When is allergy testing appropriate?

A systematic review on allergy testing in children recommends testing for allergic rhinitis if symptoms are resistant to treatment or the child is being investigated for concurrent asthma.[24] In a cross sectional study of 784 children in primary care with doctor diagnosed allergic rhinitis, 89% had a positive IgE test result for one or more allergens.[25] Allergy testing can determine a specific allergy and therefore can help to encourage avoidance of allergens and help in the recommendation of allergy specific treatment such as antihistamines or immunotherapy.[2 25]

Allergy testing is performed by either skin prick testing or measuring the levels of serum specific IgE.[26] In skin prick testing selected allergens as well as positive and negative controls (histamine and glycerol, respectively) are introduced through the skin using a needle.[2] Any wheal greater than 3 mm at 15 minutes is considered important, providing there is no response to the negative control (fig 5).[2]

Radioallergosorbent testing using radiolabelled anti-IgE is used to quantify the serum levels of IgE for a particular allergen. Testing for specific allergens is based on clinical suspicion, as with skin prick testing. Commonly, radioallergosorbent testing measures responses to house dust mites, pollen, and dander from cats, dogs, and other furred animals.[24]

Skin prick testing has a better positive predictive value than radioallergosorbent testing (48.7% v 43.5%, respectively) and provides immediate results for discussion with patients.[26] The results can, however, be influenced by the recent use of antihistamines. In practice, the choice between tests in primary care will depend on local availability.

How is allergic rhinitis treated?

The treatment of allergic rhinitis includes avoidance of allergens, nasal irrigation, drugs, and specific immunotherapy.

Allergen avoidance

Allergen control has principally focused on reducing exposure to house dust mites. However, a multicentre randomised controlled trial of 696 children found no difference between children assigned to preventive measures, which included mite impermeable mattress covers and an educational package on allergen avoidance, and those assigned to the control group.[27] Therefore the Allergic Rhinitis and its Impact on Asthma guidelines do not recommend either chemical or physical methods to reduce exposure to house dust mite.[28]

In another randomised controlled trial, symptoms of allergic rhinitis were significantly reduced in people with an allergy to cat dander who were instructed on environmental interventions compared with controls. Environmental controls included washing the cats every two weeks,

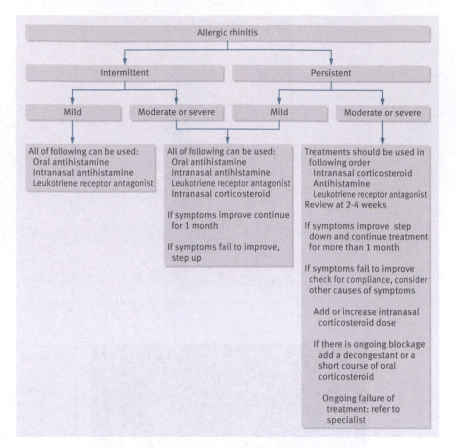

Fig 4 Treatment algorithm for allergic rhinitis[2]

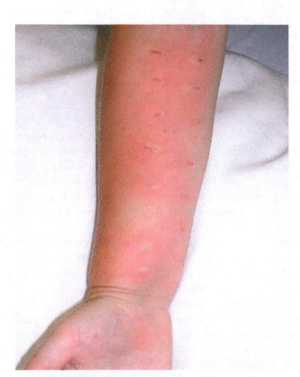

Fig 5 Result of skin prick testing on a child's arm. Marks in black correspond to different allergens being tested. Wheals are indicative of a positive test result

Additionally it recommends that patients with an allergy to mould should avoid exposure to indoor moulds.[28] Indoor moulds are associated with dampness. Exposure to moulds can be reduced by eliminating any sources of dampness and cleaning the environment thoroughly to remove the moulds.

Nasal irrigation

Nasal irrigation with saline is an inexpensive treatment for allergic rhinitis. A randomised controlled trial of 20 children with allergic rhinitis showed a considerable improvement in nasal itching and congestion, rhinorrhoea, and sneezing in those assigned to nasal irrigation using hypertonic saline (n=10) and reduced the need for antihistamines after two weeks of treatment.[30]

Saline irrigation improves mucociliary function, reducing mucosal oedema and decreasing inflammatory mediators.[30] Irrigation is generally well tolerated in children because of the preference towards finer sprays, and it can be used in infants aged 1 month or more.[31] Commercially available paediatric irrigation kits contain a nasal irrigation bottle and sachets of measured sodium chloride for adding to warm water. Alternatively, a small syringe or a bulb applicator may be used. Ideally, douching may be incorporated into a daily bathing regimen and should be continued while symptoms persist.

Drug treatment

Drugs available for treating allergic rhinitis in children are oral or intranasal antihistamines, intranasal corticosteroids, and leukotriene receptor antagonists.[2 32] Figure 4 provides an algorithm for the treatment of allergic rhinitis. The Allergic Rhinitis and its Impact on Asthma guidelines do

removing carpets from bedrooms, and washing floors regularly.[29] The 2010 update of the Allergic Rhinitis and its Impact on Asthma guidelines recommends that sensitised patients should avoid exposure to animal dander at home.[28]

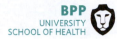

not recommend treatments in a particular order, except in persistent, moderate or severe allergic rhinitis where intranasal steroids are the preferred treatment.[2]

Antihistamines

First generation antihistamines such as chlorphenamine should be avoided in children, as their sedating action can further impair school performance.[33] Second generation H1 antihistamines, such as cetirizine, azelastine, desloratidine, levocitirizine, and loratadine, have fewer side effects than earlier formulations; in particular they are less sedating, faster acting, and have a longer duration of action.[32]

For moderately severe intermittent allergic rhinitis or mild persistent allergic rhinitis the Allergic Rhinitis and its Impact on Asthma guidelines recommend that if there is a response to antihistamines then treatment should be continued for one month and then reviewed. If there is no improvement then alternative treatments should be considered.[2] We would advise that patients are reviewed 2-4 weeks after starting treatment, or sooner if symptoms have not improved. A systematic review found that oral and intranasal preparations were equally effective in treating allergic rhinitis.[33] However, intranasal treatment has a faster onset of action than oral treatment. In a small randomised controlled trial of 46 patients, the onset of action for intranasal azelastine was 15 minutes compared with 150 minutes for oral desloratidine.[34] Treatment for ocular symptoms should be given orally; alternatively, intraocular topical treatment can be used.[32]

A multicentre randomised controlled trial consisting of 360 children showed that rupatadine, a second generation antihistamine, significantly reduced total nasal symptom scores (for severity of sneezing, rhinorrhoea, and nasal and ocular pruritus) after four weeks compared with placebo.[35] Another double blinded randomised controlled trial of 177 children showed that once daily levocitrizine in children resulted in a significant improvement in the symptoms of allergic rhinitis compared with placebo.[36] More than 80% of the children reported an improvement in symptoms with levocitrizine. None of the children discontinued treatment during the six week study period because of side effects.

Parents and patients should be informed about the possibility of drowsiness, even with second generation antihistamines, which normally improves after a few days. Other side effects include headache and gastrointestinal upset.[37] A meta-analysis of randomised controlled trials found that 24.1% of children taking fexofenadine experienced an adverse event compared with 24.4% taking placebo.[38] Headache was the commonest reported side effect, occurring in 4.3% of participants taking placebo and 5.8% of participants taking fexofenadine. No sedative effects were reported. The commonest reported adverse effect with intranasal antihistamines is bitter taste, with the rate of epistaxis and nasal discomfort being the same as for placebo.[39]

Levocitirizine, cetirizine and loratadine are all licensed for use in children over 2 years of age.[37][40]

Intranasal corticosteroids

Corticosteroids have a key role in suppressing the allergic response, and intranasal application allows high drug concentrations to be achieved locally with minimal adverse systemic effects.[32] A randomised controlled trial of 134 children aged 6-11 years with allergic rhinitis randomised to 100 µg mometasone furoate once daily had a significant reduction in total nasal symptom scores compared with children randomised to placebo, reducing scores by 39%.[41] A systematic review of 16 randomised controlled trials comprising 2267 participants (adults and children) confirmed the superiority of intranasal corticosteroids over antihistamines in allergic rhinitis.[42] Intranasal corticosteroids are more effective than antihistamines for nasal congestion and should be used if congestion predominates.[2][43] It is safe for intranasal corticosteroids to be initiated in primary care and they should be continued as long as symptoms persist. Mometasone furoate and fluticasone propionate are licensed for use in children over the age of 6 and 4 years respectively.[40] However, the European Academy of Allergy and Clinical Immunology recommends their use in children as young as 2 years.[33] Intranasal steroids should be administered with the head tilted forwards. The nozzle should be introduced into the nose and pointed along the hard palate and slightly laterally to avoid contact with the septum.

The onset of action of intranasal steroids is slower than that of intranasal antihistamines. In a randomised controlled trial of 425 patients it took 150 minutes for an effect to be noticed with mometasone compared with 30 minutes for nasal olopatadine.[44] A meta-analysis in children and adults found that the therapeutic effect of fluticasone became apparent within 12 hours, but in some of the studies this was as early as 2-4 hours.[45]

Patients and parents should be counselled about the possible side effects of intranasal steroids, including irritation of the nose and throat, epistaxis, headaches, and disturbances with smell and taste.[37] Studies suggest that the side effect profile of modern intranasal steroids is similar to that of placebo. In a subanalysis of three randomised controlled trials in children aged 6-11 years, 7% of adverse events occurred in those taking fluticasone and 8% in those taking placebo.[46] Headache was the commonest adverse event. The rate of epistaxis was 4% in both the groups.[46]

Modern intranasal glucocorticoids have low bioavailability and have not been found to impair growth.[46][47] The hypothalamic-pituitary-adrenal axis does not seem to be affected by intranasal glucocorticoids.[46][47] In a randomised controlled trial comparing mometasone furoate with placebo in 98 children, no impact on growth was found in children as young as 3 years after treatment with 100 µg of mometasone furoate once daily for one year.[48] The authors also found that it was safe to continue treatment in children who required inhaled or topical corticosteroids for asthma or atopic dermatitis.[48] Betametasone should, however, be avoided in children because of its high bioavailability and risk of growth retardation.[49]

Given that studies have not shown an effect on the hypothalamic-pituitary-adrenal axis, weaning off treatment is not required.

Other drug treatments

Leukotrienes are inflammatory mediators produced by inflammatory cells, including mast cells and eosinophils.[50] A systemic review of 11 trails found that antileukotrienes were as equally effective as antihistamines but less effective than nasal corticosteroids in improving nasal symptom scores and quality of life in patients with allergic rhinitis.[50] Antileukotrienes are recommended for all forms of intermittent allergic rhinitis as well as for mild persistent allergic rhinitis and are third line treatment for moderate or severe persistent allergic rhinitis. They are particularly useful

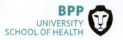

in patients with coexisting asthma and allergic rhinitis as they reduce bronchospasm and attenuate the inflammatory response.[50] Montelukast is recommended for the treatment of allergic rhinitis in children older than 6 years.[2] It is well tolerated, with a meta-analysis showing that side effects in children were similar to those of placebo.[51] Treatment should be continued while children are symptomatic, but if there is no response to treatment after 2-4 weeks then an alternative drug should be considered.

Nasal decongestants relieve nasal obstruction but are ineffective against other symptoms such as itching and sneezing.[2] Additionally, prolonged use can cause rebound congestion.[52] The Allergic Rhinitis and its Impact on Asthma guidelines do not recommend the use of nasal decongestants in children with allergic rhinitis.[30]

Immunotherapy

Immunotherapy, or desensitisation, involves exposing patients to increasing amounts of allergen to induce immunological tolerance.[2] Accurate identification of the triggering allergen by clinical history in combination with allergen testing is key.

Immunotherapy can be delivered subcutaneously or sublingually, with sublingual treatment more commonly used in children. For subcutaneous treatment, a weekly injection of allergen extract is given. Dosage is progressively increased until a maintenance dose is achieved, and thereafter monthly injections are continued for two or three years.[53] Sublingual treatment delivers the allergen extract under the tongue. As with subcutaneous treatment, the dosage is increased until a maintenance dose is achieved. After an initial dose under medical supervision, treatment may be administered at home. A meta-analysis of 22 double blinded randomised controlled trials of 979 adults and children found that immunotherapy improved symptoms scores and reduced drug use. Another meta-analysis of 10 placebo controlled double blinded randomised controlled trials in 577 children with allergic rhinitis showed sublingual treatment to be effective at reducing symptom scores in children and adolescents aged 3-18 years as well as reducing requirements for drug treatment.[54] These findings were corroborated by a Cochrane review of children and adults who received sublingual treatment.[55] In children, sublingual treatment was more effective if used for longer than 18 months.[54] The exact duration of immunotherapy in children is unknown, but it is conventionally given for three years.[33 56] In a controlled study in 23 children a significant reduction in symptoms of allergic rhinitis and sensitisation to new allergens occurred six years after cessation of immunotherapy, suggesting that the treatment has a disease modifying effect.[57]

Side effects of sublingual treatment range from localised itch, rhinitis, and mild asthma to (rarely) anaphylaxis.[2] [53] A Cochrane review found that severe side effects were rare. There were no reported cases of anaphylaxis.[55] Other adverse events included wheezing, urticaria, conjunctivitis, gastrointestinal upset, and headache. The number of reported adverse events was similar in people taking sublingual immunotherapy and placebo, except for gastrointestinal upset, which was reported by 88/630 people in the sublingual immunotherapy group and 10/561 people in the placebo group. Taking antihistamines before immunotherapy reduces both the frequency and the severity of systemic side effects.[2] Sublingual treatment avoids the morbidity of repeated injections and the need

for hospital attendance. Immunotherapy can be used in children aged more than 5 years.[2] In addition to the direct benefits of immunotherapy in children with allergic rhinitis, specific immunotherapy can also reduce the risk of asthma.[21 58] In a randomised controlled trial in 113 children with allergic rhinitis but no asthma, those in the control arm were 3.8 times more likely to develop asthma than those in the sublingual treatment arm.[59] The reduction in the risk persisted after the cessation of immunotherapy.[58] Additionally, children receiving sublingual treatment needed fewer drugs for allergic rhinitis and reported lower symptom scores.[59] Thus there is great potential for reducing the burden of disease caused by allergic rhinitis as well as for reducing the risk of asthma.

Guidelines form the British Society for Allergy and Clinical Immunology recommend that immunotherapy should be considered in patients with poorly controlled symptoms despite maximal drug treatment.[56] Contraindications include use of β blockers and perennial asthma, unless symptoms are mild and intermittent and controlled with occasional use of bronchodilators.[56]

ADDITIONAL EDUCATIONAL RESOURCES

Resources for healthcare professionals

- Bousquet J, Khaltaev N, Cruz AA, Denburg J, Fokkens WJ, Togias A, et al. Allergic rhinitis and itsimpact on asthma (ARIA). *Allergy* 2008;63:990-6—An excellent resource covering all aspects of the diagnoses and management of allergic rhinitis in children and adults
- Brozek JL, Bousquet J, Baena-Cagnani CE, Bonini S, Canonica GW, Casale TB, et al. Global Allergy and Asthma European Network; Grading of Recommendations Assessment, Development and Evaluation Working Group. Allergic Rhinitis and its Impact on Asthma (ARIA) guidelines: 2010 revision. *J Allergy Clin Immunol* 2010;126:466-76—2010 update of the ARIA guidelines
- Bousquet J, Van Cauwenberge P, Bachert C, Canonica GW, Demoly P, Durham SR, et al. European Academy of Allergy and Clinical Immunology (EAACI); Allergic Rhinitis and its Impact on Asthma (ARIA). Requirements for medications commonly used in the treatment of allergic rhinitis. *Allergy* 2003;58:192-7—Useful information on the drug management of allergic rhinitis
- Penagos M, Compalati E, Tarantini F, Baena-Cagnani R, Huerta J, Passalacqua G, et al. Efficacy of sublingual immunotherapy in the treatment of allergic rhinitis in pediatric patients 3 to 18 years of age: a meta-analysis of randomized, placebo-controlled, double-blind trials. *Ann Allergy Asthma Immunol* 2006;97:141-8—Provides evidence for the use of sublingual immunotherapy in children
- Mallol J, Crane J, von Mutius E, Odhiambo J, Keil U, Stewart A; ISAAC Phase Three Study Group. The International Study of Asthma and Allergies in Childhood (ISAAC) phase three: a global synthesis. *Allergol Immunopathol (Madr)* 2013;41:73-85—Useful epidemiological data on the prevalence of allergic rhinoconjunctivitis worldwide

Resources for patients

- Allergy UK. (www.allergyuk.org)—A good overview of allergic rhinitis, along with information on the treatments and how to administer them
- NHS. Allergic rhinitis. (www.nhs.uk/conditions/rhinitis---allergic/Pages/Introduction.aspx)—A more detailed overview of allergic rhinitis as well as additional information on diagnostic tests

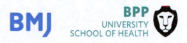

Contributors: JGB wrote the manuscript. HA-R, ATF, and CH co-wrote the manuscript. ATF provided the illustrations. CH was the senior author for the project. She is the guarantor.

Competing interests: We have read and understood the BMJ Group policy on declaration of interests and declare the following interests: ATF is a trustee of Allergy UK; a site principal investigator for a multicentre study of the sublingual immunotherapy product Grazax produced by ALK-Abello; has lectured for Medapharma, GSK, Stallergenes, and Allergy Therapeutics; and has received payment from GSK and Medapharma towards travel and accommodation costs for attendance at conferences.

Provenance and peer review: Not commissioned; externally peer reviewed.

Patient consent: Obtained.

1   Aït-Khaled N, Pearce N, Anderson HR, Ellwood P, Montefort S, Shah J; ISAAC Phase Three Study Group. Global map of the prevalence of symptoms of rhinoconjunctivitis in children: the International Study of Asthma and Allergies in Childhood (ISAAC) phase three. Allergy2009;64:123-48.

2   Bousquet J, Khaltaev N, Cruz AA, Denburg J, Fokkens W J, Togias A, et al. Allergic Rhinitis and its Impact on Asthma (ARIA) 2008. Allergy2008;63(suppl 86):8-160.

3   Meltzer EO. Quality of life in adults and children with allergic rhinitis. J Allergy Clin Immunol2001;108(1 Suppl):S45-53.

4   International Consensus Report on Diagnosis and Management of Rhinitis. International Rhinitis Management Working Group. Allergy1994;49(Suppl 19):1-34.

5   Scadding G. Optimal management of nasal congestion caused by allergic rhinitis in children: safety and efficacy of medical treatments. Paediatr Drugs2008;10:151-62.

6   Blaiss MS; Allergic Rhinitis in Schoolchildren Consensus Group. Allergic rhinitis and impairment issues in schoolchildren: a consensus report. Curr Med Res Opin2004;20:1937-52.

7   Silva CH, Silva TE, Morales NM, Fernandes KP, Pinto RM. Quality of life in children and adolescents with allergic rhinitis. Braz J Otorhinolaryngol2009;75:642-9.

8   Ghouri N, Hippisley-Cox J, Newton J, Sheikh A. Trends in the epidemiology and prescribing of medication for allergic rhinitis in England. J R Soc Med2008;101:466-72.

9   Skoner DP. Allergic rhinitis: definition, epidemiology, pathophysiology, detection, and diagnosis. J Allergy Clin Immunol2001;108(1 Suppl):S2-8.

10 Linna O, Kokkonen J, Lukin M. A 10-year prognosis for childhood allergic rhinitis. Acta Paediatrica1992;81:100-2.

11 Ciprandi G, Cirillo I, Vizzaccaro A, Tosca M, Passalacqua G, Pallestrini E, et al. Seasonal and perennial allergic rhinitis: is this classification adherent to real life? Allergy2005;60:882-7.

12 Demoly P, Allaert FA, Lecasble M, Bousquet J; PRAGMA. Validation of the classification of ARIA (allergic rhinitis and its impact on asthma). Allergy2003;58:672-5.

13 Alm B, Goksör E, Thengilsdottir H, Pettersson R, Möllborg P, Norvenius G, et al. Early protective and risk factors for allergic rhinitis at age 4½ yr. Pediatr Allergy Immunol2011;22:398-404.

14 Burbach GJ, Heinzerling LM, Edenharter G, Bachert C, Bindslev-Jensen C, Bonini S, et al. GA(2)LEN skin test study II: clinical relevance of inhalant allergen sensitizations in Europe. Allergy2009;64:1507-15.

15 Lee JH, Yu HH, Wang LC, Yang YH, Lin YT, Chiang BL. The levels of CD4+CD25+ regulatory T cells in paediatric patients with allergic rhinitis and bronchial asthma. Clin Exp Immunol2007;148:53-63.

16 Howarth PH, Salagean M, Dokic D. Allergic rhinitis: not purely a histamine-related disease. Allergy2000;55(Suppl 64):7-16.

17 Simons FE, Simons KJ. Histamine and H1-antihistamines: celebrating a century of progress. J Allergy Clin Immunol 2011;128:1139-50.

18 Leynaert B, Neukirch F, Demoly P, Bousquet J. Epidemiologic evidence for asthma and rhinitis comorbidity. J Allergy Clin Immunol2000;106(5 Suppl):S201-5.

19 Scheinmann P, Pham Thi N, Karila C, de Blic J. Allergic march in children, from rhinitis to asthma: management, indication of immunotherapy. Arch Pediatr2012;19:330-4.

20 Erbas B, Akram M, Dharmage SC, Tham R, Dennekamp M, Newbigin E, et al. The role of seasonal grass pollen on childhood asthma emergency department presentations. Clin Exp Allergy2012;42:799-805.

21 Möller C, Dreborg S, Ferdousi HA, Halken S, Høst A, Jacobsen L, et al. Pollen immunotherapy reduces the development of asthma in children with seasonal rhinoconjunctivitis (the PAT-study). J Allergy Clin Immunol2002;109:251-6.

22 Burgess JA, Walters EH, Byrnes GB, Matheson MC, Jenkins MA, Wharton CL, et al. Childhood allergic rhinitis predicts asthma incidence and persistence to middle age: a longitudinal study. J Allergy Clin Immunol2007;120:863-9.

23 Rochat MK, Illi S, Ege MJ, Lau S, Keil T, Wahn U, et al; Multicentre Allergy Study (MAS) group. Allergic rhinitis as a predictor for wheezing onset in school-aged children. J Allergy Clin Immunol2010;126:1170-5.

24 Høst A, Andrae S, Charkin S, Diaz-Vázquez C, Dreborg S, Eigenmann PA, et al. Allergy testing in children: why, who, when and how? Allergy2003;58:559-69.

25 De Bot CM, Röder E, Pols DH, Bindels PJ, van Wijk RG, van der Wouden JC, et al. Sensitisation patterns and association with age, gender, and clinical symptoms in children with allergic rhinitis in primary care: a cross-sectional study. Prim Care Respir J2013;22:155-60.

26 Tschopp JM, Sistek D, Schindler C, Leuenberger P, Perruchoud AP, Wuthrich B, et al. Current allergic asthma and rhinitis: diagnostic efficiency of three commonly used atopic markers (IgE, skin prick tests, and Phadiatop). Results from 8329 randomized adults from the SAPALDIA Study. Swiss Study on Air Pollution and Lung Diseases in Adults. Allergy1998;53:608-13.

27 Horak F Jr, Matthews S, Ihorst G, Arshad SH, Frischer T, Kuehr J; SPACE study group. Effect of mite-impermeable mattress encasings and an educational package on the development of allergies in a multinational randomized controlled birth-cohort study—24 months results of the Study of Prevention of Allergyin Children in Europe. Clin Exp Allergy2004;34:1220-5.

28 Brozek JL, Bousquet J, Baena-Cagnani CE, Bonini S, Canonica GW, Casale TB, et al. Global Allergy and Asthma European Network; Grading of Recommendations Assessment, Development and Evaluation Working Group. Allergic Rhinitis and its Impact on Asthma (ARIA) guidelines: 2010 revision. J Allergy Clin Immunol2010;126:466-76.

29 Björnsdottir US, Jakobinudottir S, Runarsdottir V, Juliusson S. The effect of reducing levels of cat allergen (Fel d 1) on clinical symptoms in patients with cat allergy. Ann Allergy Asthma Immunol2003;91:189-94.

30 Garavello W, Romagnoli M, Sordo L, Gaini RM, Di Berardino C, Angrisano A. Hypersaline nasal irrigation in children with symptomatic seasonal allergic rhinitis: a randomized study. Pediatr Allergy Immunol2003;14:140-3.

31 Iapak I, Skoupá J, Strnad P, Horník P. Efficacy of isotonic nasal wash (seawater) in the treatment and prevention of rhinitis in children. Arch Otolaryngol Head Neck Surg 2008;134:67-74.

32 Bousquet J, Van Cauwenberge P, Bachert C, Canonica GW, Demoly P, Durham SR, et al; European Academy of Allergy and Clinical Immunology (EAACI); Allergic Rhinitis and its Impact on Asthma (ARIA). Requirements for medications commonly used in the treatment of allergic rhinitis. European Academy of Allergy and Clinical Immunology (EAACI), Allergic Rhinitis and its Impact on Asthma (ARIA). Allergy2003;58:192-7.

33 Roberts G, Xatzipsalti M, Borrego LM, Custovic A, Halken S, Hellings PW, et al. Paediatric rhinitis: position paper of the European Academy of Allergy and Clinical Immunology. Allergy2013;68:1102-16.

34 Horak F, Zieglmayer UP, Zieglmayer R, Kavina A, Marschall K, Munzel U, et al. Azelastine nasal spray and desloratadine tablets in pollen-induced seasonal allergic rhinitis: a pharmacodynamic study of onset of action and efficacy. Curr Med Res Opin2006;22:151-7.

35 Potter P, Maspero JF, Vermeulen J, Barkai L, Németh I, Baillieau RA, et al. Rupatadine oral solution in children with persistent allergic rhinitis: a randomized, double-blind, placebo-controlled study. Pediatr Allergy Immunol2013;24:144-50.

36 De Blic J, Wahn U, Billard E, Alt R, Pujazon MC. Levocetirizine in children: evidenced efficacy and safety in a 6-week randomized seasonal allergic rhinitis trial. Pediatr Allergy Immunol2005;16:267-75.

37 Joint Formulary Committee. British national formulary for children. BMA, RPS, 2013.

38 Meltzer EO, Scheinmann P, Rosado Pinto JE, Bachert C, Hedlin G, Wahn U, et al. Safety and efficacy of oral fexofenadine in children with seasonal allergic rhinitis—a pooled analysis of three studies. Pediatr Allergy Immunol2004;15:253-60.

39 Shah SR, Nayak A, Ratner P, Roland P, Michael Wall G. Effects of olopatadine hydrochloride nasal spray 0.6% in the treatment of seasonal allergic rhinitis: a phase III, multicenter, randomized, double-blind, active- and placebo-controlled study in adolescents and adults. Clin Ther2009;31:99-107.

40 European Medicines Agency. 2014. www.ema.europa.eu/ema/.

41 Meltzer EO, Baena-Cagnani CE, Gates D, Teper A. Relieving nasal congestion in children with seasonal and perennial allergic rhinitis: efficacy and safety studies of mometasone furoate nasal spray. World Allergy Organ J2013;6:5.

42 Weiner JM, Abramson MJ, Puy RM. Intranasal corticosteroids versus oral H1 receptor antagonists in allergic rhinitis: systematic review of randomised controlled trials. BMJ1998;317:1624-9.

43 Bhatia S, Baroody FM, deTineo M, Naclerio RM. Increased nasal airflow with budesonide compared with desloratadine during the allergy season. Arch Otolaryngol Head Neck Surg2005;131:223-8.

44 Patel D, Garadi R, Brubaker M, Conroy JP, Kaji Y, Crenshaw K, et al. Onset and duration of action of nasal sprays in seasonal allergic rhinitis patients: olopatadine hydrochloride versus mometasone furoate monohydrate. Allergy Asthma Proc2007;28:592-9.

45 Meltzer EO, Rickard KA, Westlund RE, Cook CK. Onset of therapeutic effect of fluticasone propionate aqueous nasal spray. Ann Allergy Asthma Immunol2001;86:286-91.

46 Meltzer EO, Tripathy I, Máspero JF, Wu W, Philpot E. Safety and tolerability of fluticasone furoate nasal spray once daily in paediatric patients aged 6-11 years with allergic rhinitis: subanalysis of three randomized, double-blind, placebo-controlled, multicentre studies. Clin Drug Investig2009;29:79-86.

47 Brannan MD, Herron JM, Affrime MB. Safety and tolerability of once-daily mometasone furoate aqueous nasal spray in children. Clin Ther1997;19:1330-9.

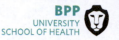

48 Schenkel EJ, Skoner DP, Bronsky EA, Miller SD, Pearlman DS, Rooklin A, et al. Absence of growth retardation in children with perennial allergic rhinitis after one year of treatment with mometasone furoate aqueous nasal spray. *Pediatrics*2000;105:E22.

49 Skoner D, Rachelefsky G, Meltzer E, Chervinsky P, Morris R, Seltzer J, et al. Detection of growth suppression in children during treatment with intranasal belcomethasone dipropionate. *Pediatrics*2000;105:e23.

50 Wilson AM, O'Byrne PM, Parameswaran K. Leukotriene receptor antagonists for allergic rhinitis: a systematic review and meta-analysis. *Am J Med*2004;116:338-44.

51 Bisgaard H, Skoner D, Boza ML, Tozzi CA, Newcomb K, Reiss TF, et al. Safety and tolerability of montelukast in placebo-controlled pediatric studies and their open-label extensions. *Pediatr Pulmonol*2009;44:568-79.

52 Johnson DA, Hricik JG. The pharmacology of alpha-adrenergic decongestants. *Pharmacotherapy*1993;13:S110-5; discussion S143-6.

53 Wilson DR, Lima MT, Durham SR. Sublingual immunotherapy for allergic rhinitis: systematic review and meta-analysis. *Allergy*2005;60:4-12.

54 Penagos M, Compalati E, Tarantini F, Baena-Cagnani R, Huerta J, Passalacqua G, et al. Efficacy of sublingual immunotherapy in the treatment of allergic rhinitis in pediatric patients 3 to 18 years of age: a meta-analysis of randomized, placebo-controlled, double-blind trials. *Ann Allergy Asthma Immunol*2006;97:141-8.

55 Radulovic S, Calderon MA, Wilson D, Durham S. Sublingual immunotherapy for allergic rhinitis. *Cochrane Database Syst Rev*2010;12:CD002893.

56 Walker SM, Durham SR, Till SJ, Roberts G, Corrigan CJ, Leech SC, et al. Immunotherapy for allergic rhinitis. *Clin Exp Allergy*2011;41:1177-200.

57 Eng PA, Reinhold M, Gnehm HP. Long-term efficacy of preseasonal grass pollen immunotherapy in children. *Allergy*2002;57:306-12.

58 Jacobsen L, Niggemann B, Dreborg S, Ferdousi HA, Halken S, Høst A, et al. (The PAT investigator group). Specific immunotherapy has long-term preventive effect of seasonal and perennial asthma: 10-year follow-up on the PAT study. *Allergy*2007;62:943-8.

59 Novembre E, Galli E, Landi F, Caffarelli C, Pifferi M, De Marco E, et al. Coseasonal sublingual immunotherapy reduces the development of asthma in children with allergic rhinoconjunctivitis. *J Allergy Clin Immunol*2004;114:851-7.

Related links

bmj.com/archive
Previous articles in this series
- Obstructive sleep apnoea (BMJ 2014;348:g3745)
- Medical management of breast cancer (BMJ 2014;348:g3608)
- Skin disease in pregnancy (BMJ 2014;348:g3489)
- Management of cutaneous viral warts (BMJ 2014;348:g3339)

bmj.com
- Get CPD/CME credits

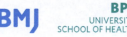

Kawasaki disease

Anthony Harnden university lecturer in general practice[1], Masato Takahashi professor of paediatrics emeritus[2], David Burgner associate professor of paediatrics[3]

[1]Department of Primary Health Care, University of Oxford, Headington, Oxford OX3 7LF

[2]University of Southern California, Keck School of Medicine, Children's Hospital, Los Angeles, 90027 CA, USA

[3]School of Paediatrics and Child Health, University of Western Australia, Child and Adolescent Health Service, GPO Box D184, Perth WA 6840, Australia

Correspondence to: A Harnden
anthony.harnden@dphpc.ox.ac.uk

Cite this as: *BMJ* 2009;338:b1514

‹DOI› 10.1136/bmj.b1514
http://www.bmj.com/content/338/bmj.b1514

Parents worry about meningitis, but few have heard of Kawasaki disease, and most doctors have never seen a case. But Kawasaki disease is an important diagnosis not to miss in febrile children because treatment within the first 10 days of illness may prevent acute and long term coronary artery damage, which on rare occasions can be fatal.[1] Diagnostic difficulty arises because many of the early clinical features of Kawasaki disease mimic other more common self limiting febrile illnesses. To make an early diagnosis of Kawasaki disease doctors should have a high index of suspicion in an irritable child with five or more days of fever, irrespective of other clinical features. This article aims to give an overview of Kawasaki disease for doctors who manage febrile children.

What is Kawasaki disease and who gets it?

Kawasaki disease is an acute febrile illness of early childhood, with about 80% of cases occurring between 6 months and 5 years. It is characterised by fever lasting at least five days and a constellation of clinical features that are used as diagnostic criteria (box 1). The clinical features are similar in all ethnic groups.[2] Kawasaki disease is an acute inflammatory vasculitis of medium sized elastic arteries that has a striking propensity to damage the coronary arteries. As a consequence, it is the leading cause of acquired heart disease in children in developed countries.

Kawasaki disease was first reported in Japan more than 40 years ago,[w1] and the condition has since been described in most populations. It is not clear if Kawasaki disease is a new disease; reports of similar clinical features are rare in Japan before the mid-20th century, whereas in Europe infantile polyarteritis nodosa, a much rarer condition that shares many features with Kawasaki disease, has been described for more than a century.[3]

SOURCES AND SELECTION CRITERIA

We searched PubMed and Cochrane databases using the keywords "Kawasaki disease" or "mucocutaneous lymph node syndrome". We reviewed abstracts from the last three international Kawasaki disease symposiums (2001, 2005, 2008). Our focus was on systematic reviews, national guidelines, and randomised controlled trials. We reviewed the reference lists of all articles retrieved together with those in our personal reference libraries. For the treatment section we looked at systematic reviews and randomised controlled trials only.

SUMMARY POINTS

- Kawasaki disease is an acute febrile illness that mainly affects children under 5
- It is the most common cause of acquired heart disease in children in the developed world
- Diagnosis is based on fever of at least five days' duration and four of five diagnostic clinical criteria
- The typical clinical features appear sequentially and are rarely all there at presentation
- The diagnosis should be considered in any child with prolonged fever, irrespective of other features
- Intravenous immunoglobulin and aspirin given 5-10 days after onset of fever reduce the incidence of coronary artery lesions from around 20% to around 5%

BOX 1 CLINICAL DIAGNOSTIC CRITERIA

- Fever of at least five days' duration and at least four of the following five clinical features:
- Polymorphous exanthema (but not petechial, bullous, or vesicular lesions)
- Bilateral non-exudative conjunctival injection
- Changes in lips and oral cavity (but not discrete oral lesions or exudates)
- Changes in the extremities, including erythema or indurative oedema, and later (in the second week of illness) membranous desquamation starting around the nail bed
- Cervical lymphadenopathy, often unilateral and large (.1.5 cm)

How common is Kawasaki disease?

The incidence of Kawasaki disease varies worldwide, and it is up to 20 times more common in North East Asians than in white people. The highest rates are reported in nationwide surveys in Japan; in 2005-6 the annual incidence reached 184 per 100000 children under 5 years.[4] Epidemiological studies report an incidence of up to 95 per 100000 in Korea,[w2] and 104 per 100000 in Taiwan in children under 5.[w3] [w4] In comparison, an analysis of hospital episode statistics in England reported an incidence that has increased over the past two decades to eight per 100000.[5] [6] The higher incidence in North East Asians persists after migration to countries with low incidence.[7] Parents of Japanese children with Kawasaki disease are more likely to have had the condition as children,[8] and the risk in siblings of children with Kawasaki disease is also significantly higher.[w5] Reports of cases in rapidly developing countries such as India have recently increased,[w3] perhaps because of improved recognition or the appearance of Kawasaki disease at a time of rapid industrialisation.[w3 w6 w7]

What causes Kawasaki disease?

Despite four decades of research, attempts to identify a causative pathogen or environmental trigger have so far been unsuccessful (see box on bmj.com). Epidemiological data suggest that one or more widely distributed infectious agent triggers an abnormal inflammatory response in a genetically predisposed child.[1] [9] [10] An infectious trigger is supported by the pronounced seasonality, with winter and spring peaks in most temperate countries[11] and summer peaks in many Asian countries,[w3] together with reported epidemics of the disease.[w8] The clinical features can initially be mistaken for severe infection. Kawasaki disease is relatively rare in the first few months of life, which suggests that most adults have been exposed to the causative agent and that protective transplacental antibodies protect the newborn infant.[w9] Supportive data are rare, however, because the infectious trigger(s) are unknown. Kawasaki disease is much less common in older children and adults and recurs in only a minority of children.[w10] We suggest that most children probably encounter the causative pathogen(s)

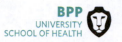

in early childhood—possibly asymptomatically—and develop protective immunity.

The role of bacterial superantigens in Kawasaki disease remains controversial.[12] Like other inflammatory diseases—such as rheumatoid arthritis, inflammatory bowel disease, and atherosclerosis—Kawasaki disease is genetically complex, with many genes contributing modest effects to the overall risk, and no single gene "causing" the disease.

How is Kawasaki disease diagnosed?

Children with Kawasaki disease are febrile and extremely irritable, much more so than children with other febrile illnesses (fig 1). No diagnostic test is available. Clear diagnostic criteria have been established by the Japanese Ministry of Health research committee and have been adopted by the American Heart Association and American Academy of Pediatrics (box 1).[13] The clinical features usually appear sequentially, and a diagnosis of Kawasaki disease should be reconsidered regularly in a young child with persistent fever. The differential diagnosis of Kawasaki disease is potentially wide, but it is most often confused with streptococcal and staphylococcal infections (including scarlet fever and toxic shock syndrome), viral infections such as measles and glandular fever, or drug reactions such as Stevens-Johnson syndrome.[1 13] Children tend to be listless and easily fatigued for four to six weeks after the acute illness, which usually lasts one to two weeks without treatment.[13] It is in the subacute phase that coronary artery aneurysms may progress. Box 2 summarises the laboratory features of Kawasaki disease.

The nature of the rash in Kawasaki disease is variable. It may be made up of pink maculopapular lesions (morbilliform rash) (fig 2), sharply demarcated red lesions (erythema multiforme), or generalised or uniform redness (scarlatiniform rash). Petechial, vesicular, or bullous lesions are not a feature and suggest an alternative diagnosis. The rash often begins in the

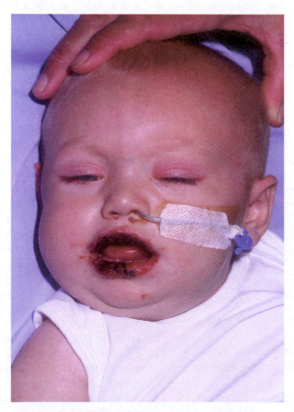

Fig 1 Eight month old boy with acute Kawasaki disease

THE PARENTS' PERSPECTIVE

When our baby was 10 months old he woke with a high temperature and seemed to have a sore throat. He wouldn't eat or drink and his breath smelled. We took him to a general practitioner, who diagnosed tonsillitis and prescribed antibiotics. He quickly got worse.

The next day I carried him, limp in my arms, to the emergency department. He was dehydrated and he had a faint rash on his legs and torso, bright red lips and eye rims, and a fever. The doctor told us it might be Kawasaki disease among other things. After he was admitted he continued to deteriorate. We were told that he did not meet all the criteria for a diagnosis of Kawasaki disease; he didn't have the peeling skin on his hands and feet and his rash was "too faint." We were told that treatment for Kawasaki disease could not begin until other illnesses such as scarlet fever and infection were ruled out. Five days after admission he was given immunoglobulin. Within hours he was smiling again and happy. After he had been home for a few days, the "missing symptom" of peeling skin appeared. Because he was treated early, he did not develop any heart abnormalities, but it was distressing having such a sick baby, not knowing what was wrong or whether he would develop long term heart problems.

BOX 2 CLINICAL INVESTIGATIONS

The following tests are often abnormal during the first 7-10 days and may support the diagnosis of Kawasaki disease, although in isolation these tests lack adequate sensitivity and specificity. Some parameters have age dependent normal ranges[1 13 14 w11]

- Haematology: Raised white blood cell count with neutrophilia (at least 50% of cases), progressive anaemia (usually normochromic and normocytic), increasing platelet count (peaking in the second or third week of illness and therefore not useful diagnostically)

- Urine analysis: The urinary sediment may contain increased numbers of white blood cells without bacteruria

- Acute phase reactants: Raised C reactive protein (>35 mg/l in 80% of cases), erythrocyte sedimentation rate (>60 mm/h in 60% of cases). The erythrocyte sedimentation rate may be even higher after intravenous immunoglobulins

- Blood chemistry: Low serum sodium, low serum protein and albumin, raised liver enzymes (specifically alanine aminotranferase), and abnormal lipid profile (which may be exacerbated by intravenous immunoglobulin)

- Cerebrospinal fluid: Pleocytosis, usually lymphocytic with normal protein and glucose

- Electrocardiography: Other than tachycardia, findings include decreased QRS voltages, flattened T waves, and prolonged rate corrected QT intervals. These findings are almost always reversible. Arrythmias including heart block may occur. In untreated large coronary artery aneurysms, electrocardiography may show signs of myocardial infarction as a result of coronary thrombosis

- Echocardiography: This may show decreased left ventricular function, mitral regurgitation, and pericardial effusion. Coronary artery dilatation begins an average of 9-10 days after onset of fever and occurs in 30-50% of cases

nappy area and spreads to the rest of the torso, extremities, and face. This nappy rash may peel during the acute illness.

A unique feature of Kawasaki disease is acute inflammation at the site of a previous BCG inoculation. The hands and feet may be swollen, erythematous, and painful to touch or on weight bearing, and the child often

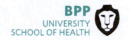

refuses to walk or crawl. In older children, desquamation of fingers and toes (fig 3), which occurs after the acute illness and is therefore not helpful diagnostically, may be the only peripheral feature. Conjunctival injection, which appears early in the illness, is not associated with purulent discharge and often spares the limbus, an avascular zone around the iris. Oropharyngeal changes may affect the lips, tongue, or pharynx, but pharyngeal exudates and ulcers are not seen. Cervical lymphadenopathy, the least frequent diagnostic feature, is more common in older children. A solitary lymph node is often non-fluctuant, firm, and mildly tender.

Rarely, there is severe peripheral vasculitis, with Raynaud's phenomenon. Severe vasculitis and vasospasm can cause distal ischaemia and result in gangrene of the fingers and toes.[w12]

Incomplete Kawasaki disease

The 15-20% of children with Kawasaki disease who have fever and fewer than four principal features may still develop coronary artery dilatation or aneurysms. They are classified as having incomplete Kawasaki disease, a particularly challenging diagnosis that is more common in infants under 6 months.[15]

The American Heart Association and American Academy of Pediatrics have published an algorithm to help in the early detection of incomplete Kawasaki disease (see bmj.com).[13] This algorithm represents expert consensus and uses commonly available laboratory tests and echocardiography, when indicated. It has been evaluated retrospectively but not yet prospectively in the clinical setting.[w13]

How is Kawasaki disease treated?

Intravenous immunoglobulin

Randomised controlled trials have shown that a single infusion of 2 g/kg of intravenous immunoglobulin given 5-10 days after the onset of fever eliminates fever in 85-90%

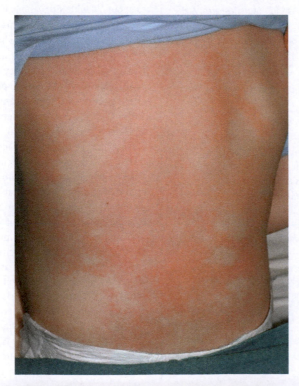

Fig 2 Morbilliform rash in young child with Kawasaki disease

of children within 36 hours and significantly reduces the risk of coronary artery aneurysms.[13 16] A single intravenous immunoglobulin infusion of 2 g/kg produces a better outcome than 400 mg/kg/day for five days.[16 17] The benefit of starting immunoglobulin before the fifth day of illness is uncertain, but treatment should be given beyond day 10 if fever or inflammation is ongoing.[13] Guidelines recommend a further dose of 2 g/kg in children who remain febrile 36 hours after the first dose of immunoglobulin.[13]

Aspirin

A Cochrane review and a meta-analysis of treatment with aspirin highlighted a lack of trial evidence,[18] although aspirin has been standard treatment for Kawasaki disease since its initial description in Japan because of its anti-inflammatory and antiplatelet activities. The American Academy of Pediatrics acknowledges that practice varies with respect to dose and duration of treatment, with most clinicians prescribing 80 mg/kg/day until the child is afebrile and 3-5 mg/kg/day thereafter until a normal echocardiogram is seen at six weeks after the onset of symptoms.[13] In Japan, however, it is common practice to give aspirin 30 mg/kg/day throughout the acute and subacute phases. Persistent coronary artery abnormalities require specialist management.

Corticosteroids

In contrast to other systemic vasculitides, which usually respond to steroids, evidence that corticosteroids reduce coronary artery abnormalities is inconclusive. A meta-analysis of trials of variable quality concluded that the addition of corticosteroids was beneficial.[w14] However, a recent well conducted, multicentre, double blinded, placebo controlled randomised trial reported no difference in coronary artery changes, days spent in hospital, and length of fever for children receiving standard treatment of intravenous immunoglobulin and aspirin plus 30 mg/kg of methylprednisolone compared with standard treatment plus placebo.[19] Although trial evidence is lacking, 30 mg/kg methylprednisolone daily for up to three days is usually recommended if there is no response to the second intravenous immunoglobulin infusion.

Other interventions

Controlled trial data are not available for other interventions such as plasma exchange, agents that block platelet receptors and tumour necrosis factor, pentoxifylline, cyclophosphamide, and statins. Live vaccines—including measles, mumps, and rubella—should be delayed after treatment with intravenous immunoglobulin, because neutralising antibodies may decrease vaccine immunogenicity.[20] The recommended interval between intravenous immunoglobulin and live vaccines varies—three months in the United Kingdom and 11 months in the United States, Canada, and Australia.

What are the cardiovascular complications of Kawasaki disease?

Clinical signs

Cardiovascular examination during acute Kawasaki disease may show tachycardia greater than expected for the patient's age and fever. Rarely, pancarditis and heart failure can occur, with muffled heart tones and gallop rhythm suggestive of either myocarditis or pericardial effusion.

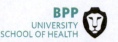

Myocarditis is thought to be common, but it rarely results in clinically relevant depression of myocardial function.[13]

Coronary artery pathology

Consensus guidelines from the American Heart Association on the diagnosis, treatment, and long term management of Kawasaki disease state that mild diffuse dilatation of coronary arteries occurs in 30-50% of cases and starts on average 10 days from onset of fever. In most cases, this dilatation is transient and regresses within six to eight

Fig 3 Membranous desquamation of fingers—a late clinical sign

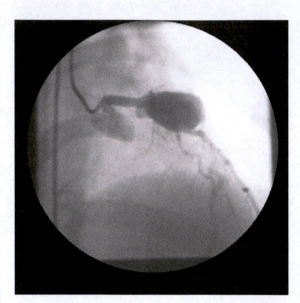

Fig 4 Selective left coronary angiogram showing a giant aneurysm of the anterior descending coronary artery

---

CURRENT RESEARCH AND KEY UNANSWERED QUESTIONS

Ongoing research

- An international collaborative project that is investigating the genetic determinants of Kawasaki disease (International Kawasaki Disease Genetics Consortium; dburgner@meddent. uwa.edu.au)
- Attempts are being made to identify viral pathogen(s) from autopsy specimens
- A global study is under way of the association between weather patterns and Kawasaki disease
- The optimal treatment for Kawasaki disease is being investigated, including the role of anti-tumour necrosis factor agents

Unanswered questions

- Does Kawasaki disease have a single infectious cause or can it be triggered by more than one type of infection? Are bacterial superantigens involved?
- Which genes are important in mediating susceptibility and outcome?
- What is the optimal way to diagnose Kawasaki disease? How does the American Heart Association algorithm perform in practice?
- Can we develop a bedside diagnostic test?
- What are the long term effects of the disease on cardiovascular health?
- Is Kawasaki disease proatherosclerotic and is this clinically important?
- What is the relation between Kawasaki disease and other inflammatory and autoimmune diseases?
- Is Kawasaki disease really increasing in incidence in countries undergoing industrialisation, and if so, why?

ADDITIONAL EDUCATIONAL RESOURCES

Resources for healthcare professionals

- Brogan PA, Bose A, Burgner D, Shingadia D, Tulloh R, Michie C, et al. Kawasaki disease: an evidence based approach to diagnosis, treatment, and proposals for future research. *Arch Dis Child* 2002;86:286-90
- Royle J, Burgner D, Curtis N. The diagnosis and management of Kawasaki disease. *J Paediatr Child Health* 2005;41:87-93

Resources for parents and families

- Patient UK (www.patient.co.uk/showdoc/23069080/)—Information sheet for patients on Kawasaki disease
- Kawasaki Disease Foundation (www.kdfoundation.org/)—A US parent led charity to raise awareness and share experiences
- Kawasaki Disease Foundation Australia (www.kdfoundation.org.au)—Group set up by families with children who have had Kawasaki disease, which provides information, social gatherings, research findings, and contact with other families affected
- Royal Children's Hospital, Melbourne (www.rch.org.au/kidsinfo/factsheets.cfm?doc_id=3731)—A succinct and sensible summary of Kawasaki disease for parents

Baker AL, Newburger JW. Kawasaki disease. *Circulation* 2008;118:e110-2

TIPS FOR NON-SPECIALISTS

- Consider the diagnosis of Kawasaki disease in a child who is irritable with a persistent fever—the classic clinical features of Kawasaki disease may not all be present
- The rash may mimic that of common infections like measles, rubella, parvovirus, and scarlet fever. It may also resemble erythema multiforme
- To reduce complications, a single infusion of 2 g/kg of intravenous immunoglobulin should be given 5-10 days after the start of fever
- All children with Kawasaki disease should have echocardiography and access to a paediatric cardiology opinion and follow-up

---

weeks of fever onset.[13] However, 20% of coronary artery lesions progress to true aneurysms, although this is reduced to about 5% with intravenous immunoglobulin treatment. In about 1% of cases, aneurysms become "giant aneurysms" (>8 mm diameter) (fig 4), which carry a poor prognosis; they may heal with stenosis and cause distal myocardial ischaemia, or more rarely they may rupture.[13 w15]

Although Kawasaki disease preferentially affects coronary arteries, other medium to large arteries may be affected. Proximal brachial arteries, femoral arteries, iliac arteries, and extraparenchymal renal arteries most often show aneurysmal changes. The aorta may show aneurysmal dilatation in postmortem specimens.[13]

An unclear vasculitic process within the coronary arteries increases endothelial activation and renders the endothelium procoagulant. In addition, the blood becomes hypercoagulable because of an increased number of activated platelets.[w16] In the presence of large aneurysms, stagnation of flow and local changes in shear stress further promote thrombosis. A large case series of Japanese children who had myocardial infarction showed that infarction as a result of occlusive thrombosis in the coronary arteries is most common during the first 6-12 months after onset.[21] The standardised mortality ratio during the convalescent stage of Kawasaki disease for Japanese children with cardiac sequelae has been reported to be as high as 2.55 in boys.[22] The in-hospital mortality rate is 0.17% in the US.[11] Cardiac arrythmias are more common after Kawasaki disease and

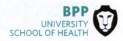

may occur independently of coronary artery involvement.[w17] Heart block and fever may occasionally be the only presenting features of Kawasaki disease.[w18]

What are the longer term implications of Kawasaki disease?

The original Japanese cohorts are now approaching middle age and are still too young for modest effects on the risk of clinically important atherosclerosis to be detected. In those with obvious changes to the coronary arteries during acute Kawasaki disease, surrogate markers of atherosclerosis are abnormal in many studies, which suggests that later cardiovascular risk may be increased.[23]

About half of patients who recover from Kawasaki disease have serum lipid abnormalities, mostly abnormally low high density lipoprotein, but some have raised low density lipoprotein or triglycerides.[w19] Patients with giant aneurysms who survive may still develop ischaemic heart disease years later because of de novo development of localised coronary stenosis.

Children with giant coronary artery aneurysms have a high probability of myocardial infarction or ischaemic events.[24] The risk of future cardiac events for children with small aneurysms or transient coronary dilatation (lasting only for 6-8 weeks) is uncertain. The American Heart Association has produced cardiovascular risk stratification guidelines for children with Kawasaki disease (see bmj.com)

Conclusion

Kawasaki disease is an important cause of fever in young children. It results in a high incidence of cardiovascular damage if not treated promptly. The diagnosis should always be considered in the young child with an unexplained and persistent fever, despite the absence of full diagnostic criteria.

Contributors: AH and DB planned the paper and all three authors contributed to the first draft. AH and DB edited and revised the draft and MT approved the final manuscript. AH is guarantor.

Competing interests: None declared

Provenance and peer review: Commissioned; externally peer reviewed.

Patient consent obtained.

1 Burns JC, Glode MP. Kawasaki syndrome. Lancet2004;364:533-44.
2 Burgner D, Harnden A. Kawasaki disease: what is the epidemiology telling us about the etiology? Int J Infect Dis2005;9:185-94.
3 Kushner HI, Bastian JF, Turner CL, Burns JC. The two emergencies of Kawasaki syndrome and the implications for the developing world. Pediatr Infect Dis J2008;27:377-83.
4 Nakamura Y, Yashiro M, Uehara R, Oki I, Watanabe M, Yanagawa H. Epidemiologic features of Kawasaki disease in Japan: results from the nationwide survey in 2005-2006. J Epidemiol2008;18:167-72.
5 Harnden A, Alves B, Sheikh A. Rising incidence of Kawasaki disease in England: analysis of hospital admission data. BMJ2002;324:1424-5.
6 Harnden A, Mayon-White R, Sharma R, Yeates D, Goldacre M, Burgner D. Kawasaki disease in England: ethnicity, urbanisation and respiratory pathogens. Pediatr Infect Dis J2009;28:21-4.
7 Holman RC, Curns AT, Belay ED, Steiner CA, Effler PV, Yorita KL, et al. Kawasaki syndrome in Hawaii. Pediatr Infect Dis J2005;24:429-33.
8 Uehara R, Yashiro M, Nakamura Y, Yanagawa H. Kawasaki disease in parents and children. Acta Paediatr2003;92:694-7.
9 Onouchi Y, Tamari M, Takahashi A, Tsunoda T, Yashiro M, Nakamura Y, et al. A genomewide linkage analysis of Kawasaki disease: evidence for linkage to chromosome 12. J Hum Genet2007;52:179-90.
10 Burgner D, Davila S, Breunis WB, Ng SB, Li Y, Bonnard C, et al. A genome-wide association study identifies novel and functionally related susceptibility loci for Kawasaki disease. PLoS Genet2009;5:e1000319.
11 Chang RK. Hospitalizations for Kawasaki disease among children in the United States, 1988-1997. Pediatrics2002;109:e87.
12 Rowley AH. The etiology of Kawasaki disease: superantigen or conventional antigen? Pediatr Infect Dis J1999;18:69-70.
13 Newburger JW, Takahashi M, Gerber MA, Gewitz MH, Tani LY, Burns JC, et al. Diagnosis, treatment, and long-term management of Kawasaki disease: a statement for health professionals from the committee on rheumatic fever, endocarditis, and Kawasaki disease, council on cardiovascular disease in the young, American Heart Association. Pediatrics2004;114:1708-33.
14 Chang FY, Hwang B, Chen SJ, Lee PC, Meng CC, Lu JH. Characteristics of Kawasaki disease in infants younger than six months of age. Pediatr Infect Dis J2006;25:241-4.
15 Rowley AH. Incomplete (atypical) Kawasaki disease. Pediatr Infect Dis J2002;21:563-5.
16 Oates-Whitehead RM, Baumer JH, Haines L, Love S, Maconochie IK, Gupta A, et al. Intravenous immunoglobulin for the treatment of Kawasaki disease in children. Cochrane Database Syst Rev2003;(4):CD004000.
17 Newburger JW, Takahashi M, Beiser AS, Burns JC, Bastian J, Chung KJ, et al. A single intravenous infusion of gamma globulin as compared with four infusions in the treatment of acute Kawasaki syndrome. N Engl J Med1991;324:1633-9.
18 Baumer JH, Love SJ, Gupta A, Haines LC, Maconochie I, Dua JS. Salicylate for the treatment of Kawasaki disease in children. Cochrane Database Syst Rev2006;(4):CD004175.
19 Newburger JW, Sleeper LA, McCrindle BW, Minich LL, Gersony W, Vetter VL, et al. Randomized trial of pulsed corticosteroid therapy for primary treatment of Kawasaki disease. N Engl J Med2007;356:663-75.
20 Miura M, Katada Y, Ishihara J. Time interval of measles vaccination in patients with Kawasaki disease treated with additional intravenous immune globulin. Eur J Pediatr2004;163:25-9.
21 Kato H, Ichinose E, Kawasaki T. Myocardial infarction in Kawasaki disease: clinical analyses in 195 cases. J Pediatr1986;108:923-7.
22 Nakamura Y, Aso E, Yashiro M, Uehara R, Watanabe M, Oki I, et al. Mortality among persons with a history of Kawasaki disease in Japan: mortality among males with cardiac sequelae is significantly higher than that of the general population. Circ J2008;72:134-8.
23 Selamet Tierney ES, Newburger JW. Are patients with Kawasaki disease at risk for premature atherosclerosis? J Pediatr2007;151:225-8.
24 Kato H, Sugimura T, Akagi T, Sato N, Hashino K, Maeno Y, et al. Long-term consequences of Kawasaki disease. A 10- to 21-year follow-up study of 594 patients. Circulation1996;94:1379-85.

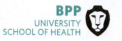

Childhood cough

Malcolm Brodlie academic clinical lecturer in paediatrics[12], Chris Graham general practitioner registrar[3], Michael C McKean consultant respiratory paediatrician[2]

[1]Institute of Cellular Medicine, Newcastle University, Newcastle upon Tyne, UK

[2]Department of Paediatric Respiratory Medicine, Great North Children's Hospital, Newcastle upon Tyne, UK

[3]Northumbria Vocational Training Scheme, Postgraduate School of Primary Care, Northern Deanery, Newcastle upon Tyne, UK, UK

Correspondence to: M Brodlie, Old Children's Outpatients Department, Royal Victoria Infirmary, Newcastle upon Tyne NE1 4LP, UK malcolm. brodlie@ncl.ac.uk

Cite this as: *BMJ* 2012;344:e1177

‹DOI› 10.1136/bmj.e1177
http://www.bmj.com/content/344/bmj.e1177

Children often present with cough,[w1] and over the counter cough remedies are among the most common drugs given to children, despite lack of evidence to support their use.[1] Questionnaire based surveys of parents suggest that the prevalence of persistent cough in the absence of wheeze in children is high and ranges from 5% to 10% at any one time.[2] Cough is an important physiological protective reflex that clears airways of secretions or aspirated material. As a symptom it is non-specific, and many of the potential causes in children are different from those in adults.[3]

Chronic cough in a child may generate parental anxiety and disrupt other family members' sleep.[4] Lessons at school may also be disturbed. For children themselves persistent coughing may be distressing and may affect their ability to sleep, study, or exercise. Parents' reports of the frequency, duration, or intensity of coughing correlate poorly with objective observations,[w2] and reported severity seems to relate most closely to the impact of coughing on parents or teachers.[w3]

Acute cough is typically defined as being of less than three weeks' duration and chronic cough is variably defined as lasting from three to 12 weeks.[5] Most children with acute cough have a viral infection of the upper respiratory tract, which is self limiting.[6] Children with an atypical history, or with chronic cough, may be more challenging to assess and are commonly incorrectly diagnosed—with asthma for example—and inappropriately treated.[7w4] Despite the wide differential diagnosis for a presenting symptom of cough in children, it is important to identify its cause and provide appropriate treatment.

We review evidence from systematic reviews and guidelines to present an overview of the causes of cough in childhood and approaches to its investigation and management, highlighting key factors that should prompt specialist referral.

SOURCES AND SELECTION CRITERIA

We based this review on British Thoracic Society guidelines published in 2008. We also consulted an evidence based review of the management of chronic non-specific cough in childhood, Cochrane reviews, and our personal archive of references. Clinical guidelines have also been published in America and Australia in recent years. All published guidelines agree on the current lack of good quality evidence on which to make evidence based statements for the diagnosis, investigation, and treatment of cough in children.

SUMMARY POINTS

- Acute cough usually resolves within three to four weeks, whereas chronic cough persists for longer than eight weeks
- Most cases of acute cough in otherwise normal children are associated with a self limiting viral infection of the upper respiratory tract
- Cough is a non-specific symptom, and in children the differential diagnosis is wide; however, careful systematic clinical evaluation will usually lead to an accurate diagnosis
- It is crucial to hear the cough because parents' reports of the nature, frequency, and duration of coughing are often unreliable
- Isolated cough without wheeze or breathlessness is rarely caused by asthma
- Adult cough algorithms are not useful when assessing children

What is the approach to assessing a child with acute cough?

Consider the potential causes of acute cough

By far the most common cause of acute cough in children is a viral infection of the upper respiratory tract that will need no specific clinical investigations.[6] Healthy children cough on a daily basis and experience upper respiratory tract infections several times a year.[8w5] A systematic review of studies set in primary care found that 24% of preschool children continue to be symptomatic two weeks after the onset of an upper respiratory tract infection.[9] A child with an acute upper respiratory tract infection will characteristically have a runny nose and sneezing.[6] A prospective cohort study of non-asthmatic preschool children presenting to primary care with acute cough investigated factors that predict future complications—defined as any new symptom, sign, or diagnosis identified by a primary care clinician at a parent initiated reconsultation or hospital admission before resolution of the cough. With a 10% pretest probability, fever, tachypnoea, or chest signs were features most likely to predict future complications.[10]

However, acute cough may also be associated with a clinically important lower respiratory tract infection, allergy, or an inhaled foreign body, or it may rarely be the presenting symptom of a serious underlying disorder, such as cystic fibrosis or a primary immunodeficiency.

Take a careful history and perform a thorough clinical examination

The figure describes factors in the history and examination that point towards a specific diagnosis in a child with acute cough. Urgent referral for specialist assessment and rigid bronchoscopy is indicated if an inhaled foreign body is suspected.[5] Foreign body aspiration is not always accompanied by an obvious history; suggestive features include sudden onset of coughing or breathlessness.

Include in the clinical examination an initial rapid assessment to judge the child's general condition, incorporating objective measurements of respiratory rate, heart rate, oxygen saturations, and temperature. The National Institute for Health and Clinical Excellence has published guidance on the assessment of feverish illness in preschool children.[11] Promptly refer any child who is acutely unwell to specialist paediatric services.[w6] Examine for signs of an upper respiratory tract infection (for example, runny nose, inflamed tympanic membranes, and throat) or effects on the lower respiratory tract (for example, crackles, wheeze, or abnormal air entry). Systematic reviews have shown that the best single finding to rule out pneumonia is the absence of tachypnoea.[12w7] Parental concern and the clinician's instinct that something is wrong remain important red flags for serious illness in settings with a low prevalence of serious infection.[12] Exclude the presence of any signs of a more chronic problem, such as poor growth or nutrition, finger clubbing, chest deformity, or atopy.

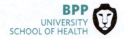

Pertussis is a cause of acute and chronic cough in children and is discussed further in the chronic cough section. In the acute setting be aware of the potential for severe disease in young and high risk infants, where it may be associated with apnoea and systemic illness.[w8]

When to consider specialist referral and further investigation

Table 1 summarises indications for performing chest radiography and considering specialist referral. Referral is especially appropriate when acute cough is progressive and severe beyond two to three weeks; if there are signs suggestive of a serious lower respiratory tract infection; if haemoptysis is present; or if the clinician suspects underlying pathology, such as cancer, tuberculosis, or an inhaled foreign body.[5]

How can acute cough be managed?

Supportive treatment only, including antipyretics as necessary and adequate intake of fluids, is indicated for viral infections of the upper respiratory tract. Antibiotics are not beneficial in the absence of signs of pneumonia, and bronchodilators are not effective for acute cough in children who do not have asthma.[13w9] A Cochrane review found no good evidence of effectiveness of over the counter drugs for acute cough, such as antihistamine or decongestant based preparations.[1w10] Young children have died from an overdose of over the counter drugs for cough, and in the United Kingdom such drugs have been withdrawn for children under 6 years.[14]

If pertussis is diagnosed, treatment with a macrolide antibiotic is indicated. Unless the diagnosis is established in the first two weeks of infection, which is clinically unlikely, the main role of these drugs is to reduce the period of infectivity.[15] There is currently no evidence to support the use of bronchodilators, steroids, or antihistamines in acute pertussis.[16]

Future unnecessary healthcare consultations may be reduced by explaining these points to parents, carefully exploring their worries, and providing them with information about what to expect.[w11] Precautionary advice about appropriate re-consultation if symptoms progress or do not improve is equally important.[12w11]

Acute cough associated with hay fever during the pollen season may be successfully treated with antihistamines or intranasal steroids.[17] Evidence based guidelines exist for the management of community acquired pneumonia,[18] bronchiolitis,[19] asthma,[20] and allergic rhinitis[17] in children.

What is the approach to assessing a child with chronic cough?

In the short to medium term most coughing in children relates to transient respiratory tract infections that will settle by three to four weeks.[9] British Thoracic Society guidelines define chronic cough as cough that lasts longer than eight weeks, with the stated caveat of a grey area of prolonged acute cough or subacute cough in children with pertussis or postviral cough that takes three to eight weeks to resolve.[5] A prospective cohort study of school aged children presenting to primary care with a cough lasting 14 days or more found that around a third had serological evidence of recent *Bordetella pertussis* infection, and nearly 90% of these children had been fully immunised.[21]

Consider the type of chronic cough

Children with chronic cough may be divided into three groups—normal children; children with specific cough and a clearly identifiable cause; and children with so called non-specific isolated cough, who are well with a persistent dry cough, no other respiratory symptoms or signs of an underlying disorder, and a normal chest radiograph.[5] Non-specific isolated cough is a label rather than a diagnosis, and such children need to be kept under careful review.[22] Children in this group have an increased frequency and severity of cough, although the specific cause has not been identified.[w12] If no specific cause can be found for the chronic cough, plan a follow-up visit to allow re-evaluation and assessment at a later date. Non-organic coughing includes habit cough and psychogenic cough. Recurrent cough refers to more than two protracted episodes of coughing a year that are not associated with a viral infection of the upper respiratory tract.[5]

History and examination

A careful history and examination will enable the clinician to identify features that may be suggestive of an important underlying disease process that requires specialist opinion or targeted intervention.

Box 1 lists points to consider when taking a history. It is vital to clarify what the child or parent means by cough. Some causes produce a characteristic cough, and it is important to hear the cough because parents' reports of respiratory symptoms such as wheeze, stridor, and nocturnal cough may not be accurate.[w3] Table 2 presents specific types of cough. Most young children do not expectorate sputum so it is important to determine the nature of the cough—wet or dry. Ask parents if they have observed phlegm in the child's vomitus. If the cough is episodic and cannot be heard at the time of consultation ask the parent to try to bring the child in during an episode. Ask about environmental factors that may contribute to cough, particularly exposure to tobacco smoke or allergens. Consider and carefully ask about psychological problems, and explore parents' concerns and expectations.

A thorough general examination should look for signs of atopy and clubbing of the fingers. Plot a growth chart and check whether the child's growth rate has recently slowed. When the child coughs feel the chest for palpable vibration owing to partial airway obstruction by retained secretions. Note any chest deformity suggestive of a chronic problem, such as increased anteroposterior diameter, sternal bowing, pectus carinatum, or Harrison's sulcus above the costal margins. Auscultate the chest listening for the quality, nature, and symmetry of air entry along with any added crackles, wheeze, or rubs. Listen for upper airway sounds and perform an ear, nose, and throat examination, particularly looking for signs of allergic rhinitis, including nasal polyps.

When should further investigation and referral be considered?

Systematic reviews and guidelines point to several red flags that should prompt swift referral to specialist care for investigation (box 2).[5 22] In particular, the presence of a chronic wet cough is abnormal and should trigger referral for investigation of chronic suppurative lung disease.

In 2007 screening was introduced for cystic fibrosis in the UK as part of the newborn bloodspot programme. This programme will not detect every child with cystic fibrosis and some will still present clinically with chronic respiratory symptoms, malabsorption, or growth faltering.[w13]

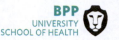

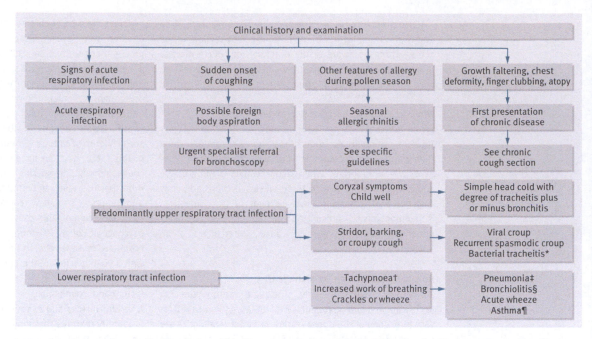

Factors that point towards a specific diagnosis in a child with acute cough. *Bacterial tracheitis is a rare but life threatening condition (croupy cough helps distinguish it from epiglottitis) that is associated with a high fever and progressive upper airway obstruction; it requires prompt specialist care—normally securing of the airway and intravenous antibiotics against *Staphylococcus aureus, Haemophilus influenzae* B, and streptococci. †Respiratory rate varies with age in children; tachypnoea is usually defined as >60 breaths/min in those under 2 months, >50 breaths/min at age 2-12 months, and >40 breaths/min in those over 1 year. ‡In the absence of stridor or wheeze, cough, fever, and signs of respiratory distress are suggestive of pneumonia. §Bronchiolitis is suggested in an infant with cough associated with crackles, with or without audible wheeze, during the winter respiratory syncytial virus season. ¶Asthma is suggested if cough is associated with wheezing plus or minus other atopic features and family history

Table 3 outlines basic investigations to be considered in a child with a chronic cough. Table 4 briefly outlines some of the potentially serious lung conditions associated with chronic coughing and the investigations performed in secondary or tertiary care that may uncover them. Persistent bacterial bronchitis in children is increasingly recognised.[23] Such children have a chronic productive wet cough but the diagnosis can be made only after underlying causes (table 4) have been excluded and a positive sputum culture result.

Do children with isolated chronic cough have asthma?

Subsequent prospective studies have supported the opinion expressed in 1994 by McKenzie that—in the absence of wheeze or dyspnoea—very few children with non-specific isolated cough have asthma.[7][24] Only a small proportion of children with non-specific isolated cough have eosinophilic airway inflammation.[25] Bronchial hyper-reactivity is associated with wheeze but not with isolated dry or nocturnal cough.[26] Children with a recurrent dry cough may, however, have genuinely increased cough sensitivity.[27]

If clinical features—such as wheeze, atopy, or a strong family history—suggest that the child has asthma, consider a trial of an inhaled corticosteroid as anti-asthma treatment.[5] Ensure the effective delivery of appropriate doses of drug, as advised by evidence based asthma management guidelines—for example, in a 6 year old child 100 µg of beclometasone dipropionate delivered twice daily via a spacer device.[20] Clearly define outcomes that will be

---

BOX 1 IMPORTANT POINTS IN THE HISTORY OF A CHILD WITH CHRONIC COUGH[5]

Nature of the cough:
- Severity
- Time course
- Diurnal variability
- Sputum production
- Associated wheeze
- Disappears during sleep?
- Any haemoptysis?
- Age of onset
- Relation to feeding and swallowing (is there a problem with aspiration?)
- Fever
- Contact with tuberculosis or HIV
- Chronic ear or nose symptoms (is there a problem with cilia function?)
- Foreign body aspiration
- Relieving factors, such as bronchodilators or antibiotics
- Exposure to cigarette smoke
- Possible allergies and triggers
- Immunisation status
- Use of drugs, such as angiotensin converting enzyme inhibitors
- Family history of atopy (is this asthma?) or chronic respiratory disorders
- General growth and development

BOX 2 RED FLAG FEATURES THAT SHOULD PROMPT SPECIALIST REFERRAL[5][22]

- Neonatal onset of the cough
- Chronic moist, wet, or productive cough
- Cough started and persisted after a choking episode
- Cough occurs during or after feeding
- Neurodevelopmental problems also present
- Auscultatory findings
- Chest wall deformity
- Haemoptysis
- Recurrent pneumonia
- Growth faltering
- Finger clubbing
- General ill health or comorbidities, such as cardiac disease or immunodeficiency

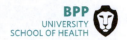

Table 1 British Thoracic Society guideline indications for performing a chest radiograph and considering specialist referral in a child with acute cough[5]

Indication	Features	Likely common diagnoses
Uncertainty about the diagnosis of pneumonia	Fever and rapid breathing in the absence of wheeze or stridor; localising signs in the chest; persistent high fever or unusual course in bronchiolitis; cough and fever persisting beyond 4-5 days	Pneumonia (chest radiograph not always indicated, see guidelines[18])
Possibility of an inhaled foreign body	Choking episode may not have been witnessed but cough of sudden onset or presence of asymmetrical wheeze or hyperinflation	Inhaled foreign body; expiratory film may be helpful but normal chest radiograph does not exclude diagnosis; bronchoscopy is the most important investigation
Pointers suggesting that this is a presentation of a chronic respiratory disorder	Growth faltering, finger clubbing, chest deformity	See chronic cough section in main text
Unusual clinical course	Cough is relentlessly progressive beyond 2-3 weeks*; recurrent fever after initial resolution	Pneumonia plus or minus associated pleural effusion or empyema; pertussis-like illness†; enlarging intrathoracic lesion; tuberculosis; inhaled foreign body; lobar collapse
Uncertainty about whether the child has true haemoptysis	To be differentiated from spitting out of blood from nose bleeds; cheek biting; or pharyngeal, oesophageal, or gastric bleeding	Acute pneumonia; underlying chronic lung disorder (such as cystic fibrosis); inhaled foreign body; tuberculosis; pulmonary haemosiderosis; tumour; arteriovenous malformation; vasculitis

*Becoming increasingly severe beyond 2-3 weeks, most acute coughs associated with infections of the upper respiratory tract should start abating in the second week.[5]

†See chronic cough section in main text.

Table 2 Characteristic cough qualities in children[22]

Quality	Possible causes
Barking or "brassy" cough	Croup, bronchomalacia, tracheomalacia, "TOF cough" after repair of a tracheo-oesophageal fistula, habit cough
Honking cough	Psychogenic
Paroxysmal cough (with or without whoop)	Pertussis
Chronic wet "fruity" cough	Suppurative lung disease

Table 3 Basic investigations in a child with chronic cough[5]

Investigation*	Rationale
Chest radiograph	Overview of the lungs (normal radiograph does not exclude serious pathology, however—for example, in bronchiectasis)
Spirometry with or without bronchodilator responsiveness or bronchial hyper-reactivity	Overview of lung volumes and airway calibre (only possible in school aged children); bronchial hyper-reactivity may not correlate with responsiveness to asthma treatment in children with chronic cough
Sputum sample	Microbiology (bacteria and viruses); differential cytology (may be difficult to obtain in young children)
Allergy testing	Skin prick or specific IgE testing

*This is not an exhaustive list of investigations and suspicion of serious underlying disease should prompt rapid referral to a paediatric respiratory specialist.

Table 4 Potentially serious disorders that are associated with chronic coughing in children[5 22]

Condition	Investigations*
Cystic fibrosis	Sweat test, genotyping
Immunodeficiency	Differential white cell count, lymphocyte subsets, immunoglobulin concentrations and subsets, functional antibody responses, neutrophil function
Primary ciliary disorders	Ex vivo studies of cilial ultrastructure and function, nasal nitric oxide, genotyping
Persistent bacterial bronchitis	Chest radiography, sputum culture, response to prolonged antibiotics and physiotherapy; high resolution computed tomography to rule out bronchiectasis
Bronchiectasis	Chest radiograph, high resolution computed tomography
Recurrent aspiration, laryngeal cleft, H-type tracheoesophageal fistula, swallowing incoordination with or without neurodevelopmental or neuromuscular disorder, gastro-oesophageal reflux	Barium swallow, video fluorosocopy, milk isotope scan, bronchoscopy, pH and impedance studies, upper gastrointestinal endoscopy, fistulography
Retained inhaled foreign body	Rigid bronchoscopy, chest radiography; high resolution computed tomography may show focal disease
Tuberculosis	Chest radiography, sputum culture, Mantoux testing, early morning gastric aspirates, bronchoscopy, interferon γ release assays
Anatomical abnormality, tracheomalacia, bronchomalacia, congenital lung malformation—for example, congenital cystic adenomatoid malformaltion	Bronchoscopy, high resolution computed tomography
Interstitial lung disease or obliterative bronchiolitis	Spirometry, chest radiography, high resolution computed tomography, lung biopsy
Cardiac disease	Chest radiography, echocardiography

*This is not an exhaustive list of investigations and suspicion of any of the above problems should prompt rapid referral to a paediatric respiratory specialist.

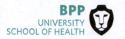

Table 5 Aspects of the management of chronic cough in children[5]

Aspect of management	Explanation
Watchful waiting in an otherwise well child	Limit to 6-8 weeks and follow by a thorough review to check that the cough has resolved and no specific features have developed
Non-specific isolated cough in an otherwise well child	Evidence is sparse and no treatments are particularly effective; parents will need to be reassured; the cough usually gradually subsides with time; careful review is needed
Removal of exposure to aeroirritants, such as tobacco smoke	Although there is limited evidence that removal of aeroirritants is helpful, there is considerable evidence that environmental exposure is associated with increased coughing, so it is sensible to remove such exposure
Trial of anti-asthma treatment	Treatment should be effectively delivered in adequate doses with clearly defined outcomes recorded over a set time period—for example, 8-12 weeks—followed by cessation of treatment
Trial of allergen avoidance and rhinosinusitis treatment	Little evidence to support in terms of respiratory symptoms, but a trial of allergen avoidance, antihistamines, and intranasal corticosteroids may be beneficial
Empirical trial of gastro-oesophageal reflux treatment	Not recommended owing to the lack of evidence in non-specific cough in children without specific diagnosis of gastro-oesophageal reflux disease
Treatment of specific cause, such as cystic fibrosis, immunodeficiency, asthma, primary ciliary dyskinesia, and tuberculosis	See condition specific evidence based guidelines
Antibiotics for persistent bacterial bronchitis	Once other conditions have been excluded, and a positive sputum culture has been obtained, persistent bacterial bronchitis may benefit from early access to prolonged courses of antibiotics and physiotherapy to prevent development of bronchiectasis in later life[23]
Behavioural approaches to psychogenic cough	Behaviour modification regimens may be helpful[w15]

recorded over a set period, such as a symptom and peak flow diary recorded over 8-12 weeks. After the trial stop the treatment to allow assessment of its effect.[5] If the child can perform spirometry or peak flow measurements, BTS asthma guidelines recommend an assessment of the reversibility of airway obstruction in response to an inhaled bronchodilator.[20] Asthma is unusual in children under 2 years of age. The clinical diagnosis of asthma in children is often challenging, and specialist referral is appropriate if there is uncertainty or symptoms are difficult to control.[20]

TIPS FOR NON-SPECIALISTS

- Most episodes of acute cough in children are related to self limiting viral upper respiratory tract infections
- In most cases, a diagnosis can be made by taking a careful history, exploring parental concerns and expectations, and conducting a systematic examination
- In a child with acute cough, signs of respiratory compromise, suggestion of foreign body aspiration or serious underlying disease should prompt swift referral to a specialist
- In children with chronic cough, quickly refer those with faltering growth, neurodevelopmental abnormalities, wet productive cough, or other signs of underlying disease
- Most children with a non-specific isolated cough will improve with time

ADDITIONAL EDUCATIONAL RESOURCES

Resources for healthcare professionals

- Shields MD, Bush A, Everard ML, McKenzie S, Primhak R. BTS guidelines: recommendations for the assessment and management of cough in children. *Thorax* 2008;63(suppl 3):iii1-15
- Harnden A. Whooping cough. *BMJ* 2009;338:b1772
- National Institute for Health and Clinical Excellence. Feverish illness in children—assessment and initial management in children younger than 5 years. 2007. www.nice.org.uk/CG047
- British Thoracic Society and Scottish Intercollegiate Guidelines Network. British guideline on the management of asthma. A national clinical guideline. 2011. www.sign.ac.uk/pdf/sign101. pdf
- Harris M, Clark J, Coote N, Fletcher P, Harnden A, McKean M, et al. British Thoracic Society guidelines for the management of community acquired pneumonia in children: update 2011. *Thorax* 2011;66(suppl 2):ii1-23
- Vance G, Lloyd K, Scadding G, Walker S, Jewkes F, Williams L, et al. The "unified airway": the RCPCH care pathway for children with asthma and/or rhinitis. *Arch Dis Child* 2011;96(suppl 2):i10-4

Resources for patients

- NHS Choices. Cough (www.nhs.uk/conditions/Cough/Pages/Introduction.aspx)—Provides a basic explanation and advice about cough
- NHS Choices. Vaccinations for kids (www.nhs.uk/Planners/vaccinations/Pages/ Vaccinesforkidshub.aspx)—A useful guide to childhood vaccinations

Is gastro-oesophageal reflux a cause of chronic cough in children?

The association between gastro-oesophageal reflux and non-specific isolated cough in children has not been fully elucidated.[28] In otherwise healthy children there is little evidence to suggest that gastro-oesophageal reflux alone is a cause of cough. Gastro-oesophageal reflux is common in infancy and is only sometimes associated with cough. An empirical trial of drugs for reflux in children with non-specific isolated cough is not currently recommended because evidence of their efficacy is lacking.[5][28]

How can psychogenic cough be recognised?

Many clinicians will be familiar with the phenomenon of a dry repetitive habit cough that persists for some time after an upper respiratory tract infection has cleared.[5] Psychogenic cough may be disruptive, bizarre, and honking, with no organic cause in an otherwise well child. Characteristically, psychogenic cough is less prominent at night or when the child is distracted and more prominent in the presence of carers or teachers. The habit may be reinforced by secondary gain derived, such as time off school. Consider Tourette's syndrome or other tic disorders, particularly if features other than an isolated cough are present.[w14]

UNANSWERED QUESTIONS AND AREAS FOR FUTURE RESEARCH

- Acute and chronic cough are common conditions in childhood; what is the real impact of cough on children, families, and society?
- Evidence from good quality research studies is needed to inform the management of cough in children
- What factors accurately predict the causes and natural course of acute and chronic cough in children?

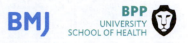

An approach to managing a child with chronic cough

Appropriate management of chronic cough in children depends on reaching an accurate diagnosis that allows targeted treatment. Treatment algorithms used for chronic cough in adults are not useful in children because the three main causes of chronic cough in adults—cough variant asthma, gastro-oesophageal reflux, and postnasal drip—are rarely relevant in children.[3] Table 5 outlines specific considerations in the management of chronic cough in children as recommended by BTS guidelines.[5]

Contributors: MB wrote the original draft of the review and collated the final version. CG and MCMcK commented on the first draft and contributed to subsequent versions. MCMcK is guarantor.

Funding: None received.

Competing interests: All authors have completed the ICMJE uniform disclosure form at www.icmje.org/coi_disclosure.pdf (available on request from the corresponding author) and declare: no support from any organisation for the submitted work; no financial relationships with any organisations that might have an interest in the submitted work in the previous three years; no other relationships or activities that could appear to have influenced the submitted work.

Provenance and peer review: Not commissioned; externally peer reviewed.

1   Smith SM, Schroeder K, Fahey T. Over-the-counter medications for acute cough in children and adults in ambulatory settings. *Cochrane Database Syst Rev*2008;1:CD001831.
2   Faniran AO, Peat JK, Woolcock AJ. Measuring persistent cough in children in epidemiological studies: development of a questionnaire and assessment of prevalence in two countries. *Chest*1999;115:434-9.
3   Chang AB. Pediatric cough: children are not miniature adults. *Lung*2010;188(suppl 1):S33-40.
4   Marchant JM, Newcombe PA, Juniper EF, Sheffield JK, Stathis SL, Chang AB. What is the burden of chronic cough for families? *Chest*2008;134:303-9.
5   Shields MD, Bush A, Everard ML, McKenzie S, Primhak R. BTS guidelines: recommendations for the assessment and management of cough in children. *Thorax*2008;63(suppl 3):iii1-15.
6   Pappas DE, Hendley JO, Hayden FG, Winther B. Symptom profile of common colds in school-aged children. *Pediatr Infect Dis J*2008;27:8-11.
7   McKenzie S. Cough—but is it asthma? *Arch Dis Child*1994;70:1-2.
8   Munyard P, Bush A. How much coughing is normal? *Arch Dis Child*1996;74:531-4.
9   Hay AD, Wilson AD. The natural history of acute cough in children aged 0 to 4 years in primary care: a systematic review. *Br J Gen Pract*2002;52:401-9.
10   Hay AD, Fahey T, Peters TJ, Wilson A. Predicting complications from acute cough in pre-school children in primary care: a prospective cohort study. *Br J Gen Pract*2004;54:9-14.
11   National Institute for Health and Clinical Excellence. Feverish illness in children—assessment and initial management in children younger than 5 years. 2007. www.nice.org.uk/CG047
12   Van den Bruel A, Haj-Hassan T, Thompson M, Buntinx F, Mant D. Diagnostic value of clinical features at presentation to identify serious infection in children in developed countries: a systematic review. *Lancet*2010;375:834-45.
13   Arroll B, Kenealy T. Antibiotics for the common cold. *Cochrane Database Syst Rev*2002;3:CD000247.
14   Medicines and Healthcare Products Regulatory Agency. Children's over-the-counter cough and cold medicines: New advice, 2010. www.mhra.gov.uk/Safetyinformation/Safetywarningsalertsandrecalls/Safetywarningsandmessagesformedicines/CON038908.
15   Health Protection Agency. Guidelines for the public health managment of pertussis. 2011. www.hpa.org.uk/webc/HPAwebFile/HPAweb_C/1287142671506
16   Bettiol S, Thompson MJ, Roberts NW, Perera R, Heneghan CJ, Harnden A. Symptomatic treatment of the cough in whooping cough. *Cochrane Database Syst Rev*2010;1:CD003257.
17   Vance G, Lloyd K, Scadding G, Walker S, Jewkes F, Williams L, et al. The "unified airway": the RCPCH care pathway for children with asthma and/or rhinitis. *Arch Dis Child*2011;96(suppl 2):i10-14.
18   Harris M, Clark J, Coote N, Fletcher P, Harnden A, McKean M, et al. British Thoracic Society guidelines for the management of community acquired pneumonia in children: update 2011. *Thorax*2011;66(suppl 2):ii1-23.
19   Scottish Intercollegiate Guidelines Network. Bronchiolitis in children. A national clinical guideline. 2006. www.sign.ac.uk/pdf/sign91.pdf
20   British Thoracic Society and Scottish Intercollegiate Guidelines Network. British guideline on the management of asthma. A national clinical guideline. 2011. www.sign.ac.uk/pdf/sign101.pdf.
21   Harnden A, Grant C, Harrison T, Perera R, Brueggemann AB, Mayon-White R, et al. Whooping cough in school age children with persistent cough: prospective cohort study in primary care. *BMJ*2006;333:174-7.
22   Gupta A, McKean M, Chang AB. Management of chronic non-specific cough in childhood: an evidence-based review. *Arch Dis Child Educ Pract Ed*2007;92:33-9.
23   Donnelly D, Critchlow A, Everard ML. Outcomes in children treated for persistent bacterial bronchitis. *Thorax*2007;62:80-4.
24   Wright AL, Holberg CJ, Morgan WJ, Taussig LM, Halonen M, Martinez FD. Recurrent cough in childhood and its relation to asthma. *Am J Respir Crit Care Med*1996;153:1259-65.
25   Gibson PG, Simpson JL, Chalmers AC, Toneguzzi RC, Wark PA, Wilson AJ, et al. Airway eosinophilia is associated with wheeze but is uncommon in children with persistent cough and frequent chest colds. *Am J Respir Crit Care Med*2001;164:977-81.
26   Chang AB. Cough, cough receptors, and asthma in children. *Pediatr Pulmonol*1999;28:59-70.
27   Chang AB, Phelan PD, Sawyer SM, Del Brocco S, Robertson CF. Cough sensitivity in children with asthma, recurrent cough, and cystic fibrosis. *Arch Dis Child*1997;77:331-4.
28   Chang AB, Lasserson TJ, Gaffney J, Connor FL, Garske LA. Gastro-oesophageal reflux treatment for prolonged non-specific cough in children and adults. *Cochrane Database Syst Rev*2011;1:CD004823.

Related links

bmj.com/archive
Previous articles in this series
- Managing retinal vein occlusion (2012;344:e499)
- New recreational drugs and the primary care approach to patients who use them (2012;344:e288)
- Diagnosis and management of Raynaud's phenomenon (2012;344:e289)
- Improving healthcare access for people with visual impairment and blindness (2012;344:e542)

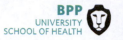

Diagnosis and management of asthma in children

Andrew Bush professor of paediatrics and head of section (paediatrics)[1] professor of paediatric respirology[2] consultant paediatric chest physician[3], Louise Fleming senior clinical lecturer[2] consultant respiratory paediatrician[3]

[1]Section of Paediatrics, Imperial College, London W2 1PG, UK

[2]National Heart and Lung Institute, Imperial College, London, UK

[3]Department of Paediatric Respiratory Medicine, Royal Brompton Harefield NHS Foundation Trust London, UK

Correspondence: A Bush a.bush@ imperial.ac.uk

Cite this as: BMJ 2015;350:h996

‹DOI› 10.1136/bmj.h996
http://www.bmj.com/content/350/
bmj.h996

Asthma is a condition characterised clinically by recurrent episodes of wheeze, cough, and breathlessness, and physiologically by variable airflow obstruction. Airway inflammation is sometimes added to the definition, but it is rarely measured in clinical practice; some groups would consider episodic viral wheeze in preschool children as a separate condition. This review gives a practical perspective on the basic steps of diagnosis and management of asthma in school age children for non-specialists in primary and secondary care.

Who gets asthma?

There is wide geographical variation in the prevalence of asthma, with wheeze in 13 and 14 year olds varying from less than 1% (Tibet) to more than 30% (New Zealand), and in 6 and 7 year olds from less than 3% (India) to nearly 40% (Costa Rica).[1] Whereas in the United Kingdom atopy is a major factor associated with asthma, this is not the case in resource poor areas. In the developed world, the risk of asthma is increased by a positive family history of asthma and atopy, maternal smoking in pregnancy, and early sensitisation to aeroallergens. Numerous "asthma genes" have been discovered, and clearly asthma is a complex polygenic disease. In the developing world, atopy is often not associated with asthma; instead, the use of biomass fuels, tobacco smoking, and viral infections seem to be more important.

What are the clinical features?

All children have intermittent respiratory symptoms, but most do not have asthma. The first prerequisite for managing asthma is knowledge of the range of normal childhood illnesses. Typically, children may have more than 10 viral related colds a year, with symptoms lasting for more than two weeks; non-specific respiratory infections may also last for two weeks or more.

The process of establishing a diagnosis of asthma should extend over at least two consultations. The first step is to

---

SOURCES AND SELECTION CRITERIA

We performed a search of PubMed using the terms "asthma" or "wheeze", with the filters "clinical trial", "published in the last 5 years", "humans", "English" activated, with the subject age range "child: birth-18 years". Additionally, we searched the Cochrane database of systematic reviews and Clinical Evidence, as well as our personal archives of references, and checked the reference lists in all the manuscripts. We selected only those manuscripts related to the diagnosis and practical management of asthma and eliminated those that studied preschool aged as well as school aged children, because the pathophysiology of wheeze and the treatment algorithms are different in these two age spans. We excluded small trials and case series if the findings had been subsumed into a meta-analysis or Cochrane review.

THE BOTTOM LINE

- In problematic cases of childhood asthma, rather than escalating treatment, a systematic approach is needed, including a review of the diagnosis; adherence, including ability to take drugs correctly; and the child's environment

- If diagnostic doubt still exists, including a failure to respond adequately to a low to medium dose of inhaled corticosteroids, referral should be made to a specialist team

- Asthma is a disease that kills, even in children with "mild" asthma, and care must be seen in that context

- Any emergency visit to hospital, regardless of whether admission occurs, is a marker of future risk, and should prompt a focused and urgent review of what trigger factors led to the attack and whether the attack was appropriately managed

- Non-adherence to treatment, overuse of bronchodilators, and underuse of inhaled corticosteroids are common problems that should be routinely tackled

- Failure of annual asthma review is a factor in asthma related deaths and for children a review should be routine at least every three months; these should be conducted by doctors or nurses with training in asthma and not seen as "tick box" exercises

- When specialist services are also involved, good communication is essential; this is particularly true after an acute asthma attack

---

BOX 1 FEATURES SUGGESTIVE OF A NON-ASTHMA DIAGNOSIS

History

- Absence of true polyphonic (musical) wheeze

- Presence of prominent upper airway symptoms such as rhinitis, snoring, and sinusitis

- Symptoms from the first day of life—these are never due to asthma, and a serious condition such as primary ciliary dyskinesia, aspiration due to incoordinate swallow, and congenital lung and airway malformations must be excluded

- Sudden onset of symptoms—suggestive of foreign body aspiration and requires immediate management. Anaphylaxis may also be a consideration, but other features such as urticarial rash and focal swelling would be expected to give clues to this diagnosis

- Presence of chronic moist cough or sputum production—if present daily for more than six weeks and has not resolved with one course of antibiotics, referral is indicated

- History of systemic illness or suggestive of immunodeficiency: severe, persistent, unusual, or recurrent infections (SPUR)

- Continuous, unremitting symptoms with no symptom-free days

Physical examination

- Systemic signs such as clubbing, weight loss, failure to thrive

- Upper airway disease–tonsillar hypertrophy, noticeable rhinitis

- Unusually severe chest deformity

- Unexpected signs on auscultation (fixed monophonic wheeze, stridor, asymmetrical signs)

- Chest palpation during coughing or forced expiratory manoeuvres—palpable secretions revealed

- Signs of cardiac or systemic disease, such as a cardiac murmur, abnormalities in heart sounds or precordial impulses, abnormal peripheral pulses, weight loss, and unusual systemic infections such as pyogenic arthritis or meningitis

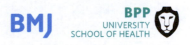

take a detailed history and carry out a physical examination, focused on excluding other causes of respiratory symptoms (box 1). Asthma is suggested by reports of wheeze, dry cough, and breathlessness. Symptoms are typically worse at night and in association with specific triggers such as viral upper respiratory tract infections, exercise, and exposure to smoke and aeroallergens. Parents use the word "wheeze" to describe a wide range of respiratory noises.[2] Parental report of wheeze correlates poorly with objectively recorded wheeze.[3] Thus until a doctor has heard and documented the presence of true polyphonic (musical) expiratory wheeze, an open mind should be kept about the nature of the sound described. A video questionnaire may be helpful to clarify what is being described.[4]

"Cough variant" asthma is a controversial topic. Although a few children may have cough and no wheeze as a manifestation of asthma, these presentations are rare. Isolated chronic dry cough in a community setting is rarely if ever due to asthma.[5] We will not diagnose asthma unless there is a history of considerable breathlessness, as well as either or both of cough and wheeze.

Box 2 lists the indications for referral to secondary care. If there are features suspicious of a non-asthmatic condition, then referral to secondary care is indicated. Referral should be expedited when children are systemically unwell or there is concern about a serious condition.

How is the diagnosis confirmed?

The figure shows a proposed diagnostic algorithm. If asthma is suspected, it is good practice to document variable airflow obstruction with a peak flow meter using the best of three attempts:

- If peak flow is below age appropriate normal ranges (www.lungfunction.org/), then improvement by 12% or more 20 minutes after administering a short acting β_2 agonist (for example, 400 µg salbutamol given with a metered dose inhaler and spacer) is a useful test to confirm variable airflow obstruction.
- If peak flow is normal, then a two week period of home monitoring may confirm the diagnosis; if the peak flow chart is a flat line (or variability is within normal limits) despite ongoing symptoms, it is difficult to attribute the findings to asthma. Peak flow variability of 15% or more is strongly suggestive of asthma; likewise, if children are given a β_2 agonist at home, an improvement by 12% or more 20 minutes later is also supportive of a diagnosis of asthma. However, it is acknowledged that compliance with peak flow monitoring is often poor.

- If peak flow is normal, consider getting children to run for 10 minutes, either on the flat or up and down steps.

None of these tests is sensitive to the diagnosis of asthma; however, it is a safe principle that the more practitioners try and fail to identify airflow obstruction, the less likely is a diagnosis of asthma. Routine chest radiography is not needed; and indeed a normal radiograph cannot exclude a serious condition.

Occasionally a blind trial of asthma treatment may be considered justifiable; in that case it is essential to have a trial period of discontinuation of treatment to ensure that any apparent benefit is related to the treatment rather than arising spontaneously. No evidence base exists to recommend a particular trial regimen; we would use a three stage protocol, preferably combined with peak flow measurements at home to document improvement:

- Initiate treatment with beclomethasone equivalent 200 µg twice daily using a metered dose inhaler and spacer
- Reassess at six weeks; if no benefit then the diagnosis is unlikely to be asthma, stop treatment and consider referral for investigations; if the symptoms have disappeared, stop treatment and reassess six weeks later
- If symptoms have recurred by six weeks, restart inhaled corticosteroid in a low dose (100 µg beclomethasone equivalent twice daily using a metered dose inhaler and spacer), and continue to adjust dose depending on response.

How is it managed?

A recent report of asthma related deaths in adults and children in the United Kingdom has highlighted that nearly half of those who died from asthma could have been saved by attention to several components of basic management (box 3).[6]

Pharmacotherapy

The basic management steps for asthma are well summarised in national and international guidelines.[7][8] All guidelines agree that first line preventive treatment should be with inhaled corticosteroids. There is no evidence to support the use of combination inhalers as first line treatment in children, indeed the reverse is the case,[9] and their increasing prescription in this role is to be discouraged. Importantly, the Best Add-on Therapy Giving Effective Responses (BADGER) study showed that the plateau of the dose-response curve to inhaled corticosteroids for most children with asthma is 200 µg/day fluticasone or equivalent, and few children benefited from a step up to 500 µg/day.[5][10] The best response was adding a long acting β_2 agonist, and some children also responded to a leucotriene receptor antagonist. We recommend that those children with asthma who do not respond to fluticasone 200 µg/day plus any one additional treatment should be managed as treatment failures and not by escalating pharmacotherapy.

No inhaled drug is effective unless delivery to the airways is optimised. Children must be shown how to use inhalers and their technique checked repeatedly. The use of spacers is particularly problematic in adolescents—the devices are often considered "babyish" and so the young person puts the metered dose inhaler straight in the mouth, with usually poor delivery of drug to the lower airway in consequence. In this case a breath actuated or dry powder device would be preferable. Spacers for school aged

---

BOX 2 WHEN TO REFER TO SECONDARY CARE

- The diagnosis is in doubt
- An age appropriate level of treatment is not working despite apparently satisfactory adherence; specifically if the child has received more than two courses of systemic corticosteroids in a year, or has not responded to British Thoracic Society Step 3 treatment (inhaled corticosteroid 400 µg/day plus long acting β_2 agonist)
- Any involved people (doctor, child, family) are unhappy with outcomes

---

BOX 3 COMPONENTS OF ASTHMA MANAGEMENT

- Institution of appropriate pharmacotherapy administered using an age appropriate inhaler device
- Attention to adverse environmental factors, especially exposure to tobacco smoke
- Attention to any comorbidities, especially dysfunctional breathing
- Provision of an asthma treatment plan
- Regular follow-up and assessment of progress

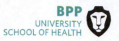

Asthma suspected in a school age child

Evidence of variable airflow obstruction?
Give inhaled short acting β2 agonist and see if peak flow increases ≥15% from baseline 20 minutes later
Give the parent or carer a peak flow meter and ask for peak flow to be measured twice daily at home, including improvement if β2 agonist is given
Check for bronchoconstriction in a field exercise test – for example, 5-10 minutes vigorous running

Yes

No

Trial of asthma treatment – for example, low dose inhaled corticosteroids

Consider alternative diagnoses

Consider blind trial of treatment – for example, low dose inhaled corticosteroids

Assess response at six week follow-up visit

Proposed diagnostic algorithm for asthma

children should always be used with a mouthpiece, not with a mask.

Adverse environmental factors

It must be highlighted that any tobacco smoking has an adverse effect on asthma outcomes.[4] [11] Cotinine levels (an objective measure of exposure to nicotine in tobacco) are just as high in those who smoke "but not in front of the children."[12] Exposure to household mould is also likely to be detrimental.[13] Skin prick testing to identify allergy to household pets should be considered. Whether sensitised people benefit from avoidance of house dust mite is controversial[14] and in the United Kingdom is not recommended in the most recent guidelines from the British Thoracic Society/Scottish Intercollegiate Guidelines Network.[7] However, multifaceted interventions may be considered in those with severe disease.[15]

Comorbidities

In childhood, comorbidities such as obesity, rhinosinusitis, food allergy, dysfunctional breathing, and psychosocial problems may contribute to respiratory symptoms. Gastro-oesophageal reflux is often found if sought, but treatment does not affect asthma outcomes.[16] It is much easier to identify obesity than to treat it; obesity may lead to breathlessness, which is not asthma related, causing confusion about the diagnosis. Whether treatment of rhinosinusitis improves

lower airway inflammation is controversial, but upper airway symptoms certainly should be treated on their independent merits.[17] Food allergy is associated with severe asthma in particular; whether allergy causes increased asthma severity.[18] Dysfunctional breathing (vocal cord dysfunction, exercise induced laryngeal obstruction) is a really important and often under-appreciated problem. It may cause stridor, and be associated with paraesthesia, sore throat, and hoarseness of the voice. It never occurs during sleep. The diagnosis may be obvious from a video of an attack; parents should be able to make a recording on their mobile phone (but clearly if children are thought to need urgent medical attention, this takes priority). Confirmation of doubtful cases can be made in specialist centres by experienced physiotherapists and laryngoscopy during exercise. Finally, psychosocial problems were identified in 26% of people with asthma who died,[6] and from our experience these are common in children with severe asthma.[19]

Provision of an asthma treatment plan

Asthma treatment plans are underused and thought to be associated with poor outcomes.[6] The purpose of a treatment plan is to guide young people and parents on maintenance treatment, asthma triggers and how to avoid them, and what to do in the event of worsening symptoms, particularly an acute asthma attack. Numerous proformas are available, and whichever is chosen should be regularly reviewed or updated. Long term, children largely do not reliably measure their peak flow twice a day, but measurement at the time of a viral cold or increased symptoms can be used to drive treatment changes and the need to seek medical attention. A major challenge is to ensure that, without causing distress, families understand that asthma can be serious. Phrases that may be helpful include "asthma is one of those conditions which can be very serious, but if properly managed should not impact on your child's life. However, if treatment is neglected, your child can become seriously ill or even worse, and we all need to remember this." An obvious adverse effect of prescribing inhalers to all patients with asthma, many of whom have a diagnosis on the weakest of grounds, is that the condition is trivialised.

Regular follow-up

As with all conditions in childhood, regular and focused follow-up is essential. Basic child health should be assessed, including height and weight, and immunisations, especially

---

BOX 4 METHODS FOR ASSESSING ADHERENCE

- Check how many prescriptions for inhaled corticosteroids have been dispensed over the previous year
- If feasible, and there is only one local pharmacist, check how many prescriptions have actually been dispensed
- Ask the child to demonstrate how the inhaler is used
- Ask questions sensitively, such as "Most patients and all doctors find it difficult to remember to take treatment; how often do you think you/your child forgets?" or "Most patients and all doctors find it difficult to remember to take treatment; do you think you forget at least once a day?", acknowledging that adherence can be difficult and encouraging patients to share their experiences
- Explore whether there are particularly difficult times for children or parents to remember the treatment, such as during the morning rush for school
- In a sensitive way, find out if carers actually supervise their children taking the drug or if it is left to the children to remember
- Consider home visits—have the drugs been removed from the wrapper, are they in date, and are they readily accessible?
- Consider electronic monitoring of treatment uptake (usually in secondary care)

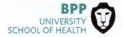

BOX 5 KEY STEPS IN RECOGNISING AND MANAGING AN ACUTE ATTACK OF ASTHMA

Children/families should be aware of the following signs of an asthma attack

- Difficulty talking or walking
- Unable to feed
- Little relief with salbutamol
- Drop in peak flow
- Hard and fast breathing
- Coughing and wheezing a lot

Personal action plan

- Give up to 10 puffs of salbutamol
- If symptoms improve see a doctor or nurse that day
- If relief lasts for four hours or less seek urgent medical attention
- If severe symptoms persist despite 10 puffs of salbutamol call an ambulance and continue to give salbutamol while waiting for the ambulance (up to 10 puffs every 15 minutes)

Moderate attack

- Able to talk in sentences
- Peripheral capillary oxygen saturation ≥92%
- Peak expiratory flow ≥50% best or predicted
- Heart rate ≤125/min in children aged >5 years (≤140/min in children aged 2-5 years)
- Respiratory rate ≤30/min in children aged >5 years (≤40/min in children aged 2-5 years)
- Mild-moderate recession and wheeze

Action plan

- Give up to 10 puffs of salbutamol through a spacer
- If poor response, add ipratropium bromide and repeat salbutamol with or without ipratropium every 20 minutes
- Prednisolone, 30-50 mg for children aged >5 years, 20 mg for children aged 2-5 years (but not if episodic viral wheeze); a three day course is usually sufficient
- Discharge with action plan when stable and requiring salbutamol 3-4 hourly
- Advise review by general practitioners within 48 hours

Severe attack

- Unable to complete sentences
- Peripheral capillary oxygen saturation <92%
- Peak expiratory flow 33-50% best or predicted
- Heart rate >125/min in children aged >5 years (>140/min in children aged 2-5 years)
- Respiratory rate >30/min in children aged >5 years (>40/min in children aged 2-5 years)
- Noticeable recession

Action plan

- High flow oxygen through a tight fitting mask or nasal cannula to achieve normal saturations (94-98%)
- Nebulised salbutamol (2.5-5 mg)
- If poor response, add nebulised ipratropium bromide (250 µg) and repeat nebulised salbutamol with or without ipratropium every 20 minutes
- Prednisolone, 30-50 mg for children aged >5 years, 20 mg for children aged 2-5 years (intravenous hydrocortisone (4 mg/kg) only if unable to tolerate oral treatment)
- Wean salbutamol to 1-2 hourly and ipratropium to 4-6 hourly, depending on clinical response
- If poor response move to life threatening algorithm

Life threatening asthma

- Peripheral capillary oxygen saturation <92%
- Peak expiratory flow <33% best or predicted (or unable to perform)
- Poor respiratory effort
- Silent chest
- Cyanosis
- Exhaustion
- Confusion
- Hypotension
- Bradycardia

Action plan

- High flow oxygen through a tight fitting mask or nasal cannula to achieve normal saturations (94-98%)
- Nebulised salbutamol (2.5-5 mg) plus ipratropium (250 µg), repeat every 20 minutes
- Obtain intravenous access
- Intravenous hydrocortisone (4 mg/kg)
- Intravenous salbutamol bolus (15 µg/kg over 10 minutes)
- Intravenous magnesium bolus (40 mg/kg, maximum 2 g)
- If response poor: aminophylline or salbutamol infusion

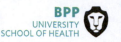

against influenza. Growth failure may be related to over-treatment with inhaled corticosteroids, poorly controlled asthma, or an unsuspected coincidental diagnosis. Day to day asthma control should be assessed, including the number of dispensed prescriptions for short acting β2 agonists and whether the child has had an emergency visit for asthma. The possibility of a missed or wrong diagnosis, no matter how eminent the health professional who initiated treatment, should always be considered. Above all, adherence to treatment, including adequacy of inhaler technique, should be checked. Assessing adherence is difficult and needs to be done with sensitivity (box 4 lists some approaches that may be useful).

Role of biomarkers
Interest is increasing in the role of biomarkers to drive asthma treatment. In children, there is as yet no evidence that any biomarker should be used to determine management. Blood eosinophil levels do not correlate well with airway eosinophilia,[20] unlike in adults; exhaled nitric oxide and airway eosinophilia have inconsistent relations over time, even within an individual[21]; and no study has yet determined a convincing role in routine practice,[22] although undoubtedly, biomarker driven treatment remains an important aspiration.

How are acute asthma attacks managed?
Asthma attacks can be immediately fatal, can be predictive of future clinical course and subsequent attacks, and may be associated with impairment in normal airway growth.[23] The term "exacerbation" has been criticised as too benign.[24] [25] Box 5 summarises the key steps in recognising and managing an acute asthma attack.

Evidence in the United Kingdom suggests that most deaths related to asthma occur in those who are not receiving specialist care.[6] Primary care clinicians must be alert to detecting patients with high risk "mild" asthma (box 6), and those with unscheduled hospital visits and admissions.

How is treatment failure managed?
A serious error of judgment is to escalate treatment in those children with asthma who are unresponsive to basic management, without due consideration of possible reasons for why this might be the case. Broadly, treatment failures can result in persistent symptoms on a daily basis or recurrent acute asthma attacks requiring oral corticosteroids, or both. The threshold for referral to specialist care depends on the experience of the treating doctor and the expertise in the clinical setting; suggested indications are given in box 2.

Persistent symptoms
The commonest causes of treatment failure are wrong diagnosis and poor compliance with treatment, and both should be reviewed, including checks of adherence and inhaler technique (box 4).[19] It is particularly important to remember symptoms of dysfunctional breathing. A check on prescription uptake is often revealing, and indeed electronic alerting of excessive β2 agonist and inadequate preventer prescription is another key recommendation of the National Review of Asthma Deaths in the United Kingdom.[6] The home environment also should be considered; a home visit by an experienced nurse, if possible, can often be illuminating.[19] The possibility that symptoms are being over-reported, and there are hidden gains, should not be forgotten.

Acute asthma attacks
A review after an acute asthma attack requires a focused response to determine whether there are ongoing reversible problems that contributed to the episode, and whether the attack itself was correctly managed.

The combination of allergic sensitisation, exposure to allergens, and viral infection is strongly predictive of asthma attacks, of which only exposure to allergens can be modulated.[26] Inhaled corticosteroids are protective of attacks in people with atopic asthma. Attention to adherence, optimising the dose of inhaled corticosteroids, and reducing exposure to environmental allergens to which the child is sensitised is essential. Poor baseline control is associated with risk of attacks, and every effort should be made to reduce this risk.

The management of the acute attack should be reviewed, regardless of whether the child was admitted. Was there an action plan in place, with documented triggers, and was it followed? Does the plan need revision in light of the attack? Has there been regular review? Was the spacer and short acting β2 agonist readily available and neither underused nor over-used? Prescription of more than one canister of a short acting β2 agonist a month, failure to prescribe or collect adequate prophylactic drugs, and prescription of long acting β2 agonists as sole treatment are red flags.

Although it is not possible to abolish asthma attacks totally, risk can be reduced and management optimised to control them.

How is episodic viral wheeze managed?
By school age, most children with asthma have many triggers leading to wheeze, including exercise, viral colds, exposure to allergens and cold air. Wheeze with viral colds as the sole trigger and with no symptoms between colds is most common in preschool children, but may occasionally be seen in school aged children. In these rare circumstances, intermittent rather than continuous treatment is permissible, but clinicians should be sure that there are no important interval symptoms.[27] If attacks are frequent and severe, then a trial of regular inhaled corticosteroids should be given. This may highlight that interval symptoms have been missed. This group needs equally careful follow-up, in particular to detect a change of symptom pattern.

How is asthma managed in adolescents?
Adolescence is a difficult time, irrespective of the presence of asthma. Risk taking behaviour, including experimenting with tobacco, e-cigarettes, and other substances of misuse is common and affects asthma control.[28] Denial of illness and symptoms is also the norm, and adolescents can be

---

BOX 6 KEY QUESTIONS FOR IDENTIFYING "AT RISK" CHILDREN

- The following information should easily be accessible electronically, and none requires special expertise. If any question cannot be answered satisfactorily, then an urgent review is mandatory
- Has the child been taken to an emergency department or admitted with asthma? If so, has there been follow-up?
- Does the child have an asthma plan and was the last annual review within the past year?
- How many prescriptions for preventive and reliever drugs are being collected for the child?
- Is the child brought to review appointments? When was the child last seen?
- Do you know what triggers this child's asthma?

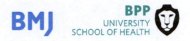

reluctant to take any treatment regularly. Spacers are often discarded and it may therefore be better to prescribe dry powder or breath activated devices to ensure adequate drug delivery. Although evidence of efficacy in paediatric practice is lacking,[29] combined budesonide and formoterol is a safer option than short acting β2 agonists as sole treatment. Time and patience are needed, and the readiness to make compromises to help young people move to safe asthma self management.

Contributors: AB wrote the first draft. AB and LF edited the manuscript, and both act as guarantors.

Competing interests: We have read and understood the BMJ policy on declaration of interests and declare the following: AB and LF are members of the BTS/SIGN asthma guideline group. LF is a member of the BTS Difficult Asthma Special Advisory Group, has performed consultancy for Chiesi, and given lectures at educational events organised by Novartis. AB was supported by the NIHR Respiratory Disease Biomedical Research Unit at the Royal Brompton and Harefield NHS Foundation Trust and Imperial College London.

Provenance and peer review: Commissioned; externally peer reviewed.

1   Lai CK, Beasley R, Crane J, Foliaki S, Shah J, Weiland S; International Study of Asthma and Allergies in Childhood Phase Three Study Group. Global variation in the prevalence and severity of asthma symptoms: phase three of the International Study of Asthma and Allergies in Childhood (ISAAC). Thorax2009;64:476-83.
2   Cane RS, Ranganathan SC, McKenzie SA. What do parents of wheezy children understand by "wheeze"? Arch Dis Child2000;82:327-32.
3   Cane RS, McKenzie SA. Parents' interpretations of children's respiratory symptoms on video. Arch Dis Child2001;84:31-4.
4   Shaw RA, Crane J, Pearce N, Burgess CD, Bremner P, Woodman K, et al. Comparison of a video questionnaire with the IUATLD written questionnaire for measuring asthma prevalence. Clin Exp Allergy1992;22:561-8.
5   Wright AL, Holberg CJ, Morgan WJ, Taussig LM, Halonen M, Martinez FD. Recurrent cough in childhood and its relation to asthma. Am J Respir Crit Care Med1996;153(4 Pt 1):1259-65.
6   Royal College of Physicians. Why asthma still kills: the national review of asthma deaths. 2014. www.rcplondon.ac.uk/sites/default/files/why-asthma-still-kills-full-report.pdf.
7   British guideline on the management of asthma. Thorax2014;69(Suppl 1):i1-i192.
8   Global Initiative for Asthma. World asthma day. 2014. www.ginasthma.org/.
9   Sorkness CA, Lemanske RF Jr, Mauger DT, Boehmer SJ, Chinchilli VM, Martinez FD, et al. Long-term comparison of 3 controller regimens for mild-moderate persistent childhood asthma: the Pediatric Asthma Controller Trial. J Allergy Clin Immunol2007;119:64-72.
10   Lemanske RF Jr, Mauger DT, Sorkness CA, Jackson DJ, Boehmer SJ, Martinez FD, et al. Step-up therapy for children with uncontrolled asthma receiving inhaled corticosteroids. N Engl J Med2010;362:975-85.
11   Cook DG, Strachan DP. Health effects of passive smoking. 3. Parental smoking and prevalence of respiratory symptoms and asthma in school age children. Thorax1997;52:1081-94.
12   Pool J, Petrova N, Russell RR. Exposing children to secondhand smoke. Thorax2012;67:926.
13   Gent JF, Kezik JM, Hill ME, Tsai E, Li DW, Leaderer BP. Household mold and dust allergens: exposure, sensitization and childhood asthma morbidity. Environ Res2012;118:86-93.
14   Nurmatov U, van Schayck CP, Hurwitz B, Sheikh A. House dust mite avoidance measures for perennial allergic rhinitis: an updated Cochrane systematic review. Allergy2012;67:158-65.
15   Morgan WJ, Crain EF, Gruchalla RS, O'Connor GT, Kattan M, Evans R III, et al. Results of a home-based environmental intervention among urban children with asthma. N Engl J Med2004;351:1068-80.
16   Gibson PG, Henry RL, Coughlan JL. Gastro-oesophageal reflux treatment for asthma in adults and children. Cochrane Database Syst Rev2000;2:CD001496.
17   Brozek JL, Bousquet J, Baena-Cagnani CE, Bonini S, Canonica GW, Casale TB, et al. Allergic Rhinitis and its Impact on Asthma (ARIA) guidelines: 2010 revision. J Allergy Clin Immunol2010;126:466-76.
18   Roberts G, Patel N, Levi-Schaffer F, Habibi P, Lack G. Food allergy as a risk factor for life-threatening asthma in childhood: a case-controlled study. J Allergy Clin Immunol2003;112:168-74.
19   Bracken MM, Fleming L, Hall P, Van SN, Bossley CJ, Biggart E, et al. The importance of nurse led home visits in the assessment of children with problematic asthma. Arch Dis Child2009;94:780-4.
20   Ullmann N, Bossley CJ, Fleming L, Silvestri M, Bush A, Saglani S. Blood eosinophil counts rarely reflect airway eosinophilia in children with severe asthma. Allergy2013;68:402-6.
21   Fleming L, Tsartsali L, Wilson N, Regamey N, Bush A. Longitudinal relationship between sputum eosinophils and exhaled nitric oxide in children with asthma. Am J Respir Crit Care Med2013;188:400-2.
22   Fleming L, Wilson N, Regamey N, Bush A. Use of sputum eosinophil counts to guide management in children with severe asthma. Thorax2012;67:193-8.
23   O'Byrne PM, Pedersen S, Lamm CJ, Tan WC, Busse WW. Severe exacerbations and decline in lung function in asthma. Am J Respir Crit Care Med2009;179:19-24.
24   Bush A, Pavord I. Following Nero: fiddle while Rome burns, or is there a better way? Thorax2011;66:367.
25   Fitzgerald JM. Targeting lung attacks. Thorax2011;66:365-6.
26   Murray CS, Poletti G, Kebadze T, Morris J, Woodcock A, Johnston SL, et al. Study of modifiable risk factors for asthma exacerbations: virus infection and allergen exposure increase the risk of asthma hospital admissions in children. Thorax2006;61:376-82.
27   Turpeinen M, Nikander K, Pelkonen AS, Syvanen P, Sorva R, Raitio H, et al. Daily versus as-needed inhaled corticosteroid for mild persistent asthma (The Helsinki early intervention childhood asthma study). Arch Dis Child2008;93:654-9.
28   Britto MT, Vockell AL, Munafo JK, Schoettker PJ, Wimberg JA, Pruett R, et al. Improving outcomes for underserved adolescents with asthma. Pediatrics2014;133:e418-27.
29   Cates CJ, Lasserson TJ. Combination formoterol and budesonide as maintenance and reliever therapy versus inhaled steroid maintenance for chronic asthma in adults and children. Cochrane Database Syst Rev2009;2:CD007313.

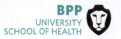

Childhood constipation

Marcus K H Auth consultant paediatric gastroenterologist, Rakesh Vora specialist registrar in paediatric gastroenterology, Paul Farrelly specialist registrar in paediatric surgery, Colin Baillie consultant paediatric general surgeon

[1]Departments of Paediatric Gastroenterology and General Surgery, Alder Hey Children's NHS Foundation Trust, Liverpool L12 2AP, UK

Correspondence to: M K H Auth
marcus.auth@alderhey.nhs.uk

Cite this as: BMJ 2012;345:e7309

‹DOI› 10.1136/bmj.e7309
http://www.bmj.com/content/345/bmj.e7309

Constipation is common in children, affecting between 5% (longer duration) and 30% (duration less than six months) of school aged children in the United Kingdom.[1][2] It accounts for 3% of general paediatric consultations and 25-30% of consultations with paediatric gastroenterologists.[1][2] Symptoms at presentation are variable, and the condition has often progressed to cause substantial discomfort, pain, and secondary effects, which require efficient and prolonged treatment.

Successful management depends on recognising common causes and excluding rare ones; explaining the functional causes, clinical diagnosis, and treatment principles to the patient and family; individual tailoring of treatment; achieving adherence; and providing personalised continuity of care. Because evidence for pathogenesis and treatment is limited, this review summarises current evidence and aims to provide practical advice in primary care.

What is childhood constipation?

The term constipation describes a collection of symptoms rather than a specific disease in childhood. Diagnosis therefore relies on the reported symptoms, accurate description of bowel habits, interpretation, and examination.[2] An international group has classified constipation among the spectrum of functional bowel disorders and provided a diagnostic definition.[3] The definition includes reduced frequency of defecation, occurrence of faecal incontinence (soiling, encopresis), stool retention (faecal impaction), painful or hard bowel movements, or large diameter stools (box 1).

How common is the problem and who gets it?

A systematic review showed a worldwide prevalence of childhood constipation of 0.7-29.6% (median 12%). Prevalence was 10-20% in the United States and UK and 20-30% in Australia, South Africa, and China.[4] Constipation can affect just one child in a family, but in some families several family members from one or different generations can be affected.[1][3][4][5]

What causes constipation?

Systematic reviews conclude that the underlying causes are functional and multifactorial in 90% of children with constipation.[1][2][3][5] Causes include problems with the autonomic and somatic nervous system, motility of the colon, muscles of the pelvic floor and anal sphincters, and the child's behaviour.[2]

Observational studies have shown that constipation may follow a change in diet, episodes of pain, febrile infections, and dehydration.[6] Observational studies found a genetic predisposition in a proportion of patients.[2] Constipation was also associated with problems with toilet training, psychological problems, major life events (parental divorce, grievance, bullying, sexual abuse), neurodevelopmental disorders and autistic spectrum, and with drugs (opiates).[2][7]

Prospective cohort studies using transit studies and manometry indicated that a proportion of children showed a delayed colonic transit time[8]; others were unable to relax the pelvic floor when attempting to defecate.[9]

Box 2 summarises the most common organic and non-organic causes of constipation, but for most children the causes are unknown.[10]

A systematic review reported that causes of stool withholding included previous passage of large, hard, or painful stools; anal fissures; serious behavioural problems; lack of time for regular toileting; and distaste for toilets other than the child's own. The review highlighted that these factors play a pivotal role in perpetuating chronic constipation (box 2).[10][11][12]

BOX 1 DEFINITION OF FUNCTIONAL CONSTIPATION[3][5]

Presence of two or more of the following criteria in the previous one to two months:

- Two or fewer defecations in the toilet each week
- At least one episode of faecal incontinence each week
- History of retentive posturing or excessive volitional stool retention
- History of painful or hard bowel movements
- Presence of a large faecal mass in the rectum
- History of large diameter stools that may obstruct the toilet

---

How do children with constipation present?

Systematic reviews indicate that children with constipation present with one or more symptoms (box 3). Large prospective trials have shown that only 75% have reduced frequency of defecation.[2] Case series from large studies showed that impaction—a large faecal mass in the abdomen or pelvis—was found in 40-100%,[2][5][9] but they also indicated that occasionally hard faeces had never been passed.[13]

According to data from several prospective studies, 75-90% of children with constipation present with faecal incontinence, which describes the involuntary passage of stools and staining in nappies (after having been toilet trained), in the underwear, or in pyjamas. The anal overflow

---

SOURCES AND SELECTION CRITERIA

We searched the Clinical Evidence Database and Cochrane Database of Systematic Reviews. We also consulted National Institute for Health and Clinical Excellence (NICE) clinical guidance 99 (updated June 2012). PubMed was used to identify peer reviewed original articles, meta-analyses, and reviews written in English, mainly published during the past 15 years, or earlier pioneering works. Empirical data are provided when evidence is lacking.

SUMMARY POINTS

- Childhood constipation is common and often associated with faecal incontinence
- An essential aim is to prevent pain associated with defecation
- Invasive investigations are not routinely needed for diagnosis
- Indications for referral are signs of organic disease and review of treatment
- Chronicity can be debilitating and has behavioural and social consequences
- The lack of evidence on causes and treatment suggests that more research is needed

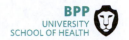

of faeces results from retained, impacted faeces leading to loss of rectal sensitivity, which can occur in smaller amounts (soiling) or larger amounts (encopresis).[2] If impaction is severe, faecal and, potentially, urinary incontinence may occur at night-time.[2] It is rare for neurological problems or anomalies of the anal sphincter to present with childhood constipation or faecal incontinence (table 1).

According to a systematic review, 35-40% of children present with retentive posturing (the position of a child attempting to avoid defecation). This can be seen as squeezing the buttocks together, extending the body, or rocking back and forth.[15]

How is functional constipation diagnosed?

According to National Institute for Health and Clinical Excellence (NICE) guidance, the diagnosis of functional constipation can usually be established by taking a comprehensive history and performing a thorough physical examination. When deciding whether to refer to a general paediatrician or specialist, it is important to recognise medical conditions, such as cows' milk protein intolerance or coeliac disease (box 2), that may require changes in diet or additional treatment, and surgical conditions that present with "red flag symptoms," such as spina bifida and Hirschsprung's disease (tables 1 and 2; fig 1).[1 2 3 16]

BOX 2 CAUSES OF CONSTIPATION BY AGE GROUP[2]

For most children the causes of constipation are unknown.[10] Common organic and non-organic causes (which may coexist) include:

For infants and toddlers

From history
- Genetic predisposition
- Nutritional change—for example, from human milk (breast feeding) to cows' milk (bottle feeding)
- Cows' milk protein allergy
- Lack of fibre in the diet
- Stool withholding behaviour
- Retentive posturing
- Coeliac disease

From examination
- Anal fissure(s)
- Spina bifida
- Anorectal malformations
- Hirschsprung's disease

For schoolchildren and adolescents

From history
- Inadequate food intake
- Toilet training coerced
- Attention-deficit disorders
- Developmental handicaps
- Toilet phobia, school bathroom avoidance
- Excessive anal interventions

From examination
- Anorexia nervosa
- Depression
- Slow transit constipation

BOX 3 COMMON SYMPTOMS AND ASSOCIATED SIGNS OF FUNCTIONAL CONSTIPATION IN CHILDHOOD[2 5 10 14]

- Faecal impaction (frequency 40-100%)[2]
- Soiling or encopresis (faecal incontinence) (75-90%)[2]
- Infrequent bowel activity (less than 3 stools/week (75%))[2]
- Large stools (75%)[2]
- Painful defecation (69%)[5]
- Withholding or straining to stop passage of stools (58%)[5]
- Abdominal mass (30-50%)[2]
- Retentive behaviour (35-45%)[2]
- Abdominal and distension (20-40%)[2]
- Enuresis or urinary tract infection (30%)[2 6]
- Poor appetite (25%)[2]
- Anorexia (10-25%)[2]
- Fissures or haemorrhoids (5-25%)[2]
- Vomiting (10%)[2]
- Rectal bleeding (7%)[5]
- Anal prolapse (3%)[2]
- Foul smelling wind and stools (empirical symptom)
- Excessive flatulence (empirical symptom)
- Occasional enormous stools or frequent small pellets (empirical symptom)
- Lack of energy, "feeling not well" (empirical symptom)
- Unhappy, angry, or irritable mood (empirical symptom)

Psychological and social problems associated with childhood constipation (20%)[2]

- Moodiness
- Disobedience, disruptive behaviour
- Attention-deficit/hyperactivity disorder
- Poor social competence and learning disabilities
- Anxiety or symptoms of depression
- Less expressive and poorly organised family environments
- Poor school performance

History

The history should include general health, evidence of systemic disease, dietary habits including introduction of cows' milk, and emotional and social aspects (table 2).[15] The use of a symptom diary and the Bristol stool scale can help determine the pattern of defecation (fig 2).[17] Elucidate the age at which first meconium was passed; when constipation, soiling, or an anal fissure with blood on the stool or toilet paper was first noticed; and the presence of any possible precipitating factors (table 2).

Type 1		Separate hard lumps, like nuts (hard to pass)
Type 2		Sausage shaped but lumpy
Type 3		Like a sausage but with cracks on the surface
Type 4		Like a sausage or snake, smooth and soft
Type 5		Soft blobs with clear cut edges
Type 6		Fluffy pieces with ragged edges, a mushy stool
Type 7		Watery, no solid pieces, entirely liquid

Fig 2 Bristol stool chart[17]

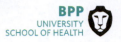

Table 1 Findings on physical examination in childhood constipation[10]

Component of history	Features suggestive of functional constipation	"Red flag" symptoms indicating an underlying disorder
Perineum	Normal appearance of anus and surrounding area; 1-2 fissures	Fistulas, bruising, multiple fissures, tight or patulous anus, anteriorly placed anus
Abdomen	Normal; soft abdominal distension; palpable faecal masses indicating impaction	Gross abdominal distension; tenderness with guarding; pathological (high pitched or absent) bowel sounds
Spine, lumbosacral area, gluteal area	Normal	Asymmetry; sacral agenesis; discoloured skin, naevi, or sinus; hairy patch; lipomas; or central pit
Lower limb	Normal gait, tone, strength, and reflex	Deformity; abnormal gait, tone, strength, or reflexes

Table 2 History taking in childhood constipation[10]

Component of history	Features suggestive of idiopathic constipation	"Red flag" symptoms indicating an underlying disorder
Onset and precipitating factors	Starts after a few weeks of life; fissure, change of diet, infections, timing of potty or toilet training, moving house, starting nursery or school, fears and phobias, major change in family, taking drugs	From birth
Passage of meconium	First stool passed with 48 hours of birth	First stool passed more than 48 hours after birth in term infants
Stool patterns	Overflow soiling—frequent loose stools alternating with infrequent hard stools; "rabbit droppings;" large, infrequent stools that can block the toilet; retentive behaviour; previous or current anal fissure	Ribbon-like stools; explosive offensive stool associated with gross abdominal distension or severe vomiting (particularly bilious)
Growth and general wellbeing	Generally well; weight and height within normal limits	Failure to thrive; evidence of maltreatment
Locomotor development	Normal neurological or locomotor development	Undiagnosed weakness in legs; locomotor delay
Diet and fluid	Changes in infant formula, poor diet, insufficient fluid intake	

Examination

Document whether the child is failing to thrive, which can indicate a systemic condition. It is often possible to detect an impacted faecal mass in the lower abdomen. Table 1 lists warnings signs for systemic or surgical conditions that can be detected on abdominal, perineal, lumbosacral, and lower limb examination.[4] As part of the neurological examination, touching the perianal and gluteal region using a Q-tip (cotton swab), the persistent lack of any perineal sensation (tickle or gluteal contraction) may indicate spinal or other neurological pathology.[15]

Rectal digital examination

NICE specifically recommends against routine digital rectal examination, unless performed by someone with expertise to interpret anatomical abnormalities or Hirschsprung's disease.[10]

Imaging

NICE recommends that abdominal imaging (radiography or ultrasound) is not indicated if the history and physical examination clearly indicate constipation.[10] [11] Although imaging may help clarify uncertainty about an abdominal mass—for example, in obese children,[2] [15] a systematic review found that sensitivity and specificity in diagnosing functional constipation are poor.[18]

Blood tests

Blood tests are not needed to confirm the diagnosis. However, blood tests are need to exclude hypothyroid disease, coeliac disease, and electrolyte disturbances in children with constipation that is resistant to treatment or is associated with other clinical symptoms.[10] Single centre reviews indicate that the prevalence of coeliac disease (1.9%) and hypothyroidism (1%) is increased in constipated children.[19] [20]

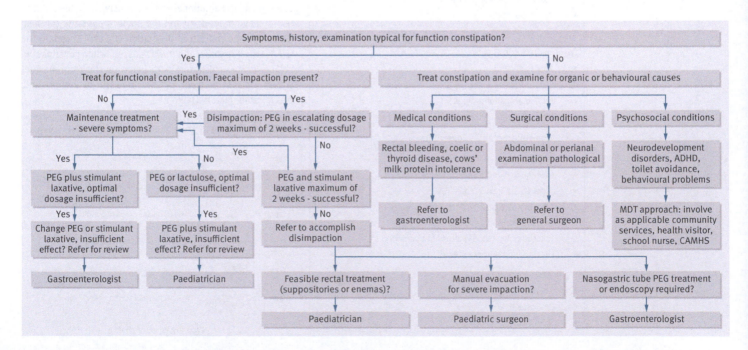

Fig 1 Suggested flow chart for management of childhood constipation. Service arrangements and pathways vary according to regional structures. ADHD=attention-deficit/hyperactivity disorder; CAMHS=child and adolescent health services; MDT=multidisciplinary team; PEG=polyethylene glycol

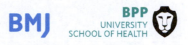

Do invasive investigations have a role?

Inform parents that small retrospective studies and systematic reviews show that it is rarely necessary to perform gastrointestinal endoscopy, anorectal manometry, or transit studies to discriminate functional constipation from other causes.[1 16 18] Referral for endoscopic investigation may be indicated to clarify the cause of rectal bleeding (for example, uncertainty or unresponsiveness to treatment for an anal fissure) or in chronic severe abdominal pain that does not respond to optimised treatment.

Treatment of constipation

The aims are to establish normal frequency and consistency of stools, to enable complete painless faecal evacuation, and to resolve any rectal bleeding or faecal incontinence. Treatment regimens should minimise invasive procedures, allow normal social interactions, and prevent relapse. The treatment principles are education, disimpaction, prevention of reaccumulation of faecal loading, and continued follow-up.[2]

Education of children and parents or guardians

Systematic reviews of four large prospective studies showed that education about constipation and toilet training, the use of a bowel habit diary (with a reward system for younger children), assessment of adherence with regular review of drugs for disimpaction and maintenance, and clear information on expected treatment duration are important for success.[1 2 10 16] It is essential that stool type is understood and recorded using the Bristol stool chart, and that the child is aware of the correlation between impacted stool and involuntary overflow. Encourage children to attempt defecation daily after each meal for five minutes, if necessary supported by a footrest to allow for active straining.[2]

Medical treatment

Oral treatment with an osmotic laxative (such as polyethylene glycol or lactulose), alone or combined with a stimulant laxative (such as bisacodyl), is indicated for all age groups of children (table 3).[21]

On the basis of systematic reviews and a meta-analysis of four well conducted trials, NICE guidance recommends polyethylene glycol (PEG) as first line treatment.[10] PEG promotes disimpaction, improves stool frequency and consistency, reduces pain at defecation and straining, and has fewer side effects than lactulose (table 3).[10] PEG increases water content in the large bowel, whereas lactulose works by promoting fermentation, which results in faecal volume expansion and accelerated transit. In contrast, stimulant laxatives increase bowel motility, whereas rectal suppositories and enemas exert their effect by local stimulation.

A medium sized randomised trial found that lactulose was more effective than senna in regulating normal stool configuration.[1 10] There is no evidence for the use of stimulant laxatives. On the basis of three systematic reviews, senna is recommended as second line combination treatment in the UK, whereas prospective data about other stimulant laxatives are lacking.[1 10 21] A systematic review found no evidence for clinical effectiveness of bulk forming laxatives in children.[10]

A recent systematic review from 14 high quality studies found that, in general, osmotic laxatives, stimulant laxatives, and faecal softeners had infrequent and mild adverse effects.[10] The side effects of PEG included abdominal pain (39%), continued (20%) or transient diarrhoea that resolved after dose adjustment (10-15%), flatulence, and vomiting. For lactulose, side effects included abdominal and rectal pain, diarrhoea, bloating, flatulence (10% each), and colic (5%). For senna they included colic (52%), diarrhoea (10%), and abdominal distension (5%).

Disimpaction

NICE concluded that faecal retention or impaction can be diagnosed by taking an appropriate history, asking the parents about the presence of overflow soiling and bowel habits, and by the detection of palpable faeces on abdominal examination.[10]

According to systematic reviews effective disimpaction is a prerequisite for successful maintenance treatment.[1 2 6 10 21] Without disimpaction, osmotic laxatives for maintenance treatment increase overflow diarrhoea.[2 10 16] One small well conducted prospective trial assessing the dose effects of PEG 3350 suggested that a dosage of 1-1.5 g/kg/day over three days resulted in efficient and safe evacuation of the impacted faeces.[10 16] NICE recommends the use of PEG 3350 plus electrolytes for all age groups in an escalating dose regimen as first line treatment, with the addition of a stimulant laxative (senna, sodium picosulfate, bisacodyl, or docusate sodium) after two weeks if disimpaction is not achieved (table 3).[10] The osmotic (PEG v lactulose) or stimulant laxative may need to be changed if problems persist. When appropriate prolonged medical treatment fails, a randomised controlled trial has shown that rectal applications can prevent complications of a megarectum by improving colonic transit time and reducing rectal distension.[12] In the UK, sodium citrate enema is usually prescribed by paediatricians and specialists when oral treatment has failed.[10]

Enemas work best if the stool is at least partly formed, so oral osmotic laxatives should be stopped during rectal treatment or started thereafter.[2 10] On the basis of a small randomised controlled trial, PEG 3350 is licensed in the UK as a bowel cleansing solution or for treatment in distal intestinal obstruction syndrome.[22] However it requires hospital admission, risk assessment for administration of a nasogastric tube, and strict control of the tube position and electrolyte control.[22]

Maintenance

Start and continue maintenance treatment immediately after disimpaction. Although the dose should be adjusted to produce a daily soft stool, it is equally important to achieve complete rectal evacuation every one to two days without straining. PEG is the recommended first line treatment (with lactulose as an alternative). Start with a maintenance dose that is about half that used for disimpaction.[10]

If PEG does not work even in optimal dosage, try combining it with a stimulant laxative. After sustained improvement (at least three months), gradually reduce the dosage over months to maintain stool consistency, frequency, and complete rectal evacuation.[10]

It is importa3nt to provide advice on the expected time scale, safety, possible side effects, and signs of undertreatment or overtreatment. Parents need reassurance that the drugs do not induce dependency but will need dose adjustment, and that adherence is essential.[2 6 10 21]

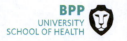

Table 3 Recommended laxatives[2 10 21]

Laxative	Dosage	Side effects
Lactulose	1 month to 1 year: 2.5 ml twice daily[10 21]	Flatulence, abdominal pain
	1-5 years: 2.5-10 ml twice daily[10 21]	
	5-18 years: 5-20 ml twice daily[10 21]	
	European guidelines: 1-3 ml/kg twice daily[2]	
PEG 3350 for disimpaction	<1 year: Movicol paediatric plain, maximum 1 sachet daily[10]	Loose stools, bad taste (PEG + electrolytes)
	1-5 years: Movicol paediatric plain, maximum of 8 sachets daily[10]	
	5-12 years: Movicol paediatric plain, maximum of 12 sachets daily[10]	
	12-18 years: Movicol (adult), maximum 8 sachets daily	
	European guidelines: 0.26-0.84 g/kg/day[2]	
PEG 3350 for maintenance	<1 year: Movicol paediatric plain, maximum of 1 sachet daily[10]	Loose stools, bloating and flatulence, nausea, vomiting
	1-12 years: Movicol paediatric plain, maximum 4 sachets daily[10]	
	12-18 years: Movicol (adult), maximum 3 sachets daily[11]	
	European guidelines: 1-1.5 g/kg/day (3-4 days)[2]	
Bisacodyl oral	4-18 years: 5-10 mg at night[10]	Abdominal cramps, abdominal pain, diarrhoea
Bisacodyl rectal	2-18 years: 5-10 mg suppositories[10]	Abdominal cramps, anal irritation, abdominal pain
Glycerin suppositories	<1 year: 1 paediatric suppository (1 g)[21]	Anal irritation
	1-12 years: 1 suppository (2 g)[21]	
	>12 years: 2 suppositories (4 g)[21]	
Docusate sodium	6 months to 2 years: 12.5 mg three times daily[10 21]	Abdominal cramps
	2-12 years: 12.5-25 mg three times daily[10 71]	
	12-18 years: up to 500 mg in divided doses[10 21]	
Sodium acid phosphate + sodium phosphate enema (Fleet)	3-7 years: 40-60 ml once daily[21]	In patients with renal problems or Hirschsprung's disease: hyperphosphataemia, electrolyte disturbance
	7-12 years: 65-100 ml once daily[21]	
	12-18 years: 90-118 ml once daily[21]	
Sodium citrate enema	3-18 years: 5-10 ml once daily[21]	Anal irritation
Sodiumlaurylsulfoacetate enema (Micro-enema)	1 month to 18 years: 5 ml once daily[21]	Anal irritation
Senna syrup (7.5 mg/5 ml)	1 month to 4 years: 2.5-10 ml once daily[10]	Abdominal cramps, melanosis coli, yellowish brown urine
	4-18 years: 2.5-20 ml once daily[10]	
Sodium picosulfate (5 mg/5 ml)	1 month to 4 years: 2.5-10 mg once at night[10]	Abdominal cramps
	4-18 years: 2.5-20 mg once at night[10]	
Lavage PEG 3350 orally or nasogastric tube	Oral: 15.5-183 ml/kg; first stool expected after 2.8 hours[2]	Nausea, vomiting, abdominal cramps, pulmonary aspiration or oedema
	Nasogastric tube: 1-1.5 g/kg/day (3-4 days); first stool expected after 1.9 days[2]	

PEG=polyethylene glycol.

Diet and lifestyle interventions

A well conducted prospective trial found that fibre has a positive effect on stool frequency and consistency and abdominal pain.[23] Ask whether the introduction of cows' milk triggered the onset of constipation. A systematic review of four prospective studies found that constipation and anal fissures were associated with a cows' milk diet and improved on elimination in a subgroup of children.[24]

A systemic review of nine prospective randomised controlled trials of limited quality that investigated non-drug based treatments of chronic childhood constipation found no significant benefits from increased fluid intake, exercise, prebiotics, probiotics, behavioural therapy, biofeedback, multidisciplinary treatment, or forms of alternative medicine.[25]

Management plan: when and where to refer

Diagnosis and management are possible within primary care services and require regular and frequent review by the general practitioner, health visitor, community nurse, or school nurse. Referral to general paediatricians is indicated for refractory constipation or to investigate secondary symptoms (such as failure to thrive) (fig 1). Hospital admission may be required to effect disimpaction.

Indications for referral to paediatric gastroenterologists or surgeons include suspected organic conditions that require a specific treatment or other problems, such as undefined rectal bleeding.

Severe chronicity of symptoms (persistent soiling) requires healthcare planning with community services, psychological services, and social services.[2]

When is surgical involvement needed in children with functional constipation?

Surgical input is needed to diagnose Hirschsprung's disease by rectal biopsy and rarely to carry out inspection and anal calibration in undiagnosed anorectal malformations. Furthermore, if examination of the spine raises suspicion of occult spinal pathology, such as tethered cord syndrome or spina bifida occulta, a surgical review is needed to correlate clinical findings and magnetic resonance imaging of the spine.[10]

One longitudinal observational study of children with faecal impaction reported the successful management of soiling in 52% of children with manual evacuation and continued enema disimpaction.[26]

When is a rectal biopsy needed?

In 80-90% of cases, Hirschsprung's disease presents in the neonatal period with bile stained vomiting and evidence of distal bowel obstruction on radiography. A large retrospective observational study indicated a low yield of positive biopsies in suspected idiopathic constipation. A rectal biopsy is always indicated for delayed passage of meconium (>48 hours), severe constipation in Down's syndrome, enterocolitic episodes, or if there is no response to an appropriate bowel management strategy.[27] Biopsy should be performed in a centre with expertise in the condition (paediatric surgeon and histopathologist).

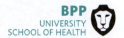

Fissure in ano
Evidence from a randomised controlled trial indicated that anal fissures have a high spontaneous healing rate with medical treatment, so interventions such as anal stretch, lateral anal sphincterotomy, or intrasphincteric injection of botulinum toxin are rarely indicated.[28]

Indications for anal procedures in functional constipation
If faecal impaction persists despite appropriate medical treatment, manual evacuation under general anaesthesia by a paediatric surgeon may be required. A double blind randomised controlled trial found no benefit for anal dilatation.[29] A small double blind randomised controlled trial found that intrasphincteric injection of botulinum toxin was as effective as internal sphincter myectomy in the management of refractory constipation.[30] [31]

Is there any evidence that functional constipation should be managed surgically?
Intervention studies suggest a role for appendicostomy or tube/button caecostomy antegrade colonic enema in cases refractory to conservative treatment after the age of 6 years.[10] Access is provided to the proximal colon via a small stoma in the lower abdomen, which is used for flushing (irrigation) the bowel with fluids using a catheter. Sizeable cohort studies show improvement in continence, soiling, quality of life scores, and management failure, as well as resolution of symptoms, albeit associated with appreciable morbidity.[31] [32] [33] Colostomy has been widely used to manage overflow soiling and megarectum with the option of eventual restoration of continuity.[34]

TIPS FOR NON-SPECIALISTS

- Children with constipation can present with a variety of symptoms, including faecal incontinence, rectal bleeding, and abdominal pain
- Treatment success depends on early recognition and administration of osmotic laxatives. The dosage and duration of treatment need to be sufficient and a combination of drugs may be needed
- Surgical treatment is appropriate and effective in a subgroup of patients

---

ADDITIONAL EDUCATIONAL RESOURCES

Resources for healthcare professionals

- National Institute for Health and Clinical Excellence. Diagnosis and management of idiopathic childhood constipation in primary and secondary care. 2010. http://publications.nice.org.uk/constipation-in-children-and-young-people-cg99
- National Institute for Health and Clinical Excellence. Constipation in children and young people (CG99). www.nice.org.uk/CG99
- NHS Evidence. CKS clinical knowledge summaries: constipation in children. Management.
- www.cks.nhs.uk/constipation_in_children/management/scenario_diagnosis_and_assessment_younger_than_1_year/view_full_scenario#467016006

Resources for patients

- NHS choices (www.nhs.uk/Conditions/Constipation/Pages/Treatment.aspx)—Advice for patients and parents on constipation and its treatment, including lifestyle advice
- National Institute for Health and Clinical Excellence (http://guidance.nice.org.uk/CG99/PublicInfo/doc/English)—Guideline for patients and carers on understanding NICE guidance CG99 on constipation in children and young people
- National Digestive Diseases Information Clearinghouse (http://digestive.niddk.nih.gov/ddiseases/pubs/constipationchild/)—US website containing information on constipation in children
- Bristol stool chart form (http://commons.wikimedia.org/wiki/File:Bristol_Stool_Chart.png)—Classifies different types of faeces by consistency and form into seven categories, using images and text, to aid clinical communication and assess the effectiveness of treatment

---

AREAS FOR FUTURE RESEARCH

- Validation of non-invasive tools to diagnose degree of faecal impaction
- Prospective studies investigating regimens for disimpaction and maintenance as monotherapy or combination treatment
- Licensing of oral medicines and rectal preparations for all age groups

---

Transit studies are useful to distinguish between pancolonic and distal motility problems, or between functional faecal incontinence with or without constipation.[18] One large observational study demonstrated spinal cord pathology in 3% of children with idiopathic constipation and normal neurological examination using magnetic resonance imaging of the spine. All children responded to medical treatment of constipation.[35]

What is the prognosis in childhood constipation?
Two large longitudinal outcome studies reported multiple relapses after the initial treatment, particularly in boys, in children under 4 years of age, in those with a background of psychosocial or behavioural problems, or when constipation was associated with encopresis.[16] [27] [36] Overall, resolution of constipation occurred in 50% of children after one year and 65-70% after two years. A third of children followed up beyond puberty continued to have severe problems.[27]

Contributors: MKHA and RV conceived the review. All authors helped planning, research, write, and edit the article. MKHA is guarantor.

Competing interests: All authors have completed the ICMJE uniform disclosure form at www.icmje.org/coi_disclosure.pdf (available on request from the corresponding author) and declare: no support from any organisation for the submitted work; no financial relationships with any organisations that might have an interest in the submitted work in the previous three years; no other relationships or activities that could appear to have influenced the submitted work.

Provenance and peer review: Commissioned; externally peer reviewed.

1 Tabbers MM, Boluyt N, Berger MY, Benninga MA. Clinical evidence BMJ overview: constipation in children. 2010 Apr 6. http://clinicalevidence.bmj.com/x/systematic-review/0303/overview.html.
2 Benninga MA, Voskuijl WP, Taminiau JA. Childhood constipation: is there new light in the tunnel? J Pediatr Gastroenterol Nutr2004;39:448-64.
3 Benninga M, Candy DC, Catto-Smith AG, Clayden G, Loening-Baucke V, Di Lorenzo C, et al. The Paris Consensus on Childhood Constipation Terminology (PACCT) Group. J Pediatr Gastroenterol Nutr2005;40:273-5.
4 Mugie SM, Benninga MA, Di Lorenzo C. Epidemiology of constipation in children and adults: a systematic review. Best Pract Res Clin Gastroenterol2011;25:3-18.
5 Boccia G, Manguso F, Coccorullo P, Masi P, Pensabene L, Staiano A. Functional defecation disorders in children: PACCT criteria versus Rome II criteria. J Pediatr2007;151:394-98.
6 Gordon M, Naidoo K, Akobeng AK, Thomas AG. Osmotic and stimulant laxatives for the management of childhood constipation (protocol). Cochrane Database Syst Rev2011;5:CD009118.
7 Pang KH, Croaker GD. Constipation in children with autism and autistic spectrum disorder. Constipation in children with autism and autistic spectrum disorder. Pediatr Surg Int 2011;27:353-8.
8 Benninga MA, Büller HA, Tytgat GN, Akkermans LM, Bossuyt PM, Taminiau JA. Colonic transit time in constipated children: does pediatric slow-transit constipation exist? J Pediatr Gastroenterol Nutr1996;23:241-51.
9 Van der Plas RN, Benninga MA, Redekop WK, Taminiau JA, Büller HA. Randomised trial of biofeedback training for encopresis. Arch Dis Child1996;75:367-74.
10 National Institute for Health and Clinical Excellence. Constipation in children and young people. Diagnosis and management of idiopathic childhood constipation in primary and secondary care. CG99. 2010, updated 2012. http://publications.nice.org.uk/constipation-in-children-and-young-people-cg99.
11 Blum NJ, Taubman B, Nemeth N. During toilet training, constipation occurs before stool toileting refusal. Pediatrics2004;113:e520-2.
12 Bekkali NL, van den Berg MM, Dijkgraaf MG, van Wijk MP, Bongers ME, Liem O, et al. Rectal fecal impaction treatment in childhood constipation: enemas versus high doses oral PEG. Pediatrics2009;124:e1108-15.

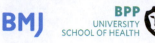

13 Keuzenkamp-Jansen CW, Fijnvandraat CJ, Kneepkens CM, Douwes AC. Diagnostic dilemmas and results of treatment for chronic constipation. *Arch Dis Child*1996;75:36-41.

14 Van Ginkel R, Reitsma JB, Buller HA, van Wijk MP, Taminiau JA, Benninga MA. Childhood constipation: longitudinal follow-up beyond puberty. *Gastroenterology*2003;125:357-63.

15 Loening-Baucke V. Functional fecal retention in childhood. *Practical Gastroenterology*2002;November:13-25. www.practicalgastro.com/pdf/Novembero2/LoeningBauckeArticle.pdf.

16 Van den Berg MM, Benninga MA, Di Lorenzo C. Epidemiology of childhood constipation: a systematic review. *Am J Gastroenterology*2006;101:2401-9.

17 Lewis SJ, Heaton KW. Stool form scale as a useful guide to intestinal transit time. *Scand J Gastroenterol*1997;32:920-4.

18 Berger MY, Tabbers MM, Kurver MJ, Boluyt N, Benninga MA. Value of abdominal radiography, colonic transit time, and rectal ultrasound scanning in the diagnosis of idiopathic constipation in children: a systematic review. *J Pediatr*2012;161:44-50.e1-2.

19 Pelleboer RA, Janssen RL, Deckers-Kocken JM, Wouters E, Nissen AC, Bolz WE, et al. Celiac disease is overrepresented in patients with constipation. *J Pediatr (Rio J)* 2012;88:173-6.

20 Bennett WE Jr, Heuckeroth RO. Hypothyroidism is a rare cause of isolated constipation. *J Pediatr Gastroenterol Nutr* 2012;54:285-7.

21 BNF for children 2011-2012. BMJ Group, 2012:64.

22 Tolia V, Lin CH, Elitsur Y. A prospective randomized study with mineral oil and oral lavage solution for treatment of faecal impaction in children. *Aliment Pharmacol Ther*1993;7:523-9.

23 Castillejo G, Bullo M, Anguera A, Escribano J, Salas-Salvado J. A controlled, randomized, double-blind trial to evaluate the effect of a supplement of cocoa husk that is rich in dietary fiber on colonic transit in constipated pediatric patients. *Pediatrics*2006;118:e641-8.

24 Anonymous. Evaluation and treatment of constipation in children: summary of updated recommendations of the North American Society for Pediatric Gastroenterology, Hepatology and Nutrition. *J Pediatr Gastroenterol Nutr*2006;43:405-7.

25 Tabbers MM, Boluyt N, Berger MY, Benninga MA. Nonpharmacologic treatments for childhood constipation: systematic review. *Pediatrics*2011;128:753-61.

26 Godbole PP, Pinfield A, Stringer MD. Idiopathic megarectum in children. *Eur J Pediatr Surg*2001;11:48-51.

27 Lewis NA, Levitt MA, Zallen GS, Zafar MS, Iacono KL, Rossman JE, et al. Diagnosing Hirschsprung's disease: increasing the odds of a positive rectal biopsy result. *J Pediatr Surg*2003;38:412-6.

28 Kenny SE, Irvine T, Driver CP, Nunn AT, Losty PD, Jones MO, et al. Double blind randomised controlled trial of topical glyceryl trinitrate in anal fissure. *Arch Dis Child*2001;85:404-7.

29 Keshtgar AS, Ward HC, Clayden GS, Sanei A. Role of anal dilatation in treatment of idiopathic constipation in children: long-term follow-up of a double-blind randomized controlled study. *Pediatr Surg Int*2005;21:100-5.

30 Freeman NV. Intractable constipation in children treated by forceful anal stretch or anorectal myectomy: preliminary communication. *J R Soc Med*1984;77(suppl 3):6-8.

31 Keshtgar AS, Ward HC, Sanei A, Clayden GS. Botulinum toxin, a new treatment modality for chronic idiopathic constipation in children: long-term follow-up of a double-blind randomized trial. *J Pediatr Surg*2007;42:672-80.

32 King SK, Sutcliffe JR, Southwell BR, Chait PG, Hutson JM. The antegrade continence enema successfully treats idiopathic slow-transit constipation. *J Pediatr Surg*2005;40:1935-40.

33 Jaffray B. What happens to children with idiopathic constipation who receive an antegrade continent enema? An actuarial analysis of 80 consecutive cases. *J Pediatr Surg*2009;44:404-7.

34 Asipu D, Jaffray B. Treatment of severe childhood constipation with restorative proctocolectomy. *Arch Dis Child*2010;95:867-70.

35 Bekkali NL, Hagebeuk EE, Bongers ME, van Rijn RR, Van Wijk MP, Liem O, et al. Magnetic resonance imaging of the lumbosacral spine in children with chronic constipation or non-retentive fecal incontinence: a prospective study. *J Pediatr*2010;156:461-5.

36 Keuzenkamp-Jansen CW, Fijnvandraat CJ, Kneepkens CM, Douwes AC. Diagnostic dilemmas and results of treatment for chronic constipation. *Arch Dis Child*1996;75:36-41.

Related links

bmj.com/archive

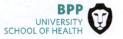

Management of bloody diarrhoea in children in primary care

M Stephen Murphy senior lecturer in paediatrics and child health, consultant paediatric gastroenterologist[12]

[1]Division of Reproductive and Child Health, Medical School, University of Birmingham, Birmingham B15 2TT

[2]Birmingham Children's Hospital NHS Foundation Trust, Birmingham B4 6NH

Correspondence to: M Stephen Murphy m.s.murphy@bham.ac.uk

Cite this as: BMJ 2008;336:1010

<DOI> 10.1136/bmj.39542.440417.BE
http://www.bmj.com/content/336/7651/1010

Bloody diarrhoea is an uncommon symptom in children, and it may indicate the presence of serious disease. This review focuses on children presenting in a primary care setting. The non-specialist should be aware of the likely causes, initial management, and indications for specialist referral. The emphasis is on children in the developed world, although traveller's diarrhoea is also considered. The epidemiology and management of this condition are different in the developing world, where infectious causes predominate. In recent years the reported incidence of inflammatory bowel disease increased greatly in the developed world and important advances have been made in its management. This diagnosis should always be considered carefully.

What are the most likely causes of bloody diarrhoea in children?

The likely diagnoses vary depending on age (box). At every age intestinal bacterial infections are an important cause. Inflammatory bowel disease may occur at any age but is more likely in older children (>1 year). In young infants non-specific (perhaps allergic) colitis is most likely. Other conditions are rarer but should be considered as they can be serious and even life threatening.

How common is infection compared with inflammatory bowel disease?

This is an important question because if it is assumed that bloody diarrhoea is caused by infection then inflammatory bowel disease will be missed. Because of this common assumption, children with inflammatory bowel disease often experience a delay in diagnosis.[1]

In the United Kingdom, the most likely causative infective agents are species of *Campylobacter*, *Salmonella*, and *Yersinia*. Much less often, *Shigella*, types of *Escherichia coli* that produce shiga toxin (such as *E coli* O157:H7), and other organisms are responsible. In the developing world other disorders including bacterial (*Shigella*) and amoebic (*Entamoeba histolytica*) dysentery are important. This should be considered in those who have recently been overseas.

Determining the incidence of infection as a cause of bloody diarrhoea is not simple, but an estimate can be made. A prospective cohort study in the UK found that 1:30 people (adults and children) presented to their general practitioner annually with gastroenteritis.[2] Bacterial gastroenteritis was confirmed in a minority of cases. The annual incidences of specific bacterial isolates (per 1000 population) were *Campylobacter* 4.14 (95% confidence interval 3.34 to 5.13), *Salmonella* 1.57 (1.19 to 2.06), *Yersinia* 0.58 (0.42 to 0.88), *Shigella* 0.27 (0.16 to 0.47), and *E coli* O157:H7 0.03 (0.01 to

---

SOURCES AND SELECTION CRITERIA

I used the Medline database to search for evidence from the literature. Randomised controlled trials, meta-analyses, and Cochrane reviews were used when relevant and available. Other sources of evidence included large case series and cohort studies. I obtained information on the incidence of specific pathogens from the UK Health Protection Agency's Centre for Infections

---

CAUSES OF BLOODY DIARRHOEA (REAL OR APPARENT) IN INFANTS AND CHILDREN

Infants aged <1 year

Common causes
- Intestinal infection
- Infant colitis
- Non-specific colitis
- Breast milk colitis
- Cow's milk colitis

Less common or rare causes
- Intestinal ischaemia
- Intussusception
- Malrotation and volvulus
- Necrotising enterocolitis
- Hirschsprung's disease
- Inflammatory bowel disease
- Crohn's colitis
- Ulcerative colitis
- Systemic vasculitis
- Factitious illness

Infants aged >1 year

Common causes
- Intestinal infection
- Inflammatory bowel disease
- Crohn's colitis
- Ulcerative colitis
- Juvenile polyp

Less common or rare causes
- Intestinal ischaemia
- Intussusception
- Malrotation and volvulus
- Mucosal prolapse syndrome
- Henoch-Schönlein purpura or other forms of systemic vasculitis
- Factitious illness

SUMMARY POINTS

- Bloody diarrhoea in infancy and childhood often indicates serious gastrointestinal disease
- Intestinal bacterial infection is the most common cause—*Campylobacter*, *Salmonella*, and *Yersinia* are important in the developed world
- Bacterial gastroenteritis is usually self limiting—antibiotics are needed only in selected cases
- Crohn's disease and ulcerative colitis often present with bloody diarrhoea and should be considered in all ages
- Children with severe bloody diarrhoea or signs of systemic illness need urgent specialist referral, as these symptoms may indicate a life threatening condition

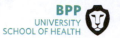

0.11). Reports to the UK Health Protection Agency's centre for infections suggest that about 15% of *Campylobacter*, 30% of *Salmonella*, and 50% of *Yersinia* infections are in children (www.hpa.org.uk). Thus, in a primary care setting the annual incidence of these bacterial infections in children may be around 1.5 per 1000. About 50-75 per 100 000 of children will develop bloody diarrhoea with these infections.

Bloody diarrhoea is a presenting symptom in about 75% of children with ulcerative colitis and 25% with Crohn's disease (table 1).[1] [3] A prospective study of paediatric inflammatory bowel disease in the UK and Ireland reported an annual incidence of 5.2 (4.8 to 5.6) per 100000.[3] Of these, 27% had ulcerative colitis and 60% Crohn's disease. The incidence of children presenting with bloody diarrhoea as a result of inflammatory bowel disease is therefore 2-3 per 100000 population.

Thus, in the developed world bloody diarrhoea in children is 15-20 times more likely to be caused by intestinal infections than by inflammatory bowel disease. In the developing world, although the true incidence of inflammatory bowel disease is unknown, bacterial and amoebic dysentery are much more likely to be the cause.

How should I investigate and manage bloody diarrhoea in primary care?

An appropriate strategy must take into account the severity and symptoms or signs of systemic illness or abdominal complications. Figure 1 outlines an approach to management, with suggested indications for specialist referral.

How should I investigate and manage intestinal infections?

Table 2 summarises the sources, clinical presentation, diagnosis, and management of various types of intestinal bacterial infections. Antibiotics are usually contraindicated. With *Campylobacter*, a meta-analysis of 11 randomised controlled trials reported that early antibiotics shortened the illness slightly,[4] but treatment is usually reserved for those with severe symptoms or impaired immunity. For *Salmonella*, a Cochrane review of 12 randomised controlled trials concluded that antibiotics provided no benefit and that treatment may prolong carriage.[5] Antibiotics are usually reserved for young infants and children with suspected bacteraemia, extraintestinal spread, or impaired immunity. Patients with *Shigella* require antibiotic treatment with, for example, ciprofloxacin. For this reason routine antibiotic treatment is given to patients with bloody diarrhoea in developing countries.

Salmonella infections generally present with diarrhoea and fever, and it usually settles within days. It is readily cultured from stool. In some patients, typically after a period of persistent diarrhoea, bloody mucoid diarrhoea develops as a result of colitis. If the organism is no longer detectable and the symptoms of colitis persist it may be difficult to distinguish from inflammatory bowel disease (fig 2). *Yersinia* is most common in children under 5 years. It may cause pain and ulceration in the terminal ileum and Crohn's disease may be wrongly suspected.

Haemolytic uraemic syndrome is a rare and life threatening condition with sudden onset of microangiopathic haemolytic anaemia, thrombocytopenia, and renal insufficiency. Most (80%) patients will have had bloody diarrhoea for three to 16 days previously. It is usually caused by shiga toxin producing *E coli*, often 0157:H7.

When should I suspect inflammatory bowel disease?

Inflammatory bowel disease is uncommon in children, but prompt diagnosis is important. The interval from onset to diagnosis is often prolonged, and this can result in avoidable morbidity.[1] [3] In a study of children presenting to a tertiary centre, even though 75% of those with ulcerative colitis had persistent or recurrent bloody diarrhoea, the mean time to diagnosis was 20 weeks (table 3).[1]

Although infection may be the first consideration, the possibility of inflammatory bowel disease should not be dismissed even in young children. Around half of children

TABLE 1   PRESENTING SYMPTOMS AND SIGNS IN INFLAMMATORY BOWEL DISEASE[1]

Symptoms	Crohn's disease (%)	Ulcerative colitis (%)
Intestinal symptoms		
Bloody diarrhoea	22	75
Non-bloody diarrhoea	42	15
Diarrhoea (overall)	64	90
Blood per rectum (no diarrhoea)	1.6	10
Abdominal pain	83	83
Anorexia and weight loss	88	56
Perianal disease	45	0
Constipation	11	0
Extraintestinal manifestations		
Clubbing	25	0
Arthralgia	8	4.7
Erythema nodosum	5	0

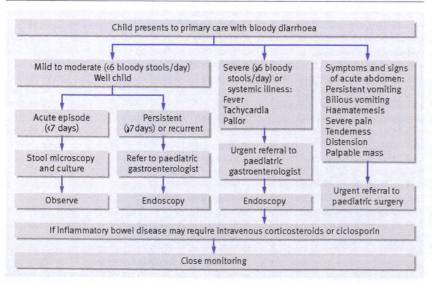

Fig 1 Strategy for initial evaluation, management, and referral of children presenting with bloody diarrhoea

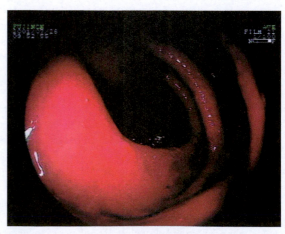

Fig 2 Ulcerative colitis resulting in mucosal inflammation with spontaneous bleeding. Patients with haemorrhagic colitis caused by *Salmonella* or other infections may present with an identical appearance

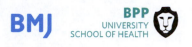

with inflammatory bowel disease present before 11 years of age, and the disease may occur even in the first year of life. If any symptoms suggest chronic gastrointestinal disease, inflammatory bowel disease should be considered (table 2). Persistent (more than seven days) or recurrent bloody diarrhoea are indications for referral to a paediatric gastroenterologist. Other important signs include impaired growth, weight loss, finger clubbing, and—in Crohn's disease—oral or perianal abnormalities. Perianal disease occurs in up to 45% of people with Crohn's disease.[1][3]

How should I screen for inflammatory bowel disease?
Screening blood tests can be helpful, but in the context of bloody diarrhoea their role is limited. In a study of children presenting to a specialist paediatric gastroenterology clinic with suspected inflammatory bowel disease the simple combination of haemoglobin and platelet count was useful.[7] Using "one or both tests abnormal" as a positive outcome gave a sensitivity of 92%, a specificity of 80%, and positive and negative predictive values of 77% and 93% for ulcerative colitis. However, another study found that haemoglobin, albumin, erythrocyte sedimentation rate, and C reactive protein were normal in 19% of children presenting with clinically mild ulcerative colitis.[8] Normal blood tests do not rule out inflammatory bowel disease in children with bloody diarrhoea. Moreover, abnormal results may be found in children with bacterial gastroenteritis. In the absence of an identified stool pathogen, endoscopic evaluation is required in children with severe or persistent symptoms (fig 1).

UNANSWERED QUESTIONS
- How can the incidence of bacterial intestinal infection be reduced?
- Given the increased incidence of inflammatory bowel disease in the developed world, what environmental factors are responsible?
- Does bacterial gastroenteritis cause irritable bowel syndrome in children, as is reported in adults?
- Are antibiotics advisable for patients with haemorrhagic colitis caused by *Escherichia coli* that produce shiga toxin?
- What are the aetiology and pathogenesis of infant colitis?

How can I recognise and manage severe colitis?
Severe bloody diarrhoea (more than five bloody stools daily) requires urgent referral to a paediatric gastroenterologist. Severe colitis is associated with an increased risk of non-response to medical treatment, progression to toxic megacolon, and colonic perforation. Early referral may reduce these risks. Intravenous corticosteroids or ciclosporin are often effective in severe disease, and children need expert monitoring for signs of deterioration. In some cases emergency colectomy may be life saving.

Which diagnoses are most likely in infants?
Infant colitis
Colonoscopy often shows mucosal inflammation and ulceration in infants who present with bloody diarrhoea. Although cows' milk allergy is usually suspected, the aetiology is often uncertain. Allergy is probably overdiagnosed.[9][10] Many infants with bloody diarrhoea are breast fed and have "breast milk colitis." In these cases, it has been proposed that small but immunologically relevant amounts of intact maternal dietary antigens might be transferred to breast milk via the mother's bloodstream. However, this hypothesis has not been confirmed. A recent study of 40 infants presenting with blood in the stool provided a useful insight.[10] The mean age at presentation was 3 months (range 1-6). The stools were watery in 38% and mucoid in 73%. Colonoscopy showed mucosal aphthae (33%), microscopic inflammation (33%), and focal eosinophilic infiltration (23%). The infants were randomly allocated to a cows' milk-free diet (n=19) or a normal diet (n=21), with breastfeeding mothers in the first group adopting a cows' milk elimination diet. They were reviewed at one and 12 months. During follow-up, bleeding was often intermittent, with an average time to the final episode of 24 days (range 1-85). All of the infants thrived. Cows' milk elimination did not affect the duration of bleeding, and re-challenge supported a diagnosis of cows' milk allergy in only 18%. The authors concluded that infant colitis is usually a benign self limiting disorder.

Table 2 Summary of bacterial intestinal infections that cause bloody diarrhoea

Pathogen	Sources	Incubation period	Clinical presentation	Diagnosis	Treatment
Campylobacter jejuni	Mainly from farm and domestic animals and animal food products, especially undercooked chicken	1-3 days (occasionally up to 10 days)	Fever and diarrhoea; bloody diarrhoea in up to 50%; usually lasts less than 1 week, with relapses in up to 25%	Stool culture; selective growth medium needed	Antibiotics reserved for those with severe symptoms or impaired immunity[4]
Salmonella species	Mainly food borne—can cause large outbreaks; farm animals (especially undercooked poultry); pets (including reptiles); person to person transmission less frequent; infants (3-5 months) especially vulnerable	6-48 hours (occasionally longer)	Gastroenteritis-like illness, often with fever lasting 3-4 days; bloody mucoid diarrhoea may follow as colitis develops; colitis may persist for 1-12 weeks	Stool culture; may stay positive for weeks	Antibiotics not usually beneficial and may prolong bacterial carriage[5]; antibiotics reserved for young infants, those with suspected bacteraemia or with extraintestinal spread, and those with impaired immunity
Yersinia enterocolitica	Farm and domestic animals; epidemics related to contaminated milk and ice cream	3-7 days	Usually presents with fever, abdominal pain, and diarrhoea; blood present in the stool in about 30%; illness usually lasts 1-3 weeks	Stool culture; organism easily missed so the laboratory should be advised of suspicion	No evidence of benefit with antibiotics, and diagnosis is often late; antibiotics reserved for those with impaired immunity or extraintestinal spread
Shiga toxin producing *Escherichia coli* (such as O157 H7)	Often caused by foods contaminated with bovine faeces, such as undercooked minced (ground) beef; large outbreaks may occur	3-9 days	Often presents with watery diarrhoea, which progresses to bloody diarrhoea; typically lasts 3-8 days; haemolytic uraemic syndrome can develop after 3-16 days	Specialised diagnostic techniques needed	Antibiotics seem to have no clinical benefit and may increase the risk of haemolytic uraemic syndrome[6]
Shigella species	Highly contagious; usually person to person transmission; occasional outbreaks from contamination of food or water; most common between 6 months and 5 years of age; more severe in adults	1-4 days	A few patients present with gastroenteritis-like illness; most experience lower abdominal pain, bloody mucoid stools, and fever; illness may be life threatening, with septicaemia	Stool microscopy shows pus cells and red cells; the organism is fastidious and requires prompt inoculation into appropriate medium for culture	Treated with antibiotics (for example, ciprofloxacin); during outbreaks or in high prevalence areas in the developing world antibiotics are given presumptively

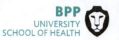

Necrotising enterocolitis

Necrotising enterocolitis is a serious disorder, rarely seen in primary care. It is characterised by diffuse or focal ulceration and necrosis in the small intestine and colon, and it may present with rectal bleeding or bloody diarrhoea. Other common features include abdominal distension, bilious vomiting, and signs of septicaemia. It mainly occurs in premature infants in the neonatal unit, although it can develop at any time up to 10 weeks of age. Moreover, up to 10% of cases are in full term infants.[11] In such cases, predisposing factors such as cardiac disease may be present.[11] [12] When necrotising enterocolitis does occur in full term infants, the onset is usually within the first week of life.[11] [13] If it is suspected then urgent hospital referral is necessary. Abdominal radiography may show features to support the diagnosis.

Hirschsprung's disease

Hirschsprung's disease (congenital absence of ganglion cells in the colon) occurs in 1:5000 live births. About 80% of affected children present in the first year of life. In more than 90% of affected infants the passage of meconium is delayed beyond the first 24 hours. The classic presentation is with constipation. However, 25% of infants present with enterocolitis causing abdominal distension, and severe watery and sometimes bloody diarrhoea.[14] This may cause hypovolaemic shock and colonic perforation, and mortality is 33% in these patients.[15] Early diagnosis is therefore essential.

What other disorders should I consider?

Any disorder that leads to mucosal ischaemia can cause bloody diarrhoea.

TIPS FOR NON-SPECIALISTS

- Children with fewer than six stools daily may be managed in primary care if they are not systemically unwell and do not have an acute abdomen
- Evidence of systemic illness includes fever, tachycardia, pallor, and shock
- Evidence of an abdominal surgical emergency includes severe pain, persistent or bilious vomiting, haematemesis, distension, tenderness, a palpable mass, and signs of septicaemia or shock
- Consider inflammatory bowel disease in children with evidence of chronic disease—persistent or recurrent bloody diarrhoea or other gastrointestinal symptoms, weight loss, or poor growth
- Severe colitis—associated with severe bloody diarrhoea—is life threatening and requires immediate referral to a paediatric gastroenterologist

---

ADDITIONAL EDUCATIONAL RESOURCES

Resources for healthcare professionals

- Health Protection Agency, Centre for Infections (www.hpa.org.uk)—Provides up to date surveillance information on the epidemiology of gastrointestinal infections in the UK

Resources for parents

- National Association for Colitis and Crohn's disease (www.nacc.org.uk)—Provides support and information for patients with ulcerative colitis and Crohn's disease
- Crohn's in Childhood Research Association (www.cicra.org)—Provides support for patients with inflammatory bowel disease, particularly children and young adults, and raises funds to support medical research into the disease

---

Table 3 Time interval from first symptoms to diagnosis of inflammatory bowel disease[1]

Diagnosis	Crohn's disease (weeks)	Ulcerative colitis
Crohn's disease	47	4 weeks to 7 years
With diarrhoea	28	4 weeks to 5 years
Without diarrhoea	66	27 weeks to 7 years
Ulcerative colitis	20	2 weeks to 3 years
Indeterminate colitis*	45	2 weeks to 2 years

*Colitis caused by inflammatory bowel disease in which it is not possible to distinguish between ulcerative colitis and Crohn's disease.

Intestinal infarction—a surgical emergency

Bloody diarrhoea can indicate a major surgical emergency. Intussusception occurs most often but not exclusively in the first year of life. The classic presentation is with episodic abdominal pain, vomiting, and the passage of blood and mucous. In some cases bloody diarrhoea is reported.[16] In infants and children with congenital gut malrotation, midgut volvulus may result in extensive intestinal gangrene. This catastrophic event typically presents with symptoms of obstruction including bilious vomiting. Again, however, bloody diarrhoea may be reported.[17]

Henoch-Schönlein purpura

Henoch-Schönlein purpura is a common form of idiopathic systemic vasculitis in children. It is associated with a characteristic rash (easily overlooked), abdominal pain, arthralgia, and overt or microscopic haematuria.[18] Overt gastrointestinal bleeding occurs in 25% of patients and bloody diarrhoea is sometimes seen.[19]

Is it really bloody diarrhoea?

Juvenile polyps

Juvenile polyps (inflammatory polyps) occur in about 1% of children (fig 3). They are usually associated with the passage of blood and mucous, but diarrhoea may be reported.[20] [21] Colonoscopy is required for diagnosis.

Mucosal prolapse syndrome and solitary rectal ulcer syndrome

Children with mucosal prolapse syndrome may report bloody diarrhoea.[22] However, the true symptom may be tenesmus—the frequent urge to defecate with just the passage of blood and mucous. In this disorder the anterior rectal mucosa is prone to prolapse, although this is often not reported by the child. The prolapse leads to mucosal injury. In some cases it is associated with the development of inflammatory cloacogenic polyps at the anorectal junction. The polyps may be detected on digital examination and are seen at endoscopy; they have a characteristic histological appearance.[23]

Solitary rectal ulcer syndrome presents with similar symptoms. The pathogenesis of this condition is uncertain, but it is probably also caused by mucosal prolapse. At endoscopy, anterior rectal ulceration is seen several centimetres above the anal canal.

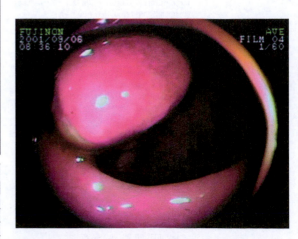

Fig 3 Typical appearance of pedunculated juvenile polyp identified at colonoscopy in the sigmoid colon. This child was said to have bloody mucoid "diarrhoea"

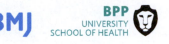

Factitious illness and illness induction

Very rarely, diarrhoea and gastrointestinal bleeding may be falsely reported either by young people or by carers.[24][25] This possibility should be considered if the clinical circumstances are bizarre or if there are other reasons for concern.

Contributors: MSM is sole author. Olivier Fontaine, of the World Health Organization (Geneva), kindly reviewed this manuscript and contributed helpful comments and advice.

Competing interests: None declared.

Provenance and peer review: Commissioned; externally peer reviewed.

1 Spray C, Debelle GD, Murphy MS. Current diagnosis, management and morbidity in paediatric inflammatory bowel disease. *Acta Paediatr* 2001;90:400-5.

2 Wheeler JG, Sethi D, Cowden JM, Wall PG, Rodrigues LC, Tompkins DS, et al. Study of infectious intestinal disease in England: rates in the community, presenting to general practice, and reported to national surveillance. The Infectious Intestinal Disease Study Executive. *BMJ* 1999;318:1046-50.

3 Sawczenko A, Sandhu BK. Presenting features of inflammatory bowel disease in Great Britain and Ireland. *Arch Dis Child* 2003;88:995-1000.

4 Ternhag A, Asikainen T, Giesecke J, Ekdahl K. A meta-analysis on the effects of antibiotic treatment on duration of symptoms caused by infection with Campylobacter species. *Clin Infect Dis* 2007;44:696-700.

5 Sirinavin S, Garner P. Antibiotics for treating salmonella gut infections. *Cochrane Database Syst Rev* 2000;(2):CD001167.

6 Wong CS, Jelacic S, Habeeb RL, Watkins SL, Tarr PI. The risk of the hemolytic-uremic syndrome after antibiotic treatment of Escherichia coli O157:H7 infections. *N Engl J Med* 2000;342:1930-6.

7 Cabrera-Abreu JC, Davies P, Matek Z, Murphy MS. Performance of blood tests in diagnosis of inflammatory bowel disease in a specialist clinic. *Arch Dis Child* 2004;89:69-71.

8 Mack DR, Langton C, Markowitz J, LeLeiko N, Griffiths A, Bousvaros A, et al. Laboratory values for children with newly diagnosed inflammatory bowel disease. *Pediatrics* 2007;119:1113-9.

9 Xanthakos SA, Schwimmer JB, Melin-Aldana H, Rothenberg ME, Witte DP, Cohen MB. Prevalence and outcome of allergic colitis in healthy infants with rectal bleeding: a prospective cohort study. *J Pediatr Gastroenterol Nutr* 2005;41:16-22.

10 Arvola T, Ruuska T, Keranen J, Hyoty H, Salminen S, Isolauri E. Rectal bleeding in infancy: clinical, allergological, and microbiological examination. *Pediatrics* 2006;117:e760-8.

11 Ostlie DJ, Spilde TL, St Peter SD, Sexton N, Miller KA, Sharp RJ, et al. Necrotizing enterocolitis in full-term infants. *J Pediatr Surg* 2003;38:1039-42.

12 Siahanidou T, Mandyla H, Anagnostakis D, Papandreou E. Twenty-six full-term (FT) neonates with necrotizing enterocolitis (NEC). *J Pediatr Surg* 2004;39:791.

13 Maayan-Metzger A, Itzchak A, Mazkereth R, Kuint J. Necrotizing enterocolitis in full-term infants: case-control study and review of the literature. *J Perinatol* 2004;24:494-9.

14 Swenson O, Sherman JO, Fisher JH. Diagnosis of congenital megacolon: an analysis of 501 patients. *J Pediatr Surg* 1973;8:587-94.

15 Swenson O, Davidson FZ. Similarities of mechanical intestinal obstruction and aganglionic megacolon in the newborn infant: a review of 64 cases. *N Engl J Med* 1960;262:64-7.

16 Macdonald IA, Beattie TF. Intussusception presenting to a paediatric accident and emergency department. *J Accid Emerg Med* 1995;12:182-6.

17 Ford EG, Senac MO, Jr, Srikanth MS, Weitzman JJ. Malrotation of the intestine in children. *Ann Surg* 1992;215:172-8.

18 Aalberse J, Dolman K, Ramnath G, Pereira RR, Davin JC. Henoch Schonlein purpura in children: an epidemiological study among Dutch paediatricians on incidence and diagnostic criteria. *Ann Rheum Dis* 2007;66:1648-50.

19 Uppal SS, Hussain MA, Al Raqum HA, Nampoory MR, Al Saeid K, Al Assousi A, et al. Henoch-Schonlein's purpura in adults versus children/adolescents: a comparative study. *Clin Exp Rheumatol* 2006;24(2 Suppl 41):S26-30.

20 Ukarapol N, Singhavejakul J, Lertprasertsuk N, Wongsawasdi L. Juvenile polyp in Thai children—clinical and colonoscopic presentation. *World J Surg* 2007;31:395-8.

21 Gupta SK, Fitzgerald JF, Croffie JM, Chong SK, Pfefferkorn MC, Davis MM, et al. Experience with juvenile polyps in North American children: the need for pancolonoscopy. *Am J Gastroenterol* 2001;96:1695-7.

22 Du Boulay CE, Fairbrother J, Isaacson PG. Mucosal prolapse syndrome—a unifying concept for solitary ulcer syndrome and related disorders. *J Clin Pathol* 1983;36:1264-8.

23 Poon KK, Mills S, Booth IW, Murphy MS. Inflammatory cloacogenic polyp: an unrecognized cause of hematochezia and tenesmus in childhood. *J Pediatr* 1997;130:327-9.

24 Mills RW, Burke S. Gastrointestinal bleeding in a 15 month old male. A presentation of Munchausen's syndrome by proxy. *Clin Pediatr (Phila)* 1990;29:474-7.

25 Libow JA. Child and adolescent illness falsification. *Pediatrics* 2000;105:336-42.

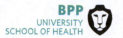

Obesity in children. Part 1: Epidemiology, measurement, risk factors, and screening

Ruth R Kipping research fellow[1], Russell Jago senior lecturer[2], Debbie A Lawlor professor of epidemiology[13]

[1]Department of Social Medicine, University of Bristol, Bristol BS8 2PS

[2]Department of Exercise, Nutrition and Health Sciences, University of Bristol, Bristol BS8 1TP

[3]MRC Centre for Causal Analysis in Translational Epidemiology, University of Bristol, Bristol BS8 2BN

Correspondence to: R Kipping ruth.kipping@bristol.ac.uk

Cite this as: BMJ 2008;337:a1824

‹DOI› 10.1136/bmj.a1824
http://www.bmj.com/content/337/bmj.a1824

References numbered w1-w34 are on bmj.com, labelled as extra

Obesity was first included in the international classification of diseases in 1948. Since then, an epidemic has developed internationally, affecting all age groups. This article describes the prevalence of obesity in children, its underlying risk factors, its consequences, and how it can be measured; it also discusses whether children should be screened for obesity. In a second article to be published next week we will discuss the prevention and management of obesity in children.[1] The terms used are defined in box 1 (where authors of cited papers use terms differently we use the authors' own words).

What is the prevalence of obesity in children?

In 2007 it was estimated that globally 22 million children under 5 years were overweight, with more than 75% of overweight and obese children living in low and middle income countries.[2] It is not only the scale of childhood obesity that is challenging, but also the speed at which the prevalence has increased. The greatest annual increases in obesity since 1970 in school children have been in North America and Western Europe.[3]

Figures 1 and 2 show trends in the prevalence of obesity in England and the United States. The data come from cross sectional surveys and use country specific growth charts. For both countries, data from the latest surveys suggest that the increase in prevalence of obesity is levelling off, but it is too early to know if the peak has been reached or if this levelling is variation around a still ongoing increase.

What are the risk factors for obesity in children?

Obesity is caused by an imbalance between energy input and energy expenditure. The relative contribution of physical activity, sedentary activity, and diet to the development of obesity in children is unclear, partly because these variables are difficult to measure and the balance of energy is complex.[6] [7] Other factors—including genetic variation, epigenetics, intrauterine exposures, and assortative mating—can also affect people's propensity to gain weight and may contribute in some populations to the epidemic (table 1).

SOURCES AND SELECTION CRITERIA

This review draws on the Foresight report, guidance from the National Institute of Health and Clinical Excellence, and a Cochrane review of preventing obesity.

In April 2008 we searched the Cochrane Library database of reviews and the Centre for Reviews and Dissemination databases using the search term "obesity". We also conducted a Medline search ((Child$ or paediatric or pediatric or adolescent) and (Obes$ or overweight)) limited to 1 January 2005 to 6 May 2008 and "review articles"; this identified 1105 articles. We read the abstracts of these articles and retrieved relevant papers. We also used articles from our own bibliographies collected over the past 10 years.

The evidence to support the measurement, prevention, and management of obesity in children is still relatively weak, with few randomised controlled trials or systematic reviews.

SUMMARY POINTS

- Population changes in physical activity and diet are probably the main drivers of the obesity epidemic
- A complex interplay of genetics; epigenetics; and intrauterine, infancy, childhood, and family non-genetic factors may also be involved
- Obesity in children and adolescents is associated with metabolic and cardiovascular abnormalities and other adverse health outcomes
- Modifiable risk factors for childhood obesity are maternal gestational diabetes; high levels of television viewing; low levels of physical activity; parents' inactivity; and high consumption of dietary fat, carbohydrate, and sweetened drinks
- Obesity is commonly measured in children by plotting body mass index on a standard growth chart to adjust for sex and age using a defined cut-off point
- Population screening for childhood obesity is not recommended

---

BOX 1 DEFINITIONS OF TERMS USED

Air displacement plethysmography system
A measurement of body composition using a unit with two chambers. The subject is in one chamber during testing and the second chamber contains instruments for measuring changes in pressure between the two chambers

Adiposity
The amount of adipose tissue present, with excessive accumulation leading to obesity

Body mass index (BMI)
Calculated as weight (kg)/height (m²)

BMI rebound
The period when a child's BMI is at its lowest, usually at age 5-6, before it starts to increase monotonically

Children
Young people aged 2-18

Densitometry
Measurement of underwater weight

Dual energy x ray absorptiometry (DEXA)
A scan that uses two x ray energies to measure the amount of x rays absorbed by the bones and tissue

Epigenetics
The study of heritable changes in genome function that occur without a change in DNA sequence

Obesity
A condition of excess body fat that may harm health

Screening
When members of a defined population are offered a test to identify who is more likely to be helped than harmed by further tests or treatment

Surveillance
The routine collection of data at a population level to be able to describe changes in disease or risk factors by person, place, and time

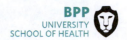

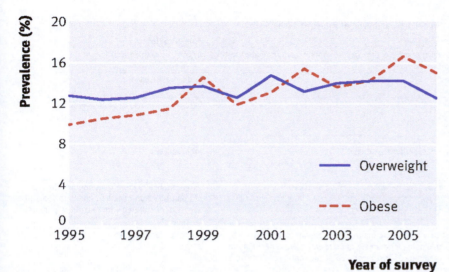

Fig 1 Prevalence of overweight and obesity in England among 2-15 year olds. Adapted from Health Survey for England 2006. The overweight category does not include those who are obese. Overweight defined as .85th and <95th UK sex specific body mass index (BMI) for age centiles; obese defined as .95th UK sex specific BMI for age centiles (1990 reference charts)

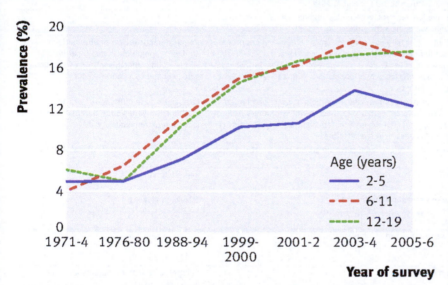

Fig 2 Prevalence of obesity in the US among 2-19 year olds. Adapted from the national health and nutrition examination survey.[4][5] Obese defined as .95th centile using US 2000 sex specific body mass index (BMI) for age growth charts from the Centers for Disease Control and Prevention

A large number of studies have reported associations between a wide variety of risk factors and overweight or obesity in children.[8][9][10] However, association does not prove causation, and confounding or reverse causality could explain these associations. Randomised controlled trials and prospective studies provide the most robust evidence for identifying causal associations,[6] but for obesity relatively little evidence comes from randomised controlled trials.

Table 1 summarises the evidence for risk factors associated with childhood obesity. Genetic variants, ethnicity, parental adiposity, birth weight, timing or rate of maturation, levels of physical activity and sedentary activity, and consumption of energy dense food are all associated with childhood obesity.[8][9][10] Some risk factors are common (prevalence >10%) but not modifiable, such as the combined effect of multiple genetic variants. Other risk factors are both common and modifiable. These include high birth weight (which is modifiable in cases of maternal diabetes mellitus); high levels of television viewing; low levels of

physical activity; parents' inactivity; and high consumption of dietary fat, carbohydrate, and sweetened drinks. Clearly these need to be the focus of prevention programmes.

How is adiposity measured in children?
Many different methods are currently used to measure adiposity in children. Direct measures, such as densitometry and scanning using dual energy x ray absorptiometry,[11] are more accurate than indirect measures but are not practical for population level surveillance or clinical management. Anthropometric methods, such as measurement of waist circumference, skinfolds, and BMI, measure adiposity indirectly. Bioelectrical impedance and air displacement plethysmography (for example, BodPod and PeaPod) provide reliable indirect estimates of adiposity and are often used in research studies.[12][13]

During adolescence, skinfold thickness is a better predictor than BMI of high adiposity in adulthood.[14] Skinfold thickness has also been associated with clustered risk of cardiovascular disease during adolescence,[15] but to our knowledge no study has found a relation between skinfold thickness in childhood and future risk of cardiovascular disease. Although BMI is an indirect measure it is practical, easy to obtain, reliable, and—to our knowledge—the only measure of adiposity in childhood that has been shown to be associated with future risk of mortality from cardiovascular disease in adulthood.[16]

Who should be classified as overweight or obese?
Internationally agreed thresholds exist for defining underweight, normal weight, overweight, and obesity in adults, but in children the effects of age, sex, and pubertal status make simple classification difficult. The assessment of obesity in children relies on plotting BMI on a standard growth chart and then defining a cut-off point for increased BMI relative to age and sex. International comparisons are difficult because countries tend to use their own standard growth charts and different cut-off points. Commonly used cut-off points for overweight and obesity include 110% or 120% of ideal weight for height; weight for height z scores (box 2) of >1 and >2; and BMI at the 85th, 90th, 95th, and 97th centiles (based on international or country specific reference populations).[3] The International Obesity Taskforce has therefore developed international BMI cut-off points for overweight and obesity according to sex and age (between 2 and 18 years). The cut-off points are defined to pass through a BMI of 25 and 30 at age 18, and are based on BMI data from six countries, which enables comparison of prevalence globally.[17]

In the UK the 1990 UK reference chart for boys and girls is used to measure BMI in children of all ages. However, the Scientific Advisory Committee on Nutrition and the Royal College of Paediatrics and Child Health recommend that the 2006 World Health Organization child growth standards for infants and children are used from 2 weeks of age to

---

BOX 2 Z SCORES

The z score is the distance from the mean in units of standard deviations. A positive z score indicates that the value is above the mean and a negative z score indicates that the value is below the mean. Z scores are often standardised by age and sometimes by sex. An age and sex standardised z score of 1.5 indicates that the value is 1.5 standard deviations above the mean for all children of the same age and sex in the population used to standardise the score.

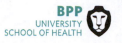

Table 1 Risk factors associated with the development of obesity in children and type of evidence available

Risk factor	Detail of risk factor	Type of evidence*
Single gene defects and obesity syndromes	Single gene defects in which obesity is the specific abnormality are related to the leptin or the melanocortin system	Reports of case series[8†]
Obesity is a manifestation of Prader-Willi, Cohen, Alström's, and Bardet-Biedl syndromes	Reports of gene studies[8†]	Endocrine disease
Hypothyroidism, Cushing's disease, Cushing's syndrome, growth hormone deficiency, growth hormone resistance, hypophosphataemic rickets, pseudohypoparathyroidism	Reports of case series[8†]	Central nervous system pathology
Hypothalamic damage can result in "hypothalamic obesity syndrome"—a severe form of obesity in children and adolescents	Review of biological and observational studies[w1]	Inheritance
Genome wide association studies have identified genetic variants that are robustly associated with greater BMIs	Twin[w2] and family[w3] studies; genome wide association studies[w4 w5]	Parental obesity more than doubles the risk of adult obesity in children under 10 years of age; 80% of children with two obese parents become obese
Cohort study[w6]	Several studies suggest that assortative mating (non-random mating driven by people of similar body size being more likely to mate with each other) may be a drive for the obesity epidemic. As the obesity epidemic continues this could become a vicious cycle	Cross sectional study[w7]
Ethnic origin	Children from the world's major regions grow similarly when their needs are met regardless of ethnic originHispanic, native American, black, and south Asian children have an increased risk of obesity compared with white children	Combined longitudinal and cross sectional study[w8]Cross sectional studies [w9 w10]
	There is increasing evidence that at a given BMI children and infants of South Asian origin have more fat mass and specifically more visceral adiposity. Recent evidence suggests these differences are present at birth	Cross sectional study[w11]
	It is unclear what contribution genetics, epigenetics, and behaviours make to patterning of adiposity between different groups	
Intrauterine exposure to gestational diabetes	In populations at high risk of obesity and diabetes (such as Pima Indians) there is good evidence that intrauterine exposure to maternal gestational diabetes results in increased risk of obesity later in life via intrauterine mechanisms, but whether this is an important risk factor for obesity in populations with a lower prevalence of diabetes and obesity is unclear	Non-systematic review of observational studies[w12]; longitudinal study that included within sibling comparison[w13]; cross sectional survey linked to a cohort study[w14]
Intrauterine exposure to maternal obesity	A study that compared obesity in children whose mothers had received bariatric surgery for extreme obesity before pregnancy to children whose mothers had surgery after pregnancy suggests that extreme maternal obesity in pregnancy is an intrauterine risk factor for obesity in the offspring	Case series with bariatric surgery as instrumental variable for maternal weight loss from extreme obesity[w15]
Birth weight	Small for gestational age babies who exhibit catch-up growth may be at risk of obesity in childhood	Systematic review (observational studies)[w16]
Higher birth weight is associated with overweight in adolescence	Non-systematic review[w17]	BMI rebound
Early BMI rebound is associated with greater risk of obesity (<5.5 years), but this may be a statistical artefact	Non-systematic review (observational studies)[w18]	Television viewing
A positive correlation exists between hours of viewing and overweight, which is stronger with increasing age	Systematic review (observational and experimental studies)[w19]	Energy expenditure
Low levels of physical activity are associated with obesity	Prospective cohort study[w20]	Children with inactive parents are more likely to be inactive
Prospective cohort studies[w21 w22]	Sleep	There is increasing evidence for an optimal sleep duration, with shorter sleep duration than is optimal associated with increased risk of obesity
Cohort study[w23]	Diet	Observational evidence suggests breast feeding may be associated with reduced risk of obesity, but detailed systematic reviews of this association suggest that much of it is explained by confounding and a recent randomised controlled trial supports this
Systematic review (observational studies)[w24]; randomised controlled trial[w25]	Evidence is emerging that dietary fat, carbohydrate, and sweetened drinks are a significant risk for obesity	Cross sectional study[w26]; prospective cohort study[w27]; systematic review (observational and experimental studies)[w28]
Parental feeding restriction has been associated with increased energy intake and bodyweight status	Non-systematic review (observational, experimental and qualitative studies)[w29]	Eating a small amount at breakfast and missing breakfast are both associated with increased risk of obesity
Cross sectional studies[w30†]	Portion size has been associated with the amount of food consumed and it seems logical that increased food consumed increases risk of obesity	Between subjects parallel group design[w31]; prospective study[w32]
Family structure	The evidence for single children or single parents being associated with obesity is inconsistent	Cohort studies[8†]
Urban versus rural	Children in urban areas are more likely to be obese than those in rural areas	Cross sectional studies[3]
Socioeconomic status	There is limited and inconclusive evidence that low socioeconomic status is associated with increased risk of childhood obesity in developed countries	Systematic review (cross sectional studies)[w33]
Treatment for leukaemia	The risk of obesity is higher after treatment for acute lymphatic leukaemia	Cohort[w34]
Medications	The role of drugs in causing weight gain in children has not been studied extensively	Report of studies[8†]

*The most recent study of highest evidence level from our review of the literature is cited for most risk factors rather than providing a comprehensive list of all studies. For some risk factors more than one reference is included when different study types, or studies in different populations are relevant.

†References cited within the study.

BMI, body mass index.

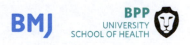

24 months and that the 1990 UK reference charts should be used only from age 2.[18] The WHO growth standards are based on babies who are exclusively or predominantly breast fed for at least four months. The WHO and UK charts begin to converge at 2 years of age, but a difference exists between the two charts at 2 years that is greater than the natural disjunction that arises because of the transition from measuring supine length to measuring height. Pilot work is currently under way to identify the most appropriate method of moving between these two charts before the new recommendations of the Scientific Advisory Committee are adopted in the UK.

The National Institute for Health and Clinical Excellence (NICE) recommends tailored clinical intervention if a child's BMI (adjusted for age and sex) is at the 91st centile or above and that assessment for comorbidities should be considered if their BMI is at the 98th centile or above, using 1990 UK reference charts. The 85th and 95th centiles are used to define overweight and obesity for surveillance purposes in the UK and the US, although until recently in the US children at or above the 95th centile were termed "overweight."

In adults, many of the health risks associated with obesity have been related to excess abdominal fat, particularly visceral fat, and in children markers of central adiposity such as waist circumference are associated with higher fasting insulin and glucose concentrations and adverse lipid profiles in cross sectional studies. Measurement of waist circumference may help identify children at risk of excess centrally located weight although, as with BMI, the correct cut-off point for defining central obesity in children is unclear. Sex specific waist centile curves for UK children aged 5-16 years have been published.[19] The International Diabetes Federation has recently suggested criteria for defining the metabolic syndrome in children and recommends a cut-off point of .90th centile of waist circumference for age, sex, and ethnic origin in children aged 6 and above for defining central adiposity.[20] However, no studies have shown an association between central adiposity or the metabolic syndrome in children and future risk of cardiovascular disease.

What are the consequences of obesity in children?

Obesity in children and adolescents is associated with a range of adverse metabolic and cardiovascular traits,[21] exacerbation of asthma,[22] poor self esteem,[23] and an increased likelihood of being obese in adulthood.[24 25 26] Table 2 shows the estimated prevalence of obesity associated metabolic and vascular characteristics in European children. However, the evidence for the consequences of childhood obesity comes from observational, often cross sectional, studies so these associations do not necessarily mean causation. Furthermore, associations found in clinically obese populations may not reflect associations in the general population, even at the same level of adiposity. It has been reported that obese children in community samples have better quality of life and self esteem than obese children from clinical samples.[28] The prevalence of raised liver enzymes, indicative of non-alcoholic fatty liver disease, is greater in obese children identified in specialist clinics than in those with similarly defined obesity who come from general population samples.[29] In a large general population sample of children, higher BMI was prospectively associated with increased risk of mortality from cardiovascular disease.[16] However, the extent to which this is the result of tracking BMI from childhood to adulthood rather than permanent changes in metabolic and vascular characteristics in childhood is unclear.

Should children be screened for obesity?

Certain criteria need to be met before a population screening programme is introduced. For example, the clinical course of the condition should be known, screening should be acceptable and valid, an effective intervention should be available for screen positive individuals, and evidence of the effectiveness of a screening programme to reduce mortality or morbidity should be available from randomised controlled trials. A systematic review of the evidence to screen primary school children concluded that most of these criteria are not met and that it is difficult to justify population screening of children for obesity.[30] In line with this, the UK National Screening Committee's policy is that, currently, not enough evidence is available to recommend screening children for obesity.

Table 2   Minimum estimated numbers of children in European Union in 2006 with obesity related disease indicators. Age range 5-17.9, unless shown otherwise[27]

Obesity related disease	Lowest estimated prevalence in obese children (%)	Lowest estimated number of obese children affected in EU 25 countries
Raised triglycerides	21.5	1.09 million
Raised total cholesterol	22.1	1.12 million
High low density lipoprotein cholesterol	18.9	0.96 million
Low high density lipoprotein	18.7	0.95 million
Hypertension	21.8	1.11 million
Impaired glucose tolerance	8.4	0.42 million
Hyperinsulinaemia	33.9	1.72 million
Type 2 diabetes	0.5	27 000
Metabolic syndrome (3+ risk factors)*	23.9	1.21 million
Metabolic syndrome (4+ risk factors)* (age 10-17.9 years)	4.6	0.13 million
Hepatic steatosis	27.9	1.42 million
Raised aminotransferase	12.8	0.65 million

*Risk factors for the metabolic syndrome were hypertension, central adiposity, low concentrations of blood high density lipoprotein cholesterol, raised blood triglycerides, raised blood glucose concentrations.

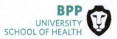

Should there be population surveillance of childhood obesity?

NICE reviewed evidence from eight longitudinal observational studies in children and concluded that opportunistic monitoring of growth charts after 2 years of age may be beneficial.[31] In 2005, an annual National Child Measurement Programme was introduced in England for surveillance (not screening) of two school year groups. In 2006-7 the programme measured 80% of children in state schools and the prevalence of obesity was 9.9% for children in reception (age 4-5) and 17.5% for children in year 6 (age 10-11) using the 95th centile on the UK 1990 reference charts.[32] The English government has introduced legislation to give parents the

results of the weight and height measurements from this surveillance programme and to allow the measurements to be used by government organisations for performance management of obesity from 2008-9. The programme is still defined as surveillance, but it treads a fine line between surveillance, screening, and performance. A qualitative study commissioned by the Department of Health in England recently found that parents would like a medical interpretation of whether their child is a healthy weight and find BMI a difficult concept to understand.[33]

In the US, Arkansas was the first state to pass legislation in 2003 for mandatory BMI assessments of children in public schools with annual reporting to parents. This approach has been followed in six other states.[34] To date, the effect of surveillance or screening programmes on the childhood obesity epidemic has not been evaluated.

Conclusion

Childhood obesity is associated with adverse health outcomes. There is a need to adopt consistent methods of measuring BMI internationally and a need for investment in research to further understand modifiable risk factors and consequences.

Contributors: All authors discussed the scope and approach to the review. RRK drafted the review. All authors helped write the paper. All authors are guarantors.

Competing interests: None declared.

Provenance and peer review: Commissioned; externally peer reviewed.

1. Kipping RR, Jago R, Lawlor DA. Obesity in children. Part 2: Prevention and management. *BMJ* 2008;337:a1848.
2. WHO. *Childhood overweight and obesity.* 2008. www.who.int/dietphysicalactivity/childhood/en/index.html.
3. Wang Y, Lobstein T. Worldwide trends in childhood overweight and obesity. *Int J Pediatr Obes* 2006;1:11-25.
4. National Centre for Health Statistics. *Prevalence of overweight among children and adolescents: United States, 2003-2004.* 2006. www.cdc.gov/nchs/products/pubs/pubd/hestats/overweight/overwght_child_03.htm#Table%201.
5. Ogden CL, Carroll MD, Flegal KM. High body mass index for age among US children and adolescents, 2003-2006. *JAMA* 2008;299:2401-5.
6. Reilly JJ, Ness AR, Sherrif A. Epidemiological and physiological approaches to understanding the etiology of pediatric obesity: finding the needle in the haystack. *Pediatr Res* 2007;61:646-52.
7. Wareham N. Physical activity and obesity prevention. *Obes Rev* 2007;8(suppl 1):109-14.
8. National Health and Medical Research Council. *Clinical practice guidelines for the management of overweight and obesity in children*

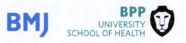

and adolescents. 2003. www.health.gov.au/internet/main/publishing.
nsf/Content/obesityguidelines-guidelines-children.htm.

9   Parsons TJ, Power C, Logan S, Summerbell CD. Childhood predictors
    of adult obesity: a systematic review. *Int J Obes Relat Metab
    Disord*1999;23(suppl 8):S1-107.

10 World Cancer Research Fund/American Institute for Cancer Research.
    *Food, nutrition, physical activity, and the prevention of cancer: a
    global perspective.* Washington, DC: AICR, 2007.

11 Dietz WH, Bellizz MC. Introduction: the use of body mass index to
    assess obesity in children. *Am J Clin Nutr*1999;70:123S-5S.

12 Goran M. Measurement issues related to studies of childhood obesity:
    assessment of body composition, body fat distribution, physical
    activity, and food intake. *Pediatrics*1998;101:505-18.

13 Ma G, Yao M, Liu Y, Lin A, Zou H, Urlando A, et al. Validation of a
    new pediatric air displacement plethysmograph for assessing body
    composition in infants. *Am J Clin Nutr*2004;79:653-60.

14 Nooyes AC, Koppes LL, Visscher TL, Twisk JW, Kemper HC, Schuit AJ, et
    al. Adolescent skinfold thickness is a better predictor of high body
    fatness in adults than is body mass index: the Amsterdam growth
    and health longitudinal study. *Am J Clin Nutr*2007;85:1533-9.

15 Andersen LB, Sardinha LB, Froberg K, Riddoch CJ, Page AS, Anderssen
    SA. Fitness, fatness and clustering of cardiovascular risk factors in
    children from Denmark, Estonia and Portugal: the European youth
    heart study. *Int J Pediatr Obes*2008;3(suppl 1):58-66.

16 Baker JL, Olsen LW, Sorensen TI. Childhood body-mass index
    and the risk of coronary heart disease in adulthood. *N Engl J
    Med*2007;357:2329-37.

17 Cole TJ, Bellizzi MC, Flegal KM, Dietz WH. Establishing a standard
    definition for child overweight and obesity worldwide: international
    survey. *BMJ*2000;320:1240.

18 Scientific Advisory Committee on Nutrition and the Royal
    College of Paediatrics and Child Health. *Application of the
    WHO growth standards in the UK.* 2007. www.rcpch.ac.uk/doc.
    aspx?id_Resource=2862.

19 McCarthy HD, Jarrett KV, Crawley HF. The development of waist
    circumference percentiles in British children aged 5.0 ±16.9 y. *Eur J
    Clin Nutr*2001;55:902-7.

20 Zimmet P, Alberti G, Kaufman F, Tajima N, Silink M, Arslanian
    S, et al. The metabolic syndrome in children and adolescents.
    *Lancet*2007;369:2059-61.

21 Lawlor DA, Riddoch CJ, Page AS, Anderssen SA, Froberg K, Harro M, et
    al. The association of birth weight and contemporary size with insulin
    resistance among children from Estonia and Denmark: findings from
    the European heart study. *Diabetic Med*2004;22:921-30.

22 Goran MI, Ball GD, Cruz J. Obesity and risk of type 2 diabetes and
    cardiovascular disease in children and adolescents. *J Clin Endocrinol
    Metab*2003;88:1417-27.

23 French SA, Story M, Perry C. Self-esteem and obesity in children and
    adolescents: a literature review. *Obes Res*1995;3:479-90.

24 Serdula MK, Ivery D, Coates RJ, Freedman DS, Williamson DF, Byers T.
    Do obese children become obese adults? A review of the literature.
    *Prev Med*1993;22:167-77.

25 Power C, Lake JK, Cole TJ. Body mass index and height from
    childhood to adulthood in the 1958 British born cohort. *Am J Clin
    Nutr*1997;66:1094-101.

26 Whitaker RC, Wright JA, Pepe MS, Seidel KD, Dietz WH. Predicting
    obesity in young adulthood from childhood and parental obesity. *N
    Engl J Med*1997;337:869-73.

27 Lobstein T, Jackson-Leach R. Estimated burden of paediatric obesity
    and co-morbidities in Europe. Part 2. Numbers of children with
    indicators of obesity-related disease. *Int J Pediatr Obes*2006;1:33-41.

28 Flodmark CE. The happy obese child. *Int J Obes (Lond)*2005;29(suppl
    2):S31-3.

29 Fraser A, Longnecker M, Lawlor DA. Prevalence of elevated alanine
    aminotransferase among US adolescents and associated factors:
    NHANES 1999-2004. *Gastroenterology*2007;133:1814-20.

30 Westwood M, Fayter D, Hartley S, Rithalia A, Butler G, Glasziou P, et
    al. Childhood obesity: should primary school children be routinely
    screened? A systematic review and discussion of the evidence. *Arch
    Dis Child*2007;92:416-22.

31 National Institute for Health and Clinical Excellence. *Obesity: the
    prevention, identification, assessment and management of overweight
    and obesity in adults and children.* 2006. www.nice.org.uk/guidance/
    index.jsp?action=byID&o=11000.

32 Information Centre. *National child measurement programme: 2006/07
    school year, headline results.* 2008. www.dh.gov.uk/en/Publichealth/
    Healthimprovement/Healthyliving/DH_083093.

33 Department of Health. *Research into parental attitudes towards
    the routine measurement of children's height and weight.* 2007.
    www.dh.gov.uk/en/Publicationsandstatistics/Publications/
    PublicationsPolicyAndGuidance/DH_080600.

34 Justus MB, Ryan KW, Rockenbach J, Katterapalli C, Card-Higginson P.
    Lessons learned while implementing a legislated school policy: body
    mass index assessments among Arkansas's public school students. *J
    School Health*2007;77:706-13.

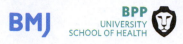

Obesity in children. Part 2: Prevention and management

Ruth R Kipping research fellow[1], Russell Jago senior lecturer[2], Debbie A Lawlor professor of epidemiology[13]

[1]Department of Social Medicine, University of Bristol, Bristol BS8 2PS

[2]Department of Exercise, Nutrition and Health Sciences, University of Bristol, Bristol BS8 1TP

[3]MRC Centre for Causal Analysis in Translational Epidemiology, University of Bristol, Bristol BS8 2BN

Correspondence to: R Kipping ruth. kipping@bristol.ac.uk

Cite this as: BMJ 2008;337:a1848

‹DOI› 10.1136/bmj.a1848
http://www.bmj.com/content/337/bmj.a1848

In the first part of this article we described how obesity in children is measured, its prevalence, whether children should be screened, and the risk factors for and consequences of obesity.[1] In this part we review the current evidence on the prevention and management of childhood obesity.

Can obesity be prevented?

A meta-analysis and Cochrane systematic review of controlled interventions to prevent childhood obesity published up to 2005 identified 61 and 22 studies, respectively.[2][3] Most studies found no strong evidence that interventions prevented weight gain or obesity, and many studies were limited in design, duration, or analysis. An update of the Cochrane review will be published in 2009.

The 2005 Cochrane review concluded that comprehensive strategies that deal with diet and physical activity, interventions with psychosocial support, and those that involved environmental change may help prevent obesity. The meta-analysis concluded that most (79%) of the large number of trials aimed at preventing childhood obesity found no effect on weight gain. The investigators pooled all studies (despite the varied types of intervention and populations) in one large meta-analysis and found a "trivial" beneficial effect on average, but marked heterogeneity between studies.

In contrast to these broad reviews of all interventions, a systematic review of controlled studies with interventions to reduce sedentary activities found that such interventions consistently reduced weight in children.[4] A systematic review of controlled trials to promote physical activity found some evidence of effect on activity levels for environmental interventions and those targeted at children from low socioeconomic backgrounds.[5] Multicomponent interventions (interventions involving school or education, family, the environment, or policy changes) increased physical activity in adolescents.

The modest effectiveness of programmes aimed at individual change to prevent obesity is similar to that found for other health behaviours.[2] Little research has evaluated the effect of interventions at the societal and political levels to prevent obesity.

The French EPODE ("ensemble, prévenons l'obésité des enfants" or "together, let's prevent obesity in children") programme has worked with families of children aged 5-12 years in 10 towns since 2004 with the aim of tackling obesity.[6] The programme involves communities in education, nutrition, and physical activity initiatives. EPODE has not been formally evaluated, but it has been adopted by the

SOURCES AND SELECTION CRITERIA

This review draws on the Foresight report, guidance from the National Institute for Health and Clinical Excellence and the Australian National Health Medical Research Council, and Cochrane review.

In April 2008 we searched the Cochrane Library database of reviews and the Centre for Reviews and Dissemination databases using the search term "obesity". We also conducted a Medline search ((Child$ or paediatric or pediatric or adolescent) and (Obes$ or overweight)) limited to 1 January 2005 to 6 May 2008 and "review articles"; this identified 1105 articles. We read the abstracts of these articles and retrieved relevant papers. We also used articles from our own bibliographies collected over the past 10 years.

The evidence to support the measurement, prevention, and management of obesity in children is still relatively weak, with few randomised controlled trials or systematic reviews. The strength of evidence is developing and the updated Cochrane review that will be published in 2009 may provide more compelling evidence for some interventions.

SUMMARY POINTS

- Few obesity prevention interventions have been shown to be effective in children
- Comprehensive strategies that tackle diet and physical activity as well as providing psychosocial support and environmental change may help prevent obesity
- Community based interventions aimed at changing activity levels, dietary knowledge, and eating behaviour may be useful but need evaluation for effectiveness and cost effectiveness
- Specialist treatment may include treatment with sibutramine or orlistat in children over 12, although long term studies are needed
- Surgery is recommended only in adolescents with extreme obesity, in limited circumstances, but the benefits need to be balanced against the possible side effects

BOX 1 SUMMARY OF HEALTHY WEIGHT, HEALTHY LIVES: A CROSS GOVERNMENT STRATEGY FOR ENGLAND[7]

The healthy growth and development of children

- Identify at risk families as early as possible
- Promote breast feeding as the norm for mothers
- Make cooking compulsory for all 11-14 year olds
- £75m (€95m; $138m) marketing programme to inform, support, and empower parents

Promoting healthier food choices

- Develop and implement a Healthy Food Code of Good Practice to reduce consumption of saturated fat, sugar, and salt
- Help local authorities to manage the proliferation of fast food outlets
- Ofcom review of restrictions on the advertising of unhealthy foods to children

Building physical activity into people's lives

- A "walking into health" campaign
- £30 million to develop "healthy towns"
- Develop tools to allow parents to manage the time that their children spend playing sedentary games
- Review approach to physical activity

Creating incentives for better health

- Develop pilot studies to explore how companies can best promote wellness among their staff
- Pilot approaches to using personal financial incentives to encourage healthy living

Personalised advice and support

- Develop the NHS Choices website to give personalised advice on diet and activity levels
- Provide extra funding for weight management services

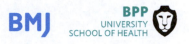

BOX 2 NATIONAL INSTITUTE FOR HEALTH AND CLINICAL EXCELLENCE RECOMMENDATIONS FOR PREVENTING OBESITY IN CHILDREN[8]

Recommendations for the public

- Children and young people should have regular meals in a pleasant, sociable environment with no distractions (such as television); parents and carers should join them as often as possible
- Gradually reduce the time children are sitting in front of a screen
- Encourage games that involve running around, such as skipping, dancing, or ball games
- Be more active as a family, by walking or cycling to school, going to the park, or swimming
- Encourage children to take part in sport inside and outside school

Recommendations for health professionals

- For families at high risk (for example, those where one or both parents are obese) offer individual counselling and ongoing support. Consider family based and individual interventions, depending on the age and maturity of the child
- In preschool settings, use a range of components. For example, offer interactive cookery demonstrations, videos, and discussions on meal planning and shopping for food and drink; in addition, offer interactive demonstrations, videos, and group discussions on physical activities, opportunities for active play, safety, and local facilities
- In family programmes to prevent obesity, provide ongoing tailored support and incorporate behaviour change techniques

Recommendations for preschool settings

- Provide regular opportunities for enjoyable active play and structured physical activity sessions
- Ensure that children eat regular healthy meals in a supervised, pleasant, sociable environment, free from distractions

Recommendations for schools

- Ensure that school policies and the whole school environment encourage physical activity and a healthy diet
- Train all staff in how to implement healthy school policies
- Create links and partnerships between sports clubs and schools
- Promote physical activities that children can enjoy outside school and into adulthood
- Ensure that children and young people eat meals in a pleasant, sociable environment, free from distractions

Recommendations for local authorities and their partners

- Work with the community to identify barriers to physical activity
- Ensure that the design of buildings and open spaces encourages people to be more active
- Encourage active travel, and promote and support physical activity schemes
- Encourage local shops and caterers to promote healthy food choices

When should interventions to prevent childhood obesity begin?

The question of when prevention should begin has to consider when increased risk for major diseases associated with obesity is established and whether it is easier to prevent obesity at some ages rather than others. We know that childhood adiposity is related to adult cardiovascular disease[9] and that childhood adiposity tracks into adulthood.[10] Greater adiposity in children has been associated with adverse metabolic risk profiles assessed at the same age; more recently, these cross sectional associations have also been found at birth—infants who have more fat tissue (particularly visceral fat) at birth have a higher fasting insulin and adverse lipid profiles at that time.[11] We also know that intrauterine factors, such as maternal gestational diabetes, are associated with increased body mass index (BMI).[12] But we do not know if the association of childhood adiposity with adult cardiovascular disease risk is fully explained by the tracking of childhood adiposity with adiposity in adulthood, or if the metabolic risks associated with obesity in infancy and childhood are reversible. The association of obesity with adverse outcomes at all ages has led most policy makers to aim to prevent obesity at all ages.

How can obesity be treated?

Much of the evidence on the treatment of obesity comes from studies of children who are extremely obese. Changes in weight (and BMI) can seem dramatic for interventions in this population compared with the general population because such children can lose large amounts of weight more easily than those in the "normal" weight range. However, such weight losses in extremely obese children may not equate to achieving a healthy weight. Interventions that are effective at treating extreme childhood obesity cannot be assumed to be suitable for treating more modest overweight or for preventing obesity. Many countries have developed guidelines for managing childhood obesity; differences in these reflect variations in the structure of health services, resources, culture, and behaviours between countries. The further educational resources section has links to guidelines from the US and Australia.[13] [14]

How can non-specialists treat obese children?

The NICE clinical guidelines provide recommendations for non-specialist clinicians (figure). Non-specialists should offer interventions to increase physical activity and encourage children and their families to eat healthily (figure).[15] The NICE quick reference guide for the NHS gives further advice about the type of interventions that are appropriate.[8]

What community programmes can non-specialists refer to?

Before considering referral to secondary care, it may be appropriate to consider community based treatment programmes. MEND (mind, exercise, nutrition . . . do it!) is the only programme provided nationwide in the United Kingdom. MEND is a twice weekly 10 week course for groups of children aged 7-13 and their parents. The course covers physical activity, behaviour change, and nutrition. To be included, children must be on or above the 91st to the 98th BMI centile (criteria vary locally). The full evaluation of MEND has yet to be published, but early data indicate that the programme has some promise as a means of reducing BMI, with the pilot evaluation reporting an average reduction of 0.24 BMI z scores.[17]

European Commission, and an EPODE European network has been established.

Policies to promote healthy eating and physical activity in schools are in place in several countries. Examples of such programmes are the National School Lunch Program in the United States and the Healthy Schools Programme in England. As with EPODE, the effect of these policies on obesity has not been evaluated. Reviews of the emerging evidence suggest that "walkable" neighbourhoods are associated with higher levels of physical activity, but there is less evidence to show links between the environment, physical activity, and obesity (A Tsouros and C Hall, personal communication).

The English cross government "healthy weight, healthy lives" strategy aims to reverse the trend in rising childhood obesity so that levels return to those of 2000 by 2020.[7] Box 1 summarises the components of the strategy. A social marketing campaign—"change4life"—will start in England in 2008. The UK National Institute for Health and Clinical Excellence (NICE) guidelines for obesity include recommendations for the public, health professionals, preschool settings, schools, and local authorities (box 2).[8]

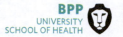

Non-specialist management

Determine degree of overweight or obesity
- Use clinical judgment to decide when to measure weight and height
- Use UK 1990 BMI charts for age to give age and sex specific information
- Do not use waist circumference routinely, although it can give information on risk of long term health problems
- Discuss with the child and family

Consider intervention or assessment
- Consider tailored clinical intervention if BMI ≥91st centile
- Consider assessing for comorbidities if BMI ≥98th centile

Assess the following
- Presenting symptoms and underlying causes of overweight or obesity
- Willingness to change
- Risk factors and comorbidities, such as hypertension, hyperinsulinaemia, dyslipidaemia, type 2 diabetes, psychosocial dysfunction, exacerbation of asthma
- Psychosocial distress—low self esteem, bullying
- Family history of overweight, obesity, and comorbidities
- Lifestyle—diet and physical activity
- Environmental, social, and family factors
- Growth and pubertal status

Management
Offer interventions including strategies to change behaviour that encourage:
- Increasing physical activity to at least 60 minutes a day of moderate activity, which can be in 10 minute sessions; reducing sedentary activities; increasing structured activity and daily exercise
- Improving eating behaviour. Interventions should be individualised, age appropriate, and aimed at reducing total energy intake to below expenditure, without using unduly restrictive diets
- Healthy eating

Consider referral to a specialist if the child has:
- Serious comorbidity or
- Complex needs such as learning or educational difficulties

Specialist management in secondary care

Assessment in secondary care
Assess comorbidities and possible aetiology; carry out investigations such as:
- Blood pressure
- Fasting lipid profile
- Fasting insulin and glucose concentrations
- Liver function tests
- Endocrine investigations

Take into account the degree of overweight or obesity, the child's age, comorbidities, family history of metabolic diseases, and possible genetic causes

Drug treatment
Consider only after dietary, exercise, and behavioural approaches have been started and evaluated
- Not recommended for children under 12 except in exceptional circumstances
- For children ≥12 years, only if they have physical comorbidities (such as sleep apnoea) or severe psychological comorbidities
- Multidisciplinary teams with appropriate expertise may prescribe a 6-12 month trial of orlistat or sibutramine with regular review

Surgery
Surgery is not generally recommended for children or young people. Consider surgery for young people only in exceptional circumstances, and if:
- They have achieved or nearly achieved physiological maturity
- They have a BMI ≥40, or a BMI between 35 and 40 and other disease (for example, type 2 diabetes, high blood pressure) that might improve if they lost weight
- All appropriate non-surgical measures have failed to achieve or maintain adequate clinically beneficial weight loss for at least 6 months
- They are receiving or will receive intensive specialist management
- They are generally fit for anaesthesia and surgery
- They commit to the need for long term follow-up

Guidance is provided on further discussions, assessment, medical evaluation, and choice of intervention

Summarised National Institute for Health and Clinical Excellence guidelines for management of overweight and obesity in children.[8] The *BMJ* clinical review of breast feeding indicates that in 2009 the 2006 WHO growth charts will need to be used for babies from 2 weeks to 2 years[16]

Children who attended the Carnegie International Camp in Leeds (England) for a mean of 29 days lost 6.0 kg on average, reduced their BMI by a mean of 2.4 units, and reduced their BMI standard deviation scores by a mean of 0.28.[18] Two free living comparison groups of overweight and normal weight children showed increases in many of these measures. This intervention needs to be evaluated by a randomised controlled trial and a cost effectiveness study. WATCH IT is a community based obesity programme provided in sports centres in Leeds, which provides individual and group sessions for children (aged 8-16 years with a BMI above the 98th centile) and their parents. To date, this programme has not been evaluated in a controlled trial.[19] The Care of Childhood Obesity programme in Bristol is a hospital based multidisciplinary service, which is being piloted for use in the community before full evaluation.[20]

Commissioners of health services face several challenges in deciding what community services they need to commission to treat obese children. Because the current number of obese children is large, treating all of them is probably beyond the capacity of secondary care. The costs of implementing community based programmes, such as those described above, need to be considered against the long term health costs of no treatment. Although there is pressure for immediate action the current evidence, particularly on cost effectiveness, is limited. Where effectiveness has been demonstrated in the short term it is difficult to know which intervention is best, and randomised comparisons of different community based programmes would be useful.

When should children be referred?

Different countries have different guidelines on when children should be referred and who they should be referred to—for example, paediatric endocrinologists, general paediatricians, dietitians, psychologists, or multidisciplinary teams. The NICE clinical guideline recommends referral to secondary care specialists if the child has serious comorbidities or complex needs, such as learning difficulties.[8]

What drug treatment is recommended for children?

Systematic reviews of randomised controlled trials in adults have shown that drugs are effective at reducing weight and associated metabolic complications, although adults do not adhere well to long term treatment with orlistat and sibutramine.[21] A non-systematic review summarised the effect of drug treatment in children and noted a mean reduction of BMI in obese adolescents of −0.86 for orlistat, −2.8 for sibutramine, and −1.38 for metformin.[22]

Treatment with orlistat or sibutramine is not recommended by NICE for children younger than 12 years unless the circumstances are exceptional.[8] It is recommended for children aged 12 years and over if they have physical or severe psychological comorbidities, and only after dietary, exercise, and behavioural approaches have been started and evaluated (figure). NICE recommends that treatment be started in secondary care (not in primary care) for six to 12 months and monitored regularly (frequency not specified in guidance) by a multidisciplinary team with expertise in drug monitoring, psychological support, and behavioural interventions. In the US, the Food and Drug Administration has approved sibutramine for patients aged 16 or more and orlistat for those aged 12 or more.[13]

Rimonabant was approved for treating obesity in adults in Europe in 2006, but it was not included in the NICE review of obesity. A meta-analysis of randomised trials suggests that the drug might increase the risk of psychiatric adverse events in patients with no previous history.[23] A Cochrane review evaluated the use of rimonabant in adults and concluded that more rigorous studies of efficacy and safety were needed.[24] In the US, the Food and Drug Administration has requested further safety data before making a licensing decision. The UK Medicines and Healthcare Products Regulatory Agency and Commission on Human Medicines reported in May 2008 that insufficient data are available to assess the risk for children under 18 years.

When is bariatric surgery recommended for children?

The two bariatric surgical approaches used for adolescents are Roux en Y gastric bypass (the more commonly performed procedure in the US) and laparoscopic adjustable gastric banding (the more commonly performed procedure in Europe and Australia).[25] In the US, the annual number of bariatric procedures carried out in adolescents increased five times between 1997 and 2003.[26] Case series of young people in Australia and the US report that, although surgery has considerable risks, larger decreases in BMI (in the order of 20.7 (37%))[27] and greater improvements in some metabolic markers are achieved with surgery than with non-surgical methods.[25] Although surgery is not generally recommended by NICE for obese children or young people, it should be considered in exceptional circumstances if certain conditions are met (figure).

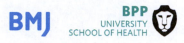

What does the future hold?

The recent Foresight report for the UK government suggested that a substantial increase in food or fuel prices, such as precipitated by climate change, might be the only scenario in which a spontaneous reversal of obesity would occur.[28] Otherwise, the Foresight report argues that a paradigm shift at societal and government levels is needed. If this shift does not occur, it is predicted that by 2050 the prevalence of obesity in under 20 year olds will be 25% in the UK.[28]

Contributors: All authors discussed the scope and approach to the review. RRK drafted the review. All authors helped write the paper. All authors are guarantors.

Competing interests: None declared.

Provenance and peer review: Commissioned; externally peer reviewed.

1. Kipping RR, Jago R, Lawlor DA. Obesity in children. Part 1: Epidemiology, measurement, risk factors, and screening. *BMJ*2008;337:a1824.
2. Stice E, Shaw H, Marti CN. A meta-analytic review of obesity prevention programs for children and adolescents: the skinny on interventions that work. *Psychol Bull*2006;132;5:667-91.
3. Summerbell CD, Waters E, Edmunds LD, Kelly S, Brown T, Campbell KJ. Interventions for preventing obesity in children. *Cochrane Database Syst Rev*2005;(3):CD001871.
4. DeMattia L, Lemont L, Meurer L. Do interventions to limit sedentary behaviours change behaviour and reduce childhood obesity: a critical review of the literature. *Obes Rev*2007;8:69-81.
5. Van Sluijs EMF, McMinn AM, Griffin SJ. Effectiveness of interventions to promote physical activity in children and adolescents: systematic review of controlled trials. *BMJ*2007;335:703.
6. Westley H. Thin living. *BMJ*2007;335:1236-7.
7. Department of Health. *Healthy weight, healthy lives: a cross government strategy for England.* London: Department of Health, 2008.
8. National Institute for Health and Clinical Excellence. *Quick reference guide 2 for the NHS obesity: the prevention, identification, assessment and management of overweight and obesity in adults and children.* 2006. www.nice.org.uk/guidance/index.jsp?action=download&o=30364.
9. Baker JL, Olsen LW, Sorensen TI. Childhood body-mass index and the risk of coronary heart disease in adulthood. *N Engl J Med*2007;357:2329-37.
10. Whitaker RC, Wright JA, Pepe MS, Seidel KD, Dietz WH. Predicting obesity in young adulthood from childhood and parental obesity. *N Engl J Med*1997;337:869-73.
11. Yajnik CS, Lubree HG, Rege SS, Naik SS, Deshpande JA, Deshpande SS, et al. Adiposity and hyperinsulinemia in Indians are present at birth. *J Clin Endocrinol Metab*2002;87:5575-80.
12. Pettitt DJ, Nelson RG, Saad MF, Bennett PH, Knowler WC. Diabetes and obesity in the offspring of Pima Indian women with diabetes during pregnancy. *Diabetes Care*1993;16:310-4.
13. Barlow SE and the Expert Committee. Expert committee recommendations regarding the prevention, assessment, and treatment of child and adolescent overweight and obesity: summary report. *Pediatrics*2007;120:S164-92.
14. National Health and Medical Research Council. *Clinical practice guidelines for the management of overweight and obesity in children and adolescents.* 2003www.health.gov.au/internet/main/publishing.nsf/Content/obesityguidelines-guidelines-children.htm.
15. Young KM. Northern JJ, Lister KM, Drummond JA, O'Brien WH. A meta-analysis of family-behavioral weight-loss treatments for children. *Clin Psychol Rev*2007;27:240-9.
16. Hoddinott P, Tappin D, Wright C. Breast feeding. *BMJ* 2008;336:881-7.

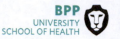

17 Sacher PM, Kolotourou M, Chadwick P, Singhal A, Cole TJ, Lawson MS. The MEND programme: effects on waist circumference and BMI in moderately obese children. *Obes Rev*2007;8(suppl 3):7-16.

18 Gately PJ, Cooke CB, Barth JH, Bewick BM, Radley D, Hill AJ. Residential weight loss programmes can work: a cohort study of acute outcomes for overweight and obese children. *Pediatrics*2005;116:73-7.

19 Rudolf M, Christie D, McElhone S, Sahota P, Dixey R, Walker J, et al. WATCH IT: a community based programme for obese children and adolescents. *Arch Dis Child*2006;91:736-9.

20 Sabin MA, Ford A, Hunt L, Jamal R, Crowne EC, Shield JP. Which factors are associated with a successful outcome in a weight management programme for obese children? *J Eval Clin Pract*2007;13:364-8.

21 Padwal R, Li SK, Lau DC. Long-term pharmocotherapy for obesity and overweight. *Cochrane Database Syst Rev*2004;(3):CD004094.

22 Freemark M. Pharmacotherapy of childhood obesity: an evidence-based, conceptual approach. *Diabetes Care*2007;30:395-402.

23 Christensen R, Kristensen PK, Bartels EM, Bliddal H, Astrup A. Efficacy and safety of the weight-loss drug rimonabant: a meta-analysis of randomised trials. *Lancet*2007;370:1706-13.

24 Curioni C, André C. Rimonabant for overweight or obesity. *Cochrane Database Syst Rev*2006;(4):CD006162.

25 Shield JPH, Crowne E, Morgan J. Is there a place for bariatric surgery in treating childhood obesity? *Arch Dis Child*2008;93:369-72.

26 Schlling PL, Davis MM, Albanese CT, Dutta S, Morton J. National trends in adolescent bariatric surgical procedures and implications for surgical centers of excellence. *J Am Coll Surg*2008;206:1-12.

27 Lawson ML, Kirk S, Mitchell T, Chen MK, Loux TJ, Daniels SR, et al, Pediatric Bariatric Study Group. One-year outcomes of Roux-en-Y gastric bypass for morbidly obese adolescents: a multicenter study from the Pediatric Bariatric Study Group. *J Pediatr Surg*2006;41:137-43; discussion 137-43.

28 Government Office for Science. Foresight. *Tackling obesities: future choices—project report*. 2nd ed. 2007. www.foresight.gov.uk/Obesity/14.pdf.

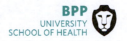

Acute leukaemia in children: diagnosis and management

Chris Mitchell consultant paediatric oncologist[1], Georgina Hall consultant paediatric haematologist[1], Rachel T Clarke foundation year 1 doctor[2]

[1]Department of Paediatric Haematology/Oncology, John Radcliffe Hospital, Oxford OX3 9DU, UK

[2]John Radcliffe Hospital, Oxford

Correspondence to: C Mitchell chris.mitchell@paediatrics.ox.ac.uk

Cite this as: BMJ 2009;338:b2285

‹DOI› 10.1136/bmj.b2285
http://www.bmj.com/content/338/bmj.b2285

Acute leukaemia is the commonest malignancy of childhood. In the United Kingdom, one in 2000 children develop the disorder, with around 450 new cases being diagnosed annually.[1] However, most general practitioners will see a case of childhood leukaemia only once or twice in their careers[2] and, since management generally takes place in tertiary referral centres, non-specialist paediatricians will encounter relatively few patients.

Compared with the 1970s, the outcome today for children with acute leukaemia has improved dramatically. Numerous high quality randomised controlled trials have shown that over 85% of children can now be cured.[3] [4] Goals for the future should focus on keeping treatment and side effects to a minimum for patients at low risk of recurrent disease, and improving the outcome for the small proportion of children at high risk of relapse.[5]

In this review, we summarise current knowledge about the presentation, diagnosis, and optimum management of children with acute leukaemia. We also suggest strategies for early diagnosis of the disease in primary care, which should minimise avoidable complications and allow for early supportive care.

What causes acute leukaemia?

Acute leukaemia arises from genetic mutations in blood progenitor cells. These mutations generate both an uncontrollable capacity for self-renewal and the developmental arrest of the progenitor cells at a particular point in their differentiation.[6] The body is therefore overwhelmed by immature cells or blasts that infiltrate the bone marrow, reticulo-endothelial system, and other extra-medullary sites. Eighty per cent of children with acute leukaemia have acute lymphoblastic leukaemia; most of the remainder have acute myeloid leukaemia.[7] Chronic leukaemia in children is extremely rare.[8]

Usually, newly diagnosed children have been previously well, with no identifiable environmental risk factors for leukaemia such as exposure to ionising radiation. In our experience, many parents therefore crave an explanation for their child's illness, asking whether it is their fault or "something in the family," particularly if an adult family member has died of leukaemia. However, the predominant leukaemia of early childhood, acute lymphoblastic leukaemia, is not inherited and is distinct from the leukaemias more

commonly seen in adults (acute myeloid leukaemia, chronic myeloid leukaemia, and chronic lymphocytic leukaemia).[9] Fewer than 5% of all cases are associated with inherited predisposing genetic syndromes such as Down's syndrome, in which there is a 20-fold increase in the risk of developing leukaemia.[10]

Acute lymphoblastic leukaemia probably arises from the interaction of environmental risk factors with a pre-existing genetic susceptibility. It is now known that a pre-natal mutation leads to the production of a pre-leukaemic clone which expands postnatally. A second mutation is required for overt disease to develop, most commonly between the ages of 2 and 5 years. What causes this second mutation is contentious. One hypothesis, that of "population mixing," suggests that when genetically susceptible children move into new, rapidly expanding towns, their immune response to unfamiliar local infections is abnormal, causing leukaemia to develop.[11] Alternatively, the "delayed infection hypothesis" suggests that susceptible children from excessively hygienic environments are protected from normal childhood infections, causing an aberrant immune response to later infections which triggers leukaemia.[12]

How does acute leukaemia present in children?

Presentations of acute leukaemia relate to three main pathological processes: bone marrow failure due to extensive infiltration by blast cells, infiltration of other tissues by blasts, and systemic effects of cytokines released by tumour cells.

Leukaemia may be strongly suspected when a child presents with classical signs of anaemia, thrombocytopenia, and pronounced hepatosplenomegaly or lymphadenopathy. However, as one high quality systematic review recently highlighted, the presenting symptoms are often vague and non-specific, mimicking those of common, self-limiting childhood illnesses.[13] In our experience, parents frequently decide to consult their GP simply because their child, in some intangible way, "is just not right," perhaps with pallor, lethargy, or malaise.

At present, there is no definitive evidence base enabling doctors, particularly GPs, to discriminate with confidence between those children for whom wait and see is appropriate practice, those for whom phlebotomy is advisable, and those who should be referred urgently to the emergency department. We failed to find any studies conducted in primary care that evaluated the positive and negative predictive value of signs and symptoms for the diagnosis of acute leukaemia, although such research is currently ongoing. Table 1, based on a wide number of case reports, review articles and our own departmental experience, outlines the range of potential presentations.[13] [14] [15] We encourage inclusion of acute leukaemia in the differential diagnosis for all children presenting with such signs and symptoms, particularly when the parent insists there is something amiss with their child.

SUMMARY POINTS

- Presentation of acute leukaemia can be non-specific, and not always have the classic signs and symptoms of anaemia, bruising, bleeding, hepatosplenomegaly, and lymphadenopathy.
- Diagnosis can be difficult, and delays can contribute to additional, sometimes life threatening problems during the period of initial treatment.
- Relatively simple, inexpensive tests—a full blood count and examination of the blood film—will diagnose acute leukaemia in most cases.
- Overall survival has risen from less than 5% in the 1960s to over 85% today.

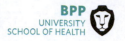

Table 1   Presentations of acute leukaemia in children

Underlying pathophysiology	Symptoms and signs
Systemic effects of cytokines	Malaise Fatigue Nausea Fever
Bone marrow infiltration	
Anaemia	Pallor Lethargy Shortness of breath Dizziness Palpitations Reduced exercise tolerance
Neutropenia	Fever Infection in general Recurrent infection Unusual infections, eg oral candida
Thrombocytopenia	Bruising Petechiae Epistaxis
Reticuloendothelial infiltration	Hepatosplenomegaly Lymphadenopathy Expiratory wheeze secondary to mediastinal mass (due to lymphadenopathy, or thymic infiltration or expansion).
Other organ infiltration	
CNS	Headaches Vomiting Cranial nerve palsies Convulsions
Testes	Testicular enlargement
Leucostasis	Headache Stroke Shortness of breath Heart failure

Leucostasis=increased plasma viscosity secondary to extremely high white cell counts, typically >100×10⁹/l

Occasionally, acute leukaemia presents with a life threatening complication requiring immediate hospital management.[16] Our experience suggests that delay in such instances may be fatal, although there is no clear evidence on this issue. We recommend that if GPs are concerned about any of these complications (table 2), they should not wait for phlebotomy and subsequent results, but rather refer immediately to the emergency department or call the on-duty haematology registrar.

How is acute leukaemia diagnosed?

When leukaemia is first suspected, the most important initial investigations are a full blood count and blood film. These quick and inexpensive tests are highly sensitive, permitting accurate diagnosis of leukaemia in most patients. Furthermore, if both are within normal ranges, acute leukaemia can be ruled out with a fair degree of confidence.

Typically, the full blood count will demonstrate pancytopenia secondary to bone marrow infiltration by blasts. Although the patient is likely to be neutropenic, millions of circulating blasts tend dramatically to elevate the overall white cell count, with blasts clearly evident on the film.

Sometimes, however, the white cell count may be only slightly raised and, if blasts remain sequestered within the bone marrow, it can even be lower than normal. Nor are clearly identifiable blasts always present. In these cases, the only clue that there is a serious underlying problem may be a few atypical cells in the blood film or the presence of leukoerythroblastic features. In our experience, any abnormal count or film, in conjunction with a suspicious clinical picture, should prompt urgent referral to a specialist centre for further investigation or, as a minimum, telephone discussion with an on-duty haematologist.

How is a child with acute leukaemia managed?

After urgent investigations and supportive care (box), the tertiary referral centre will aspirate bone marrow, usually under general anaesthetic in children, to obtain a definitive diagnosis of acute leukaemia. The aspirate provides morphological, immunological, and genetic information which, alongside clinical factors such as the child's age, sex, presenting white cell count, and initial response to chemotherapy, enables patients to be categorised according to their risk of subsequent relapse.

Simple light microscopy will usually allow classification of the diagnosis as acute lymphoblastic leukaemia or acute myeloid leukaemia. Immunophenotyping using flow cytometry identifies patterns of cell surface antigens associated with particular subtypes of acute lymphoblastic leukaemia or acute myeloid leukaemia. For example, the majority of children with acute lymphoblastic leukaemia have the precursor B cell type, which is positive for the CD10 and CD19 cell surface markers. Around 15% of children with acute lymphoblastic leukaemia will have the T cell (CD3 positive) phenotype.[3] These children tend to be male and older, with more frequent central nervous system involvement and bulkier disease, including mediastinal masses. Cytogenetic analysis identifies specific genetic abnormalities, such as the TEL/AML1 or BCR-ABL gene fusions, which correlate with a good or poor prognosis, respectively.[17]

Patients are categorised into low, standard, or high risk groups, with treatment determined, as far as possible, by risk status. For example, in both acute lymphoblastic leukaemia and acute myeloid leukaemia, very intensive treatment such as allogeneic bone marrow transplant is

---

CRITICAL POINTS IN THE MANAGEMENT OF CHILDREN WITH ACUTE LEUKAEMIA

- Early referral to specialist tertiary referral centre to provide knowledge and support to families, and to manage major complications during the first few weeks of therapy

- Urgent admission blood tests (full blood count, electrolytes, liver function tests, a coagulation screen) and chest x-ray to exclude life threatening complications such as a mediastinal mass which may compromise the airway

- Rapid institution of early supportive care: securing airway; intravenous fluids; blood products; broad spectrum antibiotics; correction of electrolyte abnormalities and hyperuricaemia or hyperphosphataemia; renal dialysis or haemofiltration

- Once patient is stable, bone marrow aspirate for precise diagnosis, categorisation of leukaemic subtype and risk stratification

- Definitive treatment and longer term plan for subsequent phases of treatment (for acute lymphoblastic leukaemia, 2-3 years of remission-induction, consolidation and maintenance therapy; for acute myeloid leukaemia, a maximum of 6 months chemotherapy)

- Allogenic bone marrow transplant is reserved for patients at especially high risk of relapse

- Management of short term adverse effects of treatment (particularly infection, but also thrombosis and avascular necrosis of bone).

- Psychosocial aspects of caring for child and family

- Management of long term adverse effects of treatment (endocrine, cardiac, respiratory, growth, fertility, neurological, and psychological)

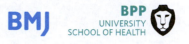

reserved for very highrisk cases (<10% of cases), protecting standard risk patients from unnecessary toxic side effects.[18] Bespoke therapy has been further refined over the last 10 years by PCR- based techniques for the assessment of "minimal residual disease." These techniques are over a hundred times more sensitive than morphological methods at identifying residual leukaemia (they can pick out one cell in 100000), enabling clinicians to predict future, as yet subclinical, relapse and plan treatment accordingly.[19]

Acute lymphoblastic leukaemia

In the UK, girls with acute lymphoblastic leukaemia currently receive two years of treatment and boys three years, because boys have an increased risk of relapse which, to some extent, can be offset by a longer period of treatment. Since the 1960s, a strategy of "total therapy" has applied: systemic therapy targets the primary disease site (the bone marrow), while intrathecal therapy is directed at leukaemic cells within the central nervous system which would otherwise evade chemotherapy.

Typically, treatment comprises four phases of chemotherapy (table 3). Most children have central venous catheters, such as Hickman lines, inserted after the first month of treatment. Much of the continuation phase of treatment is carried out locally, and children are able to pursue a relatively healthy social and academic life. Hair grows back once the intensive phase of treatment is over.

High quality randomised control trial data spanning the last four decades demonstrate a steady increase in the proportion of patients being cured and have also facilitated significant reductions in therapy, leading to fewer long term treatment related complications by demonstrating that similar outcomes can be achieved with less therapy.[3][20] For example, most patients no longer receive any cranial radiotherapy whereas in the 1980s and 1990s all patients received it.

Acute myeloid leukaemia

All children with acute myeloid leukaemia in the UK are treated with four courses of chemotherapy at roughly monthly intervals. There is no maintenance therapy afterwards, so most will have completed therapy within 6 months of diagnosis.

In the early 1980s, the outcome for acute myeloid leukaemia was poor with relapse-free survival rates at 5 years of just 18%. However, the most recent trial by the UK Medical Research Council showed a 5-year overall survival of 66%, with an event-free survival of 56%.[21] Today, patients with low risk cytogenetic abnormalities are identified at diagnosis, and have better prospects of long-term cure than patients with other abnormalities. Patients with adverse cytogenetic features or a poor response to therapy do badly even with the use of allogeneic bone marrow transplant, and fewer than 20% are cured.

What are the key complications of treatment for acute leukaemia?

The longer term side effects of the commonly used chemotherapeutic agents range from peripheral neuropathy (vincristine) and cardiotoxicity (doxorubicin) to decreased fertility (cyclophosphamide) and hepatotoxicity (cytarabine).[13] However, most children will have few, if any, long term complications of therapy, especially now that the use of cranial radiotherapy has been minimised.

By far the most important acute complication is neutropenic sepsis which, as with meningococcal sepsis, can rapidly trigger overwhelming multi-organ failure. A delay of even an hour or two in prescribing appropriate broad spectrum antibiotics (guided by local protocols) may impair the child's chances of survival.[22] Before leaving the tertiary care centre, parents are educated in the risks of subsequent fever in their child and the urgent need to visit the emergency department if, for example, they take one temperature reading over 38.5°C or two over 38.0°C. Typically, tertiary referral centres also supply parents with written guidelines about when to contact primary and secondary physicians, and secondary physicians with written protocols for how to manage complications.

Parents frequently worry about travel abroad and routine immunisations. A comprehensive review of trial evidence and expert opinion advises that no routine immunisations should be given while the child is on therapy or for 6 months afterwards. The review outlines recommended schedules for

Table 2 Life threatening early complications of acute leukaemia

Mechanism	Complication
Neutropenia	Infection: overwhelming, usually Gram-negative sepsis, with or without disseminated intravascular coagulation
Thrombocytopenia	Bleeding: stroke, pulmonary haemorrhage, gastrointestinal haemorrhage
Electrolyte imbalance	Hyperkalaemia and hyperphosphataemia secondary to blast cell lysisAcute renal failure secondary to hyperuricaemic nephropathy
Reticuloendothelial infiltration	Acute airway obstruction secondary to mediastinal thymic mass
Leucostasis	Stroke, acute pulmonary oedema, heart failure

Leucostasis=increased plasma viscosity secondary to extremely high white cell counts, typically >100×10⁹/l

Table 3 Phases of treatment for acute lymphoblastic leukaemia

Treatment phase	Goal	How goal is realised	Duration
Remission-induction	Rapid eradication of at least 99% of the initial leukaemic cell burden, leading to prompt restoration of normal haematopoiesis.	In most standard risk cases, IV administration of a 3 drug induction combination, typically dexamethasone, vincristine, and asparaginase; in high and very high risk cases, daunorubicin is added.Early assessment of marrow response: <25% leukaemic blasts in marrow is good; >25% (slow early response) requires intensification of therapy. Clinical remission (<5% leukaemic cells remaining) occurs in 96-99% of children by day 29. Early marrow response may be supplanted by day 29 assessment of minimal residual disease	4-6 weeks
Consolidation and therapy directed at central nervous system	Eradication of residual, drug-resistant leukaemic cells, reducing the risk of relapse.Reduction in risk of CNS relapse.	Stratified by risk of relapse. Slow early responders receive augmented therapyWeekly intrathecal methotrexate for 3 doses in this phase, and then subsequently every 3 months throughout continuing therapy	4-12 weeks
Intensification	Reduction in relapse risk.	Reinduction and reconsolidation mimicking the early phases of induction and consolidation.	8-12 weeks
Continuation therapy		Daily oral methotrexate and weekly oral methotrexate with monthly vincristine and dexamethasone pulses. Doses titrated to neutrophil and platelet counts, indicating degree of marrow toxicity. 2-3 years of therapy, most of which is continuation	2-3 years
Allogeneic bone marrow transplant	Elimination of residual leukaemic cells in highrisk subtypes refractory to chemotherapy.	Myeloablation, often using total body irradiation and cyclophosphamide, followed by peripheral intravenous administration of allogeneic haemopoietic stem cells. Substantial morbidity and mortality owing to overwhelming infection and graft versus host disease in particular	

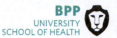

SOURCES AND SELECTION CRITERIA

We searched Medline for articles between January 1998 and December 2008 relating to the diagnosis and management of childhood acute leukaemia. Key terms used included "acute", "leukaemia", "paediatric", "diagnosis", "presentation", "management", "treatment", and "therapy". We also searched the Cochrane Library for all entries under "childhood cancer". From these searches, we identified randomised controlled trials, meta-analyses, and reviews. In addition, we drew from our personal archives of references from recognised authorities in this field.

TIPS FOR NON-SPECIALISTS

- Include acute leukaemia in the differential for any child presenting with bone pain, atypical wheeze, bruising, or petechiae.
- Consider having a lower threshold for doing a full blood count in any child with unexplained malaise, fatigue, or pallor.
- Not all children with acute leukaemia present with the obvious signs of anaemia, bleeding, and infection.
- Absence of a very high white cell count, hepatosplenomegaly, and lymphadenopathy does not rule out acute leukaemia.

ADDITIONAL EDUCATIONAL RESOURCES

- Children's Cancer and Leukaemia Group (www.cclg.org.uk)—National professional body responsible for the organisation of treatment and management of children in the UK. Coordinates national and international clinical trials, and provides information for clinicians, patients, and families.
- Institute for Cancer Research (www.icr.ac.uk)—Conducts independent research into the causes, prevention, diagnosis, and methods of treatment of all cancer, including paediatric leukaemias.
- Leukaemia Research Fund (www.lrf.org.uk)—Only charity in the UK dedicated exclusively to researching haematological malignancies, including paediatric.
- Foundation for Children with Leukaemia (www.leukaemia.org)—Campaigning charity that funds research into causes and treatments, and supports families through welfare programmes.
- Cancer and Leukaemia in Childhood Sargent (www.clicsargent.org.uk)—Offers practical support and information to families by providing specialist nurses, play specialists, family support, patient information, grants and telephone helpline.
- Cancerbackup (www.cancerbackup.org.uk)—Recently merged with Macmillan Cancer Support. Offers cancer information, practical advice and support to cancer patients and their families through online publications, telephone helpline, specialist nurses, etc.

A PATIENT AND THEIR FAMILY'S PERSPECTIVE

AH, aged 13, was diagnosed with acute lymphocytic leukaemia three years ago. After a bone marrow transplant, she remains in remission.

AH

I first felt ill when my neck became really swollen and the joints in my legs seemed really heavy. I thought it was growing pains but it wasn't, it was cancer, and so we went to the clinic. I didn't really know what was happening but my Mum was really crying so I guessed it was something bad.

I remember the doctors saying I would lose my hair and I was a bit freaked out. I didn't really know how that would happen: would I just wake up and find my hair lying on the pillow? But it came out gradually—it kept falling into my food so my Mum cut it short and then, a couple of days later, she shaved it.

I feel like I've gained a whole bunch of things. Before, I didn't know about leukaemia, I didn't even know it existed, but now I'm braver. If I have to have an injection now I get a bit teary but sometimes I don't cry. Leukaemia's not the worst thing possible—there are worse things—but it's taught me to be grateful because people who don't have it are so lucky.

AH's father

The first thing I noticed was that she was pale and she'd get tired very easily. One morning she woke up so swollen in her neck you couldn't recognise her. We went to the doctor right away and he said it could be leukaemia. We were in a state of shock. You don't want to believe it, you don't want to think this is happening to your kid. It's just a whirlwind of emotions: how serious is it? Is she going to be okay? I didn't have a clue about leukaemia. I just knew it was cancer and when someone mentions that you obviously think the worst.

She was very scared. The pain was what scared her the most. The chemo started straight away and we were amazed at the results we got instantly. The swelling went down, the pain in her bones went away, and you could see her face again.

Now, dealing with the anxiety of "what if it comes back" is really scary, especially whenever she gets pale. You can't help thinking about it. We just kind of deal with it on a day by day basis. There is always that fear.

subsequent immunisation. Unless it is particularly frequent or extensive, foreign travel is considered safe.[23]

Where should research be directed next?

- The aetiology of acute leukaemia, particularly gene-environment interactions
- Refined selection, on the basis of cytogenetic and molecular data, of patients at either very low or very high risk of relapse
- Novel immunotherapeutic agents that target specific molecular defects such as gene fusions.

In the future, standard combination chemotherapy protocols might be tailored to an individual's unique genetic profile; this approach, together with novel molecular agents directed at leukaemia specific mutations, would continue with the current goals of minimising treatment toxicity for patients at low risk of relapse while improving the outlook for patients at high risk.

Contributors: CM wrote the original draft of this paper, and all authors contributed to subsequent drafts. CM is the guarantor.

Competing interests: CM and GH participate in clinical trials of treatment for acute leukaemia supported by the Leukaemia Research Fund. CM was the chief investigator of the UK ALL97/99 trial for acute lymphoblastic leukaemia and is co-investigator for the current UK ALL2003 trial. GH runs a UK registry for children with myeloproliferative disorders.

Provenance and peer review: Commissioned; externally peer reviewed.

1 Draper GJ, Stiller CA, O'Connor CM, Vincent TJ, Elliott P, McGale P, et al. The geographical epidemiology of childhood leukaemia and non-Hodgkin lymphomas in Great Britain, 1966-83. OPCS studies on medical and population subjects, no 53. London: OPCS, 1991.
2 Feltbower RG, Lewis IJ, Picton S, Richards M, Glaser AW, Kinsey SE, et al. Diagnosing childhood cancer in primary care—a realistic expectation? Br J Cancer 2004;90:1882-4.
3 Mitchell CD, Richards SM, Kinsey SE, Lilleyman J, Vora A, Eden TO. Benefit of dexamethasone compared with prednisolone for childhood acute lymphoblastic leukaemia: results of the UK Medical Research Council ALL97 randomized trial. Br J Haematol 2005;129:734-45.
4 Matloub YH, Angiolillo A, Bostrom B, Stork L, Hunger SP, Nachman J, et al. J Clin Oncology 2007;25(18S):9511.
5 Pui C-H, Robison LL, Look AT. Acute lymphoblastic leukaemia. Lancet 2008;371:1030-43.
6 Greaves MF. Aetiology of acute leukaemia. Lancet 1997;349:344-9.
7 SEER Cancer Statistic Review, 1973-1999. Bethesda, MD: National Cancer Institute, 2000:467.
8 Ries LA, Smith MA, Gurney JG. Cancer incidence and survival among children and adolescents: United States SEER Program 1975-1995. SEER Pediatric Monograph.
9 Horwitz M. The genetics of familial leukemia. Leukemia 1997;11:1347-59.
10 Hasle H, Clemmensen IH, Mikkelsen M. Risks of leukaemia and solid tumours in individuals with Down's syndrome. Lancet 2000;355:165-9.
11 Kinlen LJ. Infections and immune factors in cancer; the role of epidemiology. Oncogene 2004;23:6341-8.
12 Greaves M. Infection, immune responses and the aetiology of childhood leukaemia. Nat Rev Cancer 2006;6:193-203.
13 Redalli A, Laskin BL, Stephens JM, Boteman MF, Pashos CL. A systematic literature review of the clinical and epidemiological burden of acute lymphoblastic leukaemia (ALL). Eur J Cancer Care 2005;14:53-62.
14 Alvarez Y, Caballin MR, Gaitan S, Perez A, Bastida P, Ortega JJ, et al. Presenting features of 201 children with acute lymphoblastic leukemia: comparison according to presence or absence of ETV6/RUNX1 rearrangement. Cancer Genet Cytogenet 2007;177:161-3.
15 Chessells JM. Pitfalls in the diagnosis of childhood leukaemia. Br J Haematology 2001;114:506-11.
16 Frankfurt O, Tallman M. Emergencies in acute lymphoblastic leukaemia. In: Estey EH, Faderl SH, Kantarjian HM, eds. Hematologic malignancies: acute leukaemias. Berlin: Springer, 2008:281-8.
17 Harrison CJ, Kempski H, Hammond DW, Kearney L. Molecular cytogenetics in childhood leukemia. Methods Mol Med 2003;91:123-37.
18 Rubnitz JE, Evans WE. Pathobiology of acute lymphoblastic leukaemia. In: Hoffman R, Benz Jr EJ, Shattil SJ, Furie B, Cohen HJ, Silberstein LE, et al eds. Hematology, basic principles and practice. New York: Churchill Livingstone, 2000:1052-60.
19 Campana D. Role of minimal residual disease evaluation in leukaemia therapy. Current Hematologic Malignancy Reports 2008;3:155-60.
20 Eden OB, Harrison G, Richards S, Lilleyman JS, Bailey CC, Chessells JM, et al. Long-term follow-up of the United Kingdom Medical Research Council protocols for childhood acute lymphoblastic leukaemia, 1980-1997. Leukemia 2000;14:2307-20.

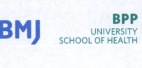

21 Hann IM, Webb DK, Gibson BE, Harrison CJ. MRC trials in childhood acute myeloid leukaemia. *Annals Hematol* 2004;83:S108-12.
22 Pizzo P. Management of fever in patients with cancer and treatment-induced neutropenia. *N Engl J Med* 1993;328:1323-32.
23 Royal College of Paediatrics and Child Health. Immunisation of the immunocompromised child. Best practice statement. 2002. www.rcpch.ac.uk/doc.aspx?id_Resource=1768.

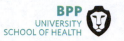

Identifying brain tumours in children and young adults

S H Wilne consultant paediatric oncologist[1], R A Dineen clinical associate professor[2], R M Dommett National Institute for Health Research clinical lecturer[3], T P C Chu research fellow in epidemiology[2], D A Walker professor of paediatric oncology[2]

[1]Department of Paediatric Oncology, Nottingham University Hospitals NHS Trust, Queens Medical Centre, Nottingham NG7 2UH, UK

[2]Faculty of Medicine and Health Sciences, University of Nottingham, Nottingham, UK

[3]School of Clinical Sciences, University of Bristol, Bristol, UK

Correspondence to: S H Wilne
sophie.wilne@nuh.nhs.uk

Cite this as: BMJ 2013;347:f5844

‹DOI› 10.1136/bmj.f5844
http://www.bmj.com/content/347/bmj.f5844

Healthcare professionals caring for children need to promptly identify the child or young person with a serious underlying condition from the majority who present with minor self limiting illness. Recognising when a child might have cancer can be particularly difficult. Despite the perception that cancer is rare in children, an average general practice will see a child or young person with a new cancer every six years, and a quarter of the tumours will be brain tumours (personal communication, Patricia O'Hare, 2013).[1] Early diagnosis can be crucial—evidence from cohort studies shows that it can improve short term and long term outcomes.[2] [3] [4] [5] This review summarises current evidence on the presentation and recognition of brain tumours in children and young adults and provides an overview of the treatment and long term care strategies for this population.

What brain tumours occur in children?

The term "brain tumour" encompasses a large number of different tumour types that have different cells of origin and clinical course (table 1). The most common brain tumours in children and young people are pilocytic astrocytomas, medulloblastomas, ependymomas, high grade gliomas, and germ cell tumours.[6] [7] Histologically, brain tumours are assigned a World Health Organization grade of 1-4 according to features suggesting malignancy, such as pleomorphic nuclei, high mitotic rate, and vascular invasion. Grades 1 and 2 are regarded as benign and 3 and 4 as malignant,[8] although the correlation between histological grade and patient outcome is poor. A low grade tumour that is not susceptible to treatment and is in a crucial area of the brain, such as the brain stem, is more likely to be fatal than

certain high grade tumours that are resectable and sensitive to chemoradiotherapy.[9] [10]

What are the risk factors for brain tumours in children?

As is true for most childhood cancers, no cause or trigger can be identified for most brain tumours. Several genetic syndromes, however, are associated with an increased risk of brain tumours (table 2)[7]

The development of some childhood brain tumours is related to changes in the local tumour (brain) environment that are linked to age. Children with neurofibromatosis type 1 have a 10-20% risk of developing an intracranial pilocytic astrocytoma, particularly in the optic pathways, owing to loss of neurofibromin 1 (the product of the *NF1* gene), which is a negative regulator of cell growth through the mitogen activated protein kinases/extracellular signal regulated kinases pathway. Not every child with neurofibromatosis type 1 develops an optic pathway glioma, and almost all children with the condition who develop one are under the age of 7 years. Therefore there is an interaction between germline *NF1* mutations, the age of the child, and another unknown factor that results in the development of an optic pathway glioma in some but not all children with the condition.

Studies in mouse models of neurofibromatosis type 1 have shown that reduced cAMP production in the brain is needed for the development of tumours. Mouse and human tissue studies have shown that cAMP levels vary with polymorphisms in cAMP regulators,[11] and that cAMP levels in the optic pathway are lower in young children than in older ones. These findings explain why optic pathway gliomas occur in only some young children with neurofibromatosis type 1.

Intracranial germ cell tumours provide another less well understood example. With the exception of mature teratomas, intracranial germ cell tumours are very rare in young children but are much more common as adolescence proceeds, in parallel with the onset of puberty. Presumably, this is a result of the hormonal drive to gonadal development interacting with potential tumour cells within the brain.

Case-control and cohort studies have shown that exposure to ionising radiation is the only environmental factor associated with brain tumours.[7] Brain or central nervous system radiotherapy for a previous cancer is the most common cause of exposure to high doses of ionising radiation, and secondary high grade gliomas and meningiomas have been reported in these populations.[12] Children who undergo computed tomography (CT) also have a risk of radiation induced cancer. A recently published epidemiological study found 608 excess cancers (of which 147 were brain tumours) in 680 211 patients who had a CT scan between the ages of 0 and 19 years, with children less than 5 years being particularly at risk.[13]

SOURCES AND SELECTION CRITERIA

We searched Medline, Embase, and the Cochrane Library for review articles. Key words were brain tumour(s), brain tumor(s), and diagnosis. Articles were restricted to English language and all children. We also used personal reference libraries and consulted experts.

SUMMARY POINTS

- Each week in the United Kingdom, 10 children and young people are diagnosed with a brain tumour
- An average general practice sees a new childhood cancer every six years; a quarter of these will be brain tumours
- Earlier diagnosis of brain tumours in children and young adults improves long term outcomes
- Diagnosis requires recognition of the specific combinations of symptoms and signs seen with tumours in different areas of the brain and with raised intracranial pressure, followed by brain imaging
- The developmental stage of the child affects tumour presentation; young children may not be able to describe visual abnormalities and headache
- Include a focused history (looking for corroborative symptoms and risk factors) and assessment of vision, motor skills, growth, and puberty in children or young people who present with symptoms or signs suggestive of a brain tumour

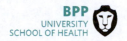

How do brain tumours present in children and young people?

The symptoms and signs of brain tumours are varied and determined by the part of the brain affected, the developmental stage and ability of the child or young person, and whether or not intracranial pressure is raised. There is usually a clinical evolution in the time period between initial symptom onset and diagnosis. In a retrospective four centre cohort study of 139 children with a brain tumour, an average of one symptom or sign was reported at symptom onset, but this increased to six at the time of diagnosis.[14]

Figure 1 shows the combinations of symptoms and signs at diagnosis caused by tumours developing in different parts of the brain and the frequency with which they occur.[15] This information was obtained from a meta-anlysis of the presenting symptoms and signs in 4171 children who were newly diagnosed with a brain tumour. Recognition of these specific combinations of symptoms and signs is an essential step towards diagnosis. Cerebellar tumours present with ataxia, nystagmus, head tilt, and poor coordination (www.youtube.com/watch?v=SwcQoTv_4Vw). At least 75% of cerebellar tumours obstruct the flow of cerebrospinal fluid through the aqueduct and into the fourth ventricle so also present with symptoms and signs of raised intracranial pressure (headache, vomiting, lethargy, increasing head circumference, papilloedema, reduced level of consciousness).

Central brain tumours present with reduced visual acuity and fields, wandering or roving eye movements in young children (owing to loss of visual fixation), and damage to the hypothalamic-pituitary axis.

This last feature leads to abnormal pubertal progression (precocious, arrested, or delayed), growth failure, diabetes insipidus, and diencephalic syndrome in young children (emaciation despite normal energy intake). Central tumours may also obstruct the flow of cerebrospinal fluid, leading to symptoms and signs of raised intracranial pressure.

Brain stem tumours present with swallowing difficulties, facial asymmetry and squint (owing to lower cranial nerve damage), hemiplegia, poor coordination, and abnormal gait (owing to long tract involvement). Cerebral hemisphere tumours are least likely to cause neurological signs and often present with focal seizures; they can also cause hemiplegia or a more focal motor weakness.

The developmental stage and ability of the child can also alter the presentation of tumours. For example, at least 20% of midline tumours cause visual impairment owing to compression of the optic chiasm and optic tracts. Older children can recognise that visual loss is abnormal and have the language skills to express this. Younger children lack this ability and are good at navigating familiar environments, so they can develop marked loss before this is recognised. Similarly, raised intracranial pressure causes headache. Older children can describe this, but younger children are often not good at localising pain and don't have the language skills to describe headache; instead, they may appear unsettled, lethargic, or withdrawn. Table 3 shows the most common symptoms and signs of brain tumours in different age groups.

Red flag symptoms

Attempts to reduce delays in diagnosis of tumours have identified "red flag" symptoms and signs that trigger referral to a "fast track" investigation and diagnostic service in secondary care. A population based case-control study determined the predicative value of such symptoms and signs in identifying children with a subsequent diagnosis of cancer presenting to primary care.[16] The red flags were taken from National Institute for Health and Care Excellence (NICE) referral guidelines for suspected cancer.[17] Just over a quarter of patients diagnosed as having cancer had any red flag symptom recorded in the previous three months, and a third in the preceding year.

However, red flag symptoms also occurred in children and young people who did not have a tumour (1.4% in three months and 5.4% in 12 months). Occurrence of a red flag symptom or sign increased the likelihood of a cancer diagnosis from 0.35 to 5.5 in 10 000 children at three months and from 1.4 to 7.0 in 10 000 children over a year. Symptoms and signs with the highest predictive value for brain tumours were abnormal movement, visual symptoms, vomiting, headache, pain, and seizures.

Thus, red flag symptoms and signs do occur in brain tumours, but their lack of specificity limits their usefulness in identifying children and young people requiring rapid brain imaging to diagnose or exclude a brain tumour. Further evidence for this is provided by the routes to diagnosis study of all patients diagnosed as having cancer in England between 2006 and 2008, which found that only 2% of all childhood cancers were diagnosed through a "two week" wait referral.[18]

Cohort and case-control studies have shown an association between frequency of consultation and subsequent tumour diagnosis. The specificity of consultation frequency alone is low, but it is improved if combined with a red flag symptom. For example, of 10 000 children attending their GP with visual symptoms within a three month period, six would be diagnosed as having cancer, but if they had consulted on three or more occasions (for any reason), this number increases to 23.[19] Referral should therefore be carefully considered for children with repeated consultations and a red flag symptom.

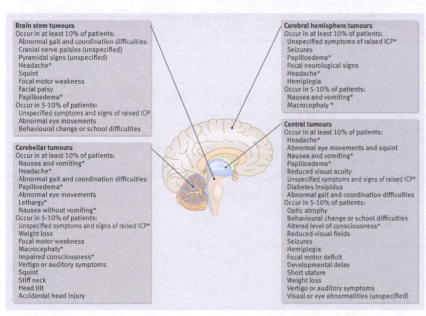

Brain stem tumours
Occur in at least 10% of patients:
 Abnormal gait and coordination difficulties
 Cranial nerve palsies (unspecified)
 Pyramidal signs (unspecified)
 Headache*
 Squint
 Focal motor weakness
 Facial palsy
 Papilloedema*
Occur in 5-10% of patients:
 Unspecified symptoms and signs of raised ICP
 Abnormal eye movements
 Behavioural change or school difficulties

Cerebellar tumours
Occur in at least 10% of patients:
 Nausea and vomiting*
 Headache*
 Abnormal gait and coordination difficulties
 Papilloedema*
 Abnormal eye movements
 Lethargy*
 Nausea without vomiting*
Occur in 5-10% of patients:
 Unspecified symptoms and signs of raised ICP*
 Weight loss
 Focal motor weakness
 Macrocephaly*
 Impaired consciousness*
 Vertigo or auditory symptoms
 Squint
 Stiff neck
 Head tilt
 Accidental head injury

Cerebral hemisphere tumours
Occur in at least 10% of patients:
 Unspecified symptoms of raised ICP*
 Seizures
 Papilloedema*
 Focal neurological signs
 Headache*
 Hemiplegia
Occur in 5-10% of patients:
 Nausea and vomiting*
 Macrocephaly *

Central tumours
Occur in at least 10% of patients:
 Headache*
 Abnormal eye movements and squint
 Nausea and vomiting*
 Papilloedema*
 Reduced visual acuity
 Unspecified symptoms and signs of raised ICP*
 Diabetes insipidus
 Abnormal gait and coordination difficulties
Occur in 5-10% of patients:
 Optic atrophy
 Behavioural change or school difficulties
 Altered level of consciousness*
 Reduced visual fields
 Seizures
 Hemiplegia
 Focal motor deficit
 Developmental delay
 Short stature
 Weight loss
 Vertigo or auditory symptoms
 Visual or eye abnormalities (unspecified)

Fig 1 Brain tumour presentation according to tumour location. *Symptom or sign caused by raised intracranial pressure (ICP)

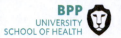

Table 1 Classification of brain tumours that occur in children and young people

Tumour group	Tumour	Location	WHO* grade	Approximate frequency (%)
Embryonal tumours: arise from transformation of undifferentiated and immature neuroepithelial cells	Medulloblastoma	Cerebellum	4	20
	Central primitive neuroectodermal tumour	Cerebral hemispheres	4	5
	Atypical teratoid or rhabdoid tumour	Throughout the brain	4	1
Glial tumours: arise from glial (supporting) cells	Astrocytoma	Throughout the brain	Pilocytic astrocytomas: 1; pilomyxoid astrocytomas: 2; anaplastic astrocytomas: 3; glioblastoma multiforme: 4	45
	Oligodendroglioma	Cerebral hemispheres	Oligodendroglioma: 2; anaplastic oligodendroglioma: 3	4
	Ependymoma	Throughout the ventricular system	Ependymoma: 2; anaplastic ependymoma: 3	10
	Choroid plexus tumours	Choroid plexus (within lateral ventricle)	Choroid plexus papilloma: 1; choroid plexus carcinoma: 3	2
Neuronal and glioneuronal tumours: arise from nerve cells	Ganglioglioma	Throughout the brain	1	3
	Dysembryoplastic neuroepithelial tumour	Cerebral hemispheres	1	2
Pineal parenchymal tumours: arise from melatonin secreting cells in the pineal glands (pineocytes)	Pineoblastoma	Pineal gland	2	1
	Pineocytoma	Pineal gland	4	1
Germ cell tumours: arise from germ cells that have become mislocated during embryonic development	Germinomas	Throughout the midline brain—for example, pituitary and pineal regions, hypothalamus, and third ventricle	Not included in WHO grading	4
	Teratomas			
	Embryonal carcinoma and yolk sac tumours			
Other developmental tumours	Craniopharyngioma	Epithelial tumour of sellar region (arises from Rathke's pouch epithelium)		
Meningiomas: arise from meningeal cells	Meningioma	Throughout the meninges	Meningioma: 1; atypical meningiomas: 2; anaplastic meningiomas: 3	2

*WHO=World Health Organization.

Table 2 Genetic syndromes associated with brain tumours in children and young people

Syndrome*	Prevalence (UK newborns)	Associated brain tumour	Clinical characteristics
Neurofibromatosis type 1	1/2500-3000	Astrocytomas; meningiomas; schwannomas	Skin: cafe au lait patches, axillary freckles, neurofibromas; bones: scoliosis, pseudarthrosis; learning and behavioural difficulties; peripheral nerve sheath tumours
Tuberous sclerosis	1/6000	Subependymal giant cell astrocytoma	Skin: hypomelanic nodules, angiofibromas, shagreen patch, ungula fibromas; heart: rhabdomyomas; Brain: cortical tubers, subependymal nodules, epilepsy; kidneys: angiomyolipomas; learning and behavioural difficulties
Neurofibromatosis 2	1/25 000	Schwannomas; meningiomas; ependymomas	Schwannomas (bilateral vestibular schwannomas); cataracts
Von Hippel-Lindau disease	1/36 000	Haemangioblastomas	Cerebellar and retinal haemangioblastoma, phaeochromocytoma, renal cysts, renal carcinoma, pancreatic cysts, pancreatic carcinoma, endolymphatic sac tumours
Li-Fraumeni syndrome	Unknown, rare	Astrocytomas; choroid plexus carcinoma	Early onset soft tissue sarcomas; leukaemia; osteosarcoma; melanoma; cancer of the breast, colon, pancreas, adrenal cortex, and brain
Turcot syndrome	Unknown, rare	Astrocytomas; medulloblastoma	Multiple adenomatous polyps, colorectal cancer and central nervous system tumours

Table 3 Brain tumour presentation according to age*

Pre-school (<5 years)	Primary school (5-11 years)	Secondary school (12-18 years)
Persistent or recurrent vomiting	Persistent or recurrent headache†	Persistent or recurrent headache†
Problems with balance, coordination, or walking	Persistent or recurrent vomiting	Persistent or recurrent vomiting
Abnormal eye movements	Problems with balance, coordination, or walking	Problems with balance, coordination, or walking
Behavioural change (particularly lethargy)	Abnormal eye movements	Abnormal eye movements
Fits or seizures (not with a fever)	Blurred or double vision†	Blurred or double vision†
Abnormal head position such as wry neck, head tilt, or persistent stiff neck	Behavioural change	Behavioural change
Progressively increasing head circumference†	Fits or seizures	Fits or seizures
	Abnormal head position such as wry neck, head tilt, or persistent stiff neck	Delayed or arrested puberty, slow growth†

*Based on a systematic review,[15] combined with clinical expertise and experience.
†Symptoms that differ according to age group.

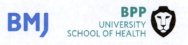

What should I do if I suspect that a child has a brain tumour?

Include a brain tumour in the (often very wide) differential diagnosis of any child or young person presenting with the symptoms and signs shown in fig 1. Their presence should trigger a focused history (including family history and any predisposing genetic factors) and examination to look for corroborative findings (particularly the symptom and sign clusters associated with tumours in specific locations). Include motor and visual assessment, pubertal staging, and comparison of the child's height and weight with previous growth and age appropriate norms in the examination. It can be difficult to assess the visual function of pre-school children, so if necessary refer them to community optometry or ophthalmology. Children who present with symptoms of critical raised intracranial pressure (persistent headache and vomiting, confusion, drowsiness, reduced consciousness level) require urgent imaging of the central nervous system so, if in primary care, refer them the same day to local paediatric services.

The much harder management decision in both primary and secondary care is for children who appear reasonably well at assessment but who have a symptom or sign that could be caused by a brain tumour. In this situation, the clinician must decide whether no further action is needed and the family can be reassured; whether a period of watchful waiting and subsequent review is needed; or whether symptoms, signs, and additional examination findings are specific enough to merit referral for secondary care review or imaging.

A short period of watchful waiting can be helpful because symptoms and signs often evolve with time in children with brain tumours. Brain tumours however can progress rapidly, so review children who present with headache within four weeks and those with all other symptoms and signs within two weeks. Tell parents and carers to return sooner if their child deteriorates. Book a follow-up appointment for young people at their initial consultation because they tend to be less reliable at returning with persisting symptoms.

NHS evidence endorsed clinical guidelines advising on assessment and indications for referral and imaging of children and young people who may have a brain tumour have been published.[20] The guidelines and other information sources are available on the HeadSmart website (www.headsmart.org.uk), which also advises on specific clinical situations where reassurance, review, or referral is an appropriate action.

How is a brain tumour confirmed?

Imaging of the central nervous system is needed to confirm or refute the diagnosis of a brain tumour. Imaging is used to confirm the presence of an intracranial mass lesion and to identify complications that require urgent intervention, such as the presence of a large mass effect or hydrocephalus. Both CT and magnetic resonance imaging (MRI) are suitable for this purpose. The widespread availability, ease of access, and speed of CT mean that this modality is widely used as first line imaging in children with suspected brain tumours. CT is particularly useful for emergency scanning of children who present in extremis, where time does not allow MRI, or for young children who would otherwise require general anaesthesia to undergo MRI in centres where access to general anaesthesia is limited.

However, in centres with good access to paediatric MRI services, MRI is used in preference to CT for children with suspected brain tumours. A brief protocol consisting of axial T2 weighted imaging can be used to effectively exclude a large intracranial mass lesion and takes around five minutes to perform. Full tumour MRI protocols may take more than an hour but provide both accurate anatomical localisation (including neuroaxis dissemination) and additional biological information, such as chemical composition, cellularity, and vascularity.

How are brain tumours treated in children and young people?

Brain tumours require multidisciplinary management, and the care of children and young people with brain tumours should be coordinated by their regional paediatric neurosurgery and neuro-oncology service. Treatment will be determined by the tumour type and location as well as the age of the child; it may involve surgery, chemotherapy, and radiotherapy. Research in paediatric neuro-oncology requires international collaboration, and patients are offered participation in clinical trials when available; our experience is that most families and young people welcome this opportunity.

Sequential clinical trials have led to great improvements in survival for many children and young people with brain tumours (fig 2).[21] [22] However, survival varies greatly between different tumour types and locations. Recent progress in biotechnology has enabled identification of novel pathway aberrations in multiple tumour types and led to the search for novel anti-tumour agents that can act on these pathways.[23] [24] [25] Treatment of young children is particularly challenging because brain directed treatment can have a serious impact on the child's subsequent development.

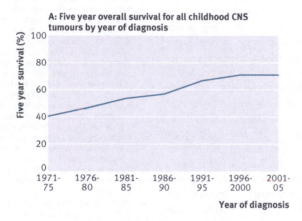

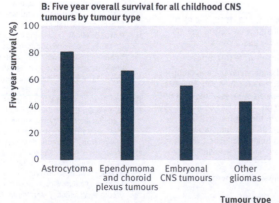

Fig 2 Five year overall survival for childhood (age 0-15 years) brain tumours by year of diagnosis (A) and tumour type (B). Data from the national registry of childhood tumours and the Office for National Statistics[21] [22]

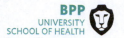

ADDITIONAL EDUCATIONAL RESOURCES

Resources for healthcare professionals

- HeadSmart (www.headsmart.org.uk)—Guidance on the identification and management of children and young people presenting with signs or symptoms that could be caused by a brain tumour

- Royal College of General Practitioners (http://elearning.rcgp.org.uk/course/info.php?id=99)—Education module using case illustrations to educate healthcare professionals about the presentation of childhood brain tumours

- BMJ Learning (http://learning.bmj.com/learning/module-intro/sarcomas-brain-tumours-children.html?moduleId=10042893&locale=en_GB)—Education module using case illustrations to educate healthcare professionals about the presentation of childhood brain and bone tumours

- National Institute for Health and Care Excellence. Referral for suspected cancer. CG27. www.nice.org.uk/cg027

- Neuro Foundation (www.nfauk.org/)—Information about neurofibromatosis, including advice on managing children and young people with the condition

- Tuberous Sclerosis Association (www.tuberous-sclerosis.org/)—Clinical guidelines for the management of people with tuberous sclerosis

Resources for patients and families

- HeadSmart (www.headsmart.org.uk)—Information on how brain tumours present and what to do if you are concerned that you or your child could have a brain tumour

- Neuro Foundation (www.nfauk.org/)—Information about neurofibromatosis including cause, potential complications, and management; also a source of advice and support

- Tuberous Sclerosis Association (www.tuberous-sclerosis.org/)—Information about tuberous sclerosis including cause, potential complications, and management; also a source of advice and support

- Brain Tumour Charity (www.thebraintumourcharity.org/)—The largest UK brain tumour charity. Provides information about brain tumours, including diagnosis and treatment options, plus support and a helpline

Current clinical strategies used to minimise the side effects of treatment include the use of intraventricular chemotherapy and proton radiotherapy.[26][27][28]

Rehabilitation and support for reintegration into education and society are essential. Children and young people should be assessed by neuropsychology, physiotherapy, occupational therapy, and speech and language services at diagnosis and ongoing care provided if needed. Return to education can be particularly challenging, and early communication with the child or young person's education provider to obtain advice on what support is likely to be needed facilitates this process. Children and young people treated with chemoradiotherapy for brain tumours often develop cognitive difficulties, particularly with the speed of processing, and it is important that this is recognised and supportive strategies implemented.[29][30] Children often require lifelong additional care, so early engagement with primary care is essential.

Contributors: SHW drafted the initial version. RAD, TPCC, and RMD provided advice on specific sections. All authors reviewed and contributed to subsequent versions. SHW is guarantor.

Funding: The authors received no funding to write this article.

Competing interests: We have read and understood the BMJ Group policy on declaration of interests and declare the following interests: RMD, RAD, TPCC have none. DAW is an expert witness in the field of clinical practice in childhood brain tumours, codirector of a university research centre related to children's brain tumour research and principal investigator for the "HeadSmart Be Brain Tumour Aware" campaign, which is a Health Foundation funded collaborative national project. SHW is one of the coinvestigators for the "HeadSmart Be Brain Tumour Aware" campaign.

Provenance and peer review: Not commissioned; externally peer reviewed.

1 Cancer Research UK. Cancer incidence by age. www.cancerresearchuk.org/cancer-info/cancerstats/incidence/age/.

2 Batchelder P, Foreman N, Madden J, Wilkinson C, Handler M. Catastrophic presentations in pediatric brain tumors [abstract]. Neuro oncology 2010;12:ii76.

3 Reimers T, Ehrenfels S, Mortensen E, Schmiegelow M, Sonderkaer S, Carstensen H, et al. Cognitive deficits in long-term survivors of childhood brain tumours: identification of predictive factors. Med Pediatr Oncol 2003;40:26-34.

4 Yule S, Hide T, Cranney M, Simpson E, Barrett A. Low grade astrocytomas in the west of Scotland 1987-96: treatment, outcome and cognitive function. Arch Dis Childhood 2001;84:61-4.

5 Chou S, Digre K. Neuro-ophthalmic complications of raised intracranial pressure, hydrocephalus and shunt malfunction. Neurosurg Clin N Am 1999;10:587-608.

6 Stiller C, Allen M, Eatock E. Childhood cancer in Britain: the national registry of chidhood tumours and incidence rates 1978-1987. Eur J Cancer 1995;31:2028-34.

7 Stiller C, Bleyer W. Epidemiology. In: Taylor R, Walker D, Perilongo G, Punt J, eds. Brain and spinal tumours of childhood. Arnold, 2004:35-49.

8 Louis D, Ohgaki H, Wiestler O, Cavenee W, Burger P, Jouvet A, et al. The 2007 WHO classification of tumours of the central nervous system. Acta Neuropathol 2007;114:97-109.

9 Korones D, Fisher P, Kretschmar C, Zhou T, Chen Z, Kepner J, et al. Treatment of children with diffuse intrinsic brian stem glioma with radiotherapy, vincristine and oral VP-16: a children's oncology group phase II study. Pediatr Blood Cancer 2008;50:227-30.

10 Packer R, Gajjar A, Vezina G, Rorke-Adams L, Burger P, Robertson P, et al. Phase III study of craniospinal radiation therapy followed by adjuvant chemotherapy for newly diagnosed average-risk medulloblastoma. J Clin Oncol 2006;25:4202-8.

11 Warrington N, Woerner M, Daginakatte G, Dasgupta B, Perry A, Gutmann DH, et al. Spatiotemporal differences in CXCL 12 expression and cyclic AMP underlie the unique pattern of optic pathway glioma growth in neurofibromatosis type 1. Cancer Res 2007;67:8588-95.

12 Banerjee J, Paakko E, Harila M, Herva R, Tuominen J, Koivula A, et al. Radiation-induces meningiomas: a shadow in the sucess story of childhood leukaemia. Neurooncology 2009;11:543-9.

13 Matthews JD, Forsythe AV, Brady Z, Butler MW, Georgen SK, Byrnes GB, et al. Cancer risk in 680 000 people exposed to computer tomography scans in childhood or adolescence: data linkage study of 11 million Australians. BMJ 2013;346:f2360.

14 Wilne S, Collier J, Kennedy C, Jenkins A, Grout J, Mackie S, et al. Progression from first symptoms to diagnosis in childhood brain tumours. Eur J Pediatr 2011;71:87-93.

15 Wilne S, Collier J, Kennedy C, Grundy R, Wlaker D. Presentation of childhood CNS tumours: a systematic review and meta-analysis. Lancet Oncol 2007;8:685-95.

16 Dommett R, Redaniel M, Stevens M, Hamilton W, Martin RM. Features of childhood cancer in primary care: a population-based case-control study. Br J Cancer 2012;106:982-7.

17 National Institute for Health and Care Excellence. Referral for suspected cancer. CG27. 2005. www.nice.org.uk/CG27.

18 Ellis-Brookes L, McPhail S, Ives A, Greenslade M, Shelton J, Hiorn S, et al. Routes to diagnosis for cancer—determining the patient journey using multiple routine data sets. Br J Cancer 2012;107:1220-6.

19 Dommett R, Redaniel T, Stevens M, Martin R, Hamilton W. Risk of childhood cancer with symptoms in primary care: a population-based case control study. Br J Gen Pract 2013;63:22-9.

20 Wilne S, Koller K, Collier J, Kennedy C, Grundy R, Walker D. The diagnosis of brain tumours in children: a guideline to assist healthcare professionals in the assessment of children who may have a brain tumour. Arch Dis Child 2010;95:534-9.

21 Childhood Cancer Research Group. Survival from childhood cancer, Great Britain, 1971-2005. 2010. www.ccrg.ox.ac.uk/datasets/survivalrates.shtml.

22 Cancer Research UK. Childhood cancer survival statistics. www.cancerresearchuk.org/cancer-info/cancerstats/childhoodcancer/survival/ .

23 Franz D, Belousova E, Sparagana S, Bebin M, Frost M, Kuperman R, et al. Efficacy and safety of everolimus for subependymal giant cell astrocytomas associated with tuberous sclerosis complex (EXIST-1): a multicentre, randomised, placebo-controlled phase 3 trial. Lancet 2013;381:125-32.

24 Picard D, Miller S, Hawkins C, Bouffet E, Rogers HA, Chan TS, et al. Markers of survival and metastatic potential in childhood CNS primitive neuro-ectodermal brain tumours: an integrative genomic analysis. Lancet Oncol 2012;13:838-48.

25 Low J, Sauvage F. Clinical experience with hedgehog pathway inhibitors. J Clin Oncol 2010;28:5321-26.

26 Von Bueren A, von Hoff K, Pietsch T, Gerber N, Warmuth-Metz M, Deinlein F, et al. Treatment of young children with localised medulloblastoma by chemotherapy alone: results of the multicentretrial HIT 2000 confirming the porgnostic impact of radiotherapy. Neurooncology 2011;13:669-79.

27 Merchant T, Hua C, Shukla H, Ying X, Nill S, Oelfke U. Proton versus photon radiotherapy for common pediatric brain tumors: comparison of models of dose characteristics and their relationships to cognitive function. Pediatr Blood Cancer 2008;51:110-17.

28 Brodin N, Vogelius I, Maraldo M, Munck A, Rosenschold P, Aznar M, et al. Life years lost—comparing potentially fatal late complications after radiotherapy for pediatric medulloblsatoma on a common scale. Cancer 2012;118:5432-40.

29 Pruitt D, Ayyanger R, Craig K, White A, Neufeld J. Pediatric brain tumor rehabilitation. J Pediatr Rehabil Med 2011;4:59-70.

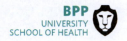

30   Nazemi K, Butler R. Neuropsychological rehabilitation for survivors
      of childhood and adolescent brain tumors: a view of the past and a
      vision for a promising future. *J Pediatr Rehabil Med* 2011;4:37-46.

Related links

bmj.com
- Get Cleveland Clinic CME creditrs for this article

bmj.com/archive
- Gout (*BMJ* 2013;347:f5648)
- Testicular germ cell tumours (*BMJ* 2013;347:f5526)
- Managing cows' milk allergy in children (*BMJ* 2013;347:f5424)
- Personality disorder (*BMJ* 2013;347:f5276)
- Dyspepsia (*BMJ* 2013;347:f5059)

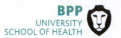

Managing and preventing depression in adolescents

Anita Thapar professor of child and adolescent psychiatry[1], Stephan Collishaw senior lecturer in developmental psychopathology[1], Robert Potter consultant child and adolescent psychiatrist [2], Ajay K Thapar general practitioner[3]

[1]Department of Psychological Medicine and Neurology, Cardiff University School of Medicine, Cardiff CF14 4XN

[2]Trehafod Child and Family Clinic (Cwm Taf NHS Trust), Cockett, Swansea SA2 0GB

[3]Taff Riverside Practice, Riverside, Cardiff CF11 9SH

Correspondence to: A Thapar
thapar@cf.ac.uk

Cite this as: BMJ 2010;340:c209

‹DOI› 0.1136/bmj.c209
http://www.bmj.com/content/340/
bmj.c209

Depressive disorder affects 1-6% of adolescents each year worldwide,[1][2] and early onset heralds a more severe and persistent illness in adult life.[3] Effective treatment is available, but best treatment practice is controversial because of concerns about the use of antidepressants in young people and inconsistencies in evidence. This review provides guidance for non-specialists on the assessment and management of adolescent unipolar depression and considers emerging evidence on prevention strategies.

Why is it important to identify adolescent depression?

Evidence from prospective community studies suggests that rates of underdiagnosis and undertreatment of depression are higher in adolescents than in adults.[4] Large scale, longitudinal population based and clinical cohort studies have consistently shown that rates of depression rise sharply after puberty, especially in girls, with immediate and long term risks.[5][6] Clinical depression adversely affects schooling, educational attainment, and relationships,[7] and it has long term negative consequences on adult physical health and functioning.[8] Although most affected adolescents show initial remission, 50-70% of them will have a recurrence within five years of initial diagnosis.[5] Large prospective studies have also shown that adolescent depression is associated with a raised risk of suicide (odds ratio 11 to 27),[9] and suicide represents the third leading cause of death in this age group (aged 14-19 years).[10]

SOURCES AND SELECTION CRITERIA

We searched for papers published between 1990 and 2009 using key index terms (adolescent depression, treatment, and prevention) on PubMed (Medline and life science journals). In addition, we consulted the Institute of Medicine report "Preventing mental, emotional and behavioral disorders among young people: progress and possibilities" (published by National Academies Press 2009), NICE guidelines on adolescent depression, Cochrane systematic reviews, and BMJ Clinical Evidence. This was supplemented by reviews and our own knowledge.

SUMMARY POINTS

- Depression affects 1-6% of adolescents each year worldwide
- Diagnostic criteria for depression are the same as for adults, but the primary presenting concern may be different (for example, behavioural problems, refusal to go to school)
- For mild depression, cognitive behavioural therapy seems to be effective. Because such treatment is a scarce resource, less specialised supportive treatment and guided self help can be used initially
- For moderate-severe depression, fluoxetine and routine specialist (child and adolescent mental health service) clinical care or fluoxetine plus cognitive behavioural therapy is recommended
- Suicidal risk must be carefully monitored
- Parental depression needs to be treated

Which adolescents are most at risk of developing a depressive disorder?

Evidence from clinical and epidemiological studies shows that three groups are at increased risk of developing a depressive disorder. Firstly, adolescents who have raised levels of depressive symptoms but fall below the diagnostic threshold have a two to three times greater risk of developing future depressive episodes than those without such symptoms.[8] Secondly, the adolescent offspring of parents with a history of depression are three to four times more likely than those of parents with no psychiatric history to develop depression.[11] Thirdly, in adolescents who have previously had depression, recurrence rates are high.[8]

How is adolescent depression diagnosed?

Diagnostic criteria from either ICD-10 (international classification of diseases, 10th revision) (box) or the *Diagnostic and Statistical Manual of Mental Disorders*, fourth edition (DSM-IV) are currently used; these two sets of criteria are similar.

CRITERIA FOR DEPRESSIVE EPISODE, ACCORDING TO ICD-10

Two of the first three symptoms listed below must be present. In addition, at least four symptoms (for mild episode), six symptoms (for moderate episode), or eight symptoms (for severe episode) must be present during the same two week period.

- Depressed mood for most of the day and almost every day
- Loss of interest or pleasure in activities
- Decreased energy or increased fatigability
- Loss of confidence or self esteem
- Unreasonable feelings of self reproach or excessive inappropriate guilt
- Recurrent thoughts of death or suicide, or any suicidal behaviour
- Reduced ability to think or concentrate
- Change in psychomotor activity, agitation, or retardation
- Sleep disturbance
- Change in appetite with corresponding weight change

The criteria for depression in adolescents are the same as for adults (although the DSM-IV criteria allow "irritable" (easily annoyed and provoked to anger) instead of "depressed" mood in children and adolescents). Thus the clinical questioning approach with adolescents should be similar to that used in adults. In this age group, it is helpful to question both the adolescent and the parent(s) about specific symptoms and to check whether the symptoms of depression are associated with impairment—for example, an adolescent with depression may stop going out with friends or show deterioration in school work. Irritability may be a prominent symptom. In this age group, comorbidity

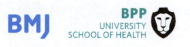

with other psychiatric disorders—notably disruptive behaviour disorders (20-40%) and anxiety disorders—is common (occurring in 30-75% of cases), as is association with deliberate self harm and suicidality (odds ratio 51).[12] Depression may be missed if the primary reported features are behavioural problems, substance misuse, anxiety symptoms, refusal to go to school, academic failure, or unexplained physical symptoms—especially musculoskeletal pains[13]—all of which are significantly associated with adolescent depression (reported odds ratios 10 to 29).[14]

Questionnaires can be used for screening and monitoring changes in the depression symptom score. The Mood and Feelings Questionnaire (MFQ; http://devepi.duhs. duke.edu/mfq.html) is one of the most well established screening instruments for adolescent depression,[15] and it has been validated in clinical and community samples. If a parent raises the initial concerns, their reports on the adolescent can be helpful as a first screen, and the above questionnaire has both a parent version and a child version. Other questionnaires are also available.[16] It is important to ask the adolescent about suicidal thoughts and intent.

Which treatments work for adolescent depression?

Inconsistent evidence and guidelines have made best treatment practice of depression in adolescents controversial.[17] [18] Most published evaluation studies have focused on the short term effectiveness of newer generation antidepressant drugs or cognitive behavioural therapy (CBT), or both. Evidence on long term efficacy and prevention of relapse is lacking.

Psychological treatments
The two most commonly investigated treatments are CBT and interpersonal psychotherapy. The evidence on CBT is mixed. One meta-analysis suggests that CBT is effective for adolescent depression, although effect sizes are modest (0.3).[19] A recent systematic review and meta-analysis also shows that CBT is modestly effective for adolescent depression, but that effect sizes are smaller in more recent better designed studies and in more complicated cases.[20] In contrast, a large randomised controlled trial (TADS) from the United States found that in moderate-severe depression, CBT alone was no better than placebo,[21] and that it provided benefits only in combination with fluoxetine.

Interpersonal psychotherapy has been shown to be effective in treating adolescent depression in three randomised controlled trials.[22] However, good quality psychological treatments for adolescents are not widely available in many countries.

Taken together, the evidence on psychological treatments can be summarised as follows:
- CBT alone is probably most useful for mild depression
- Interpersonal psychotherapy, if available, is worthwhile.

Drugs
The effectiveness of selective serotonin reuptake inhibitors for children and adolescents has been systematically reviewed.[23] Two systematic reviews suggest that fluoxetine is an effective treatment for adolescent depression (41-61% response to fluoxetine v 20-35% response to placebo, relative risk 1.86; treatment effect in terms of depression symptom scores −5.63). Consistent good quality evidence on other newer generation antidepressants is currently lacking.

Treating mild depression in non-specialist settings
In most countries, including the United Kingdom, primary care plays a key part in the detection and initial management of adolescent depression, but few treatment studies are based in this setting. One randomised controlled trial in the US suggested that organisational changes in primary care through trained care managers who enhanced access to evidence based treatments (CBT and antidepressants) significantly reduced symptoms of adolescent depression in the short term.[24]

Simple, non-specific psychosocial strategies might also be helpful as an initial treatment, although good quality evidence on these is lacking. Such first line pragmatic approaches deserve proper evaluation because specialised resources such as CBT are limited. Suggested strategies include providing parental support; recognising and treating parental mental illness; educating patients about depression (this may include the use of educational leaflets); problem solving; attending to recent family or peer group conflicts; dealing with comorbidity; and liaising with schools and other agencies while monitoring mental state and using an empathic reflective approach.[25] Advice on nutrition and diet, exercise (45 minutes to one hour three times week), sleep hygiene, and anxiety management, along with guided self help and non-directive supportive counselling are also recommended.[17]

Treating moderate-severe depression
Clinical guidelines on the treatment of adolescent depression differ between Europe and the US, and some guidance is based on consensus opinion rather than evidence. Currently, evidence on the best available treatment for moderate-severe adolescent depression comes from two randomised controlled treatment versus placebo trials. One study was based on UK NHS patients (ADAPT),[25] had no sponsorship from a drug company, and found a significant treatment effect at 12 weeks. It compared fluoxetine alone (61% "much or very much improved" by 28 weeks) with CBT plus fluoxetine (53% much or very much improved); all patients received routine specialist clinical care. The other study (TADS) was from the US, and it compared 12 weeks of CBT alone (43% response), fluoxetine alone with no psychosocial care (61% response), and CBT plus fluoxetine (71% response) with placebo (35% response).[21] The evidence on treating moderate-severe depression can be summarised as follows:
- Fluoxetine is an effective treatment for adolescent depression[21] [23] [25]
- Evidence on the benefits of adding CBT to fluoxetine is mixed. The US study suggested that it accelerated the response to treatment and reduced suicidality,[21] whereas the UK study found no benefits.[25] This might have been because the UK study included more severe clinic derived cases and all patients received routine specialist care
- Consistent effectiveness data on newer generation antidepressants other than fluoxetine are lacking,[23] and they are currently not approved for use in patients under 18 years in the UK and Europe. Escitalopram has been approved by the US Food and Drug Administration, but consistent evidence on its effectiveness in adolescence is still limited.

Only around 60% of adolescents with depression show remission after treatment, so what about those who fail to respond to initial treatment? One large US randomised control trial of adolescents who had not responded to two

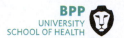

months of initial treatment with a first selective serotonin reuptake inhibitor suggested that adding CBT and switching to another one of these drugs (paroxetine or citalopram) results in a higher response rate (54.8%) than switching drugs only (40.5%).[26] A switch to venlafaxine was not recommended because of adverse side effects.

Suicidal risk

One of the major concerns has been that new generation antidepressants seem to be associated with greater suicidal risk in adolescents than in adults.[27] Caution is needed in interpreting results, however, because untreated adolescent depression can itself lead to suicidality and the evidence is mixed.[23] [27] A recent pooled analysis of 27 published and unpublished randomised placebo controlled trials of newer generation antidepressants in children and adolescents found that the benefits of antidepressants (number needed to treat 10) were greater than the risk of suicidal ideation and suicide attempts (number needed to harm 143).[27] Overall, the evidence supports careful monitoring for suicidal risk in adolescents with depression, regardless of treatment choice.

Can we prevent or delay onset of depression in adolescents?

Given the serious burden of depression, the poor prognosis when onset is early, and the limited treatment options available, it is increasingly being argued that preventing, or at least delaying, the onset of depression in children and adolescents is a major public health and clinical priority.

A meta-analysis of the evidence on this topic suggests that prevention strategies are likely to be effective only when given to high risk groups of adolescents rather than to the whole population.[28]

What sorts of prevention strategies might be useful?

The most promising prevention programme has been targeted at three high risk groups—those with raised depression symptoms, a previous episode of depression, and whose parents have a history of depression. It consists of a group based CBT approach delivered to parents and children.[29] A recent high quality randomised controlled trial in the US found that this type of intervention resulted in significantly fewer depressive episodes at one year (21.4% v 32.7% in controls).[29] However, the intervention was less effective if the parents had current depression. This could simply reflect higher inherited risk for depression in the adolescents, but it could mean that adolescent depression can arise from the direct and indirect risk effects of being exposed to current parental depression. In support of current maternal depression being an important target, the largest treatment trial of adult depression, STAR*D, found that successfully treating depression in mothers improved the mental health of children.[30] However, this finding requires confirmation. Nevertheless, these results highlight the importance of effectively monitoring and treating maternal depression and better integrating adult and child services. They also suggest future possibilities for prevention programmes.

Conclusion

Depression in adolescents is common, severe, and leads to immediate and long term morbidity and mortality. It is important for clinicians who deal with young people and families to be aware of the problem, so that high

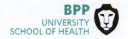

risk adolescents can be screened, assessed, and offered appropriate treatment. Prevention strategies in high risk groups are likely to become increasingly important.

Contributors: AT, AKT, and SC reviewed the literature. RP consulted guidelines and web resources. All authors helped interpret papers and write the article. AT is guarantor.

Funding: The authors' research on depression is supported by Sir Jules Thorne Medical Trust.

Competing interests: AT accepted fees from drug companies for speaking and organising educational events and received an educational grant for attention deficit hyperactivity disorder before 2006. All other authors have none to declare.

Provenance and peer review: Commissioned; externally peer reviewed.

Parental consent obtained.

1. Green H, McGinnity A, Meltzer H, Ford T, Goodman R. Mental health of children and young people in Great Britain, 2004. Palgrave Macmillan, 2005.
2. Costello EJ, Erkanli A, Angold A. Is there an epidemic of child or adolescent depression? *J Child Psychol Psychiatry* 2006;47:1263-71.
3. Lewinsohn PM, Clarke GN, Seeley JR, Rohde P. Major depression in community adolescents: age at onset, episode duration, and time to recurrence. *J Am Acad Child Adolesc Psychiatry* 1994;33:809-18.
4. Leaf PJ, Alegria M, Cohen P, Goodman SH, Horwitz SM, Hoven CW, et al. Mental health service use in the community and schools: results from the four-community MECA study. Methods for the epidemiology of child and adolescent mental disorders study. *J Am Acad Child Adolesc Psychiatry* 1996;35:889-97.
5. Lewinsohn PM, Rohde P, Seeley JR, Klein DN, Gotlib IH. Natural course of adolescent major depressive disorder in a community sample: predictors of recurrence in young adults. *Am J Psychiatry* 2000;157:1584-91.
6. Kessler RC, Avenevoli S, Ries Merikangas K. Mood disorders in children and adolescents: an epidemiologic perspective. *Biol Psychiatry* 2001;49:1002-14.
7. Birmaher B, Ryan ND, Williamson DE, Brent DA, Kaufman J, Dahl RE, et al. Childhood and adolescent depression: a review of the past 10 years. Part I. *J Am Acad Child Adolesc Psychiatry* 1996;35:1427-39.
8. Lewinsohn PM, Rohde P, Seeley JR. Major depressive disorder in older adolescents: prevalence, risk factors, and clinical implications. *Clin Psychol Rev* 1998;18:765-94.
9. Gould MS, Greenberg T, Velting DM, Shaffer D. Youth suicide risk and preventative interventions: a review of the past 10 years. *J Am Acad Child Adolesc Psychiatry* 2003;42:386-405.
10. Centers for Disease Control and Prevention. National Center for Injury Prevention and Control. Web-based injury statistics query and reporting system (WISQARS). 2009. http://webappa.cdc.gov/sasweb/ncipc/leadcaus10.html.
11. Rice F, Harold G, Thapar A. The genetic aetiology of childhood depression: a review. *J Child Psychol Psychiatry* 2002;43:65-79.
12. Foley DL, Goldston DB, Costello EJ, Angold A. Proximal psychiatric risk factors for suicidality in youth: the Great Smoky Mountains study. *Arch Gen Psychiatry* 2006;63:1017-24.
13. Egger HL, Costello EJ, Erkanli A, Angold A. Somatic complaints and psychopathology in children and adolescents: stomach aches, musculoskeletal pains, and headaches. *J Am Acad Child Adolesc Psychiatry* 1999;38:852-60.
14. Costello EJ, Mustillo S, Erkanli A, Keeler G, Angold A. Prevalence and development of psychiatric disorders in childhood and adolescence. *Arch Gen Psychiatry* 2003;60:837-44.
15. Daviss WB, Birmaher B, Melhem NA, Axelson DA, Michaels SM, Brent DA. Criterion validity of the mood and feelings questionnaire for depressive episodes in clinic and non-clinic subjects. *J Child Psychol Psychiatry* 2006;47:927-34.
16. Williams SB, O'Connor EA, Eder M, Whitlock EP. Screening for child and adolescent depression in primary care settings: a systematic evidence review for the US Preventive Services Task Force. *Pediatrics* 2009;123:e716-35.
17. National Institute for Health and Clinical Excellence. Depression in children and young people: identification and management in primary, community and secondary care. 2005. Clinical guideline CG28. guidance.nice.org.uk/CG28.
18. Birmaher B, Brent D, Bernet W, Bukstein O, Walter H, et al; AACAP Work Group on Quality Issues. Practice parameter for the assessment and treatment of children and adolescents with depressive disorders. *J Am Acad Child Adolesc Psychiatry* 2007;46:1503-26.
19. Weisz JR, McCarty CA, Valeri SM. Effects of psychotherapy for depression in children and adolescents: a meta-analysis. *Psychol Bull* 2006;132:132-49.
20. Klein JB, Jacobs RH, Reinecke MA. Cognitive-behavioral therapy for adolescent depression: a meta-analytic investigation of changes in effect-size estimates. *J Am Acad Child Adolesc Psychiatry* 2007;46:1403-13.
21. Treatment for Adolescents with Depression Study (TADS) Team. The treatment for adolescents with depression study (TADS): outcomes over 1 year of naturalistic follow-up. *Am J Psychiatry* 2009;166:1141-9.
22. Mufson L, Dorta KP, Wickramaratne P, Nomura Y, Olfson M, Weissman MM. A randomized effectiveness trial of interpersonal psychotherapy for depressed adolescents. *Arch Gen Psychiatry* 2004;61:577-84.
23. Hetrick S, Merry S, McKenzie J, Sindahl P, Proctor M. Selective serotonin reuptake inhibitors (SSRIs) for depressive disorders in children and adolescents. *Cochrane Database Syst Rev* 2007;(3):CD004851.
24. Asarnow JR, Jaycox LH, Duan N, LaBorde AP, Rea MM, Murray P, et al. Effectiveness of a quality improvement intervention for adolescent depression in primary care clinics: a randomized controlled trial. *JAMA* 2005;293:311-9.
25. Goodyer I, Dubicka B, Wilkinson P, Kelvin R, Roberts C, Byford S, et al. Selective serotonin reuptake inhibitors (SSRIs) and routine specialist care with and without cognitive behaviour therapy in adolescents with major depression: randomised controlled trial. *BMJ* 2007;335:142.
26. Brent D, Emslie G, Clarke G, Wagner KD, Asarnow JR, Keller M, et al. Switching to another SSRI or to venlafaxine with or without cognitive behavioural therapy for adolescents with SSRI-resistant depression: the TORDIA randomized controlled trial. *JAMA* 2008;299:901-13.
27. Bridge JA, Yengar S, Salary CB, Barbe RP, Birmaher B, Pincus HA, et al. Clinical response and risk for reported suicidal ideation and suicide attempts in pediatric antidepressant treatment: a meta-analysis of randomized controlled trials. *JAMA* 2007;63:332-9.
28. Stice E, Shaw H, Bohon C, Marti CN, Rohde P. A meta-analytic review of depression prevention programs for children and adolescents: factors that predict magnitude of intervention effects. *J Consult Clin Psychol* 2009;77:486-503.
29. Garber J, Clarke GN, Weersing VR, Beardslee WR, Brent DA, Gladstone TR, et al. Prevention of depression in at-risk adolescents: a randomized controlled trial. *JAMA* 2009;301:2215-24.
30. Weissman MM, Pilowsky DJ, Wickramaratne PJ, Talati A, Wisniewski SR, Fava M, et al. Remissions in maternal depression and child psychopathology: a STAR*D-child report. *JAMA* 2006;295:1389-98.

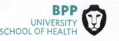

Use and misuse of drugs and alcohol in adolescence

Paul McArdle consultant child and adolescent psychiatrist

¹Fleming Nuffield Unit, Northumberland Tyne and Wear NHS Trust, Newcastle upon Tyne NE2 3AE

Correspondence to: Paul McArdle mcardlep@btinternet.com

Cite this as: *BMJ* 2008;337:a306

‹DOI› 0.1136/bmj.a306
http://www.bmj.com/content/337/bmj.a306

Substance misuse is one of a group of linked behaviours that has recently become more common among young people in westernised societies.[w1] This rise has paralleled increasing rates of anxiety and depressive symptoms and of deaths related to substance misuse.[1] [w1-w3] Substance use disorders are potentially treatable and should be managed as chronic, relapsing diseases of complex origin.[2] This review examines the scale of these disorders among young people and how healthcare practitioners can intervene.

Method

We searched Medline, Google, and the websites of the UK National Treatment Agency, US National Institute on Drug Abuse, and European Monitoring Centre for Drugs and Drug Addiction for suitable evidence based material. We also consulted colleagues working with young people with substance misuse, as well as consulting young people themselves and their carers.

BOX 1 DEFINITIONS OF MISUSE AND DEPENDENCE*

Substance misuse

Substance misuse is a maladaptive pattern of use leading to clinically important impairment or distress, manifested by one or more of the following over 12 months:

- Failure to fulfil major obligations at work, school, or home
- Use of a substance in situations in which it is physically hazardous
- Persistent or recurrent use of the substance despite persistent or recurrent social or interpersonal problems caused or exacerbated by the effects of the substance
- Persistent or recurrent use despite legal problems related to use of the substance

Substance dependence

Substance dependence is broadly equivalent to addiction and generally suggests physiological changes related to chronic drug administration. Dependence is associated with three or more of the following over 12 months:

- Tolerance
- Withdrawal
- Taking larger amounts than intended
- Unsuccessful efforts to cut down
- Spending a great deal of time obtaining or using the substance
- Giving up important activities because of use
- Continued use despite physical or psychological problems likely to have been caused or exacerbated by the substance

*Based on the Diagnostic and Statistical Manual of Mental Disorders[w4]

SUMMARY POINTS

- Substance misuse or dependence is a form of chronic, relapsing, debilitating illness
- International survey findings from a range of countries found that parental knowledge of their child's whereabouts protected against substance use, though this may be the result of a confiding parent-child relationship
- Without always consciously doing so, healthcare staff can exert substantial psychological "healing" and stabilisation, which can be valuable to troubled young people
- Healthcare organisations should actively engage young people through alliances with youth services, outreach, and continuity of care

---

BOX 2 EVIDENCE FOR A NEUROLOGICAL EXPLANATION OF DEPENDENCE

- A series of imaging studies of adults dependent on cocaine have shown abnormal responses in the prefrontal cortex and basal ganglia, including the nucleus accumbens and related structures. The studies showed that the "high" experienced by the participants coincided with rapid saturation of dopamine transporters in the basal ganglia.[3] [w5-w7]

- Increased extracellular dopamine in the basal ganglia also motivates (or in animal studies prompts) the "emission of behaviours" in the pursuit of anticipated rewards such as food.[w8] Commonly misused substances seem to trigger this mechanism, which leads to the person seeking reward.

- As use progresses to dependence there is pressure to avoid uncomfortable withdrawals.[w7] This system seems to be the physiological basis for dependence or addiction, a condition in which the person's life becomes organised not by what we regard as rational considerations but by the largely subcortical drive to obtain the substance.

What constitutes substance misuse?

Substance misuse and dependence are a subset of "substance use," which includes phenomena such as experimentation and intermittent recreational use. "Substances" include alcohol as well as illicit or (if deliberately misused) prescribed drugs. See box 1 and 2 for definitions. (Substance misuse is also referred to as substance abuse—for example, by the *Diagnostic and Statistical Manual of Mental Disorders*.)

Is substance use increasing?

Drugs

Serial data from the European school survey project on alcohol and other drugs (n=103 000 in 2003) showed a broadly stable rate of 40% lifetime use of cannabis in 15 year olds in the United Kingdom up to 2003.[4] A more recent English school survey of 8200 schoolchildren aged 11-15 years showed an overall decline in drug use from 11% in 2005 to 9% in 2007[5] but also showed that 4% of 11 year olds had used illicit drugs in the past month, compared with 0% in 1998, when comparable data were first obtained.

Some southern (Cyprus, Malta, Greece) and northern (Norway, Sweden) European countries report rates for adolescents of ‹10% lifetime use of any illicit drug.[4] However, other regions with previously low rates such as eastern Europe have shown considerable catch-up in lifetime use. In the United States, daily use of cannabis by 15 year olds has dropped from 6% to 5% but remains well above the 2% of the early 1990s.[w9]

Alcohol

According to survey data,[4] regular drinking is common among UK and Irish adolescents and has increased among 15 and 16 year olds from 22% in 1995 to 27% in 2003. This rise results partly from an increase from 20% to 29% in

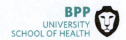

binge drinking among young females and an increase in self reported consumption of "alcopops" (fizzy, flavoured alcoholic drinks) among 15-16 year old girls. Reported rates of drinking among 11-13 year old boys and 14 year old girls have trebled since 1990.[5]

What do we know about rates of misuse and dependence?

Few large scale studies directly examine this question. However, survey data suggest that 10% of UK 15-16 year olds reported "problems" linked with substance use.[4] A diagnostic study of a representative sample of 3021 Munich adolescents and young adults found that 18% exhibited substance misuse or dependence.[6][w10] At age 18 years, 20% of a New Zealand birth cohort of 1265 children were misusing alcohol and 6% were dependent. The corresponding figures for cannabis were 12% and 5%.[7]

Two large US cross sectional population studies of young adults showed that rates of cannabis dependence increased between 1991 and 2001.[w11] The authors attributed this rise to more potent varieties of cannabis; the rise also paralleled the increase in cannabis use during that decade.

Does substance misuse impair the developing brain?

Recent research supports the view that early adolescence is a potential "critical period" during which the long term direction of biopsychosocial development can be altered.[8] Substance use in the early teenage years may prove to have serious long term consequences.

Two studies of representative samples of over 43 000 US adults found that those who reported their first alcoholic drink before age 14 or their first drug use before age 15 were three times more likely to develop alcohol or drug dependence than those whose first use of alcohol or drugs was at age 15 or older.[9][w12] Regular use of cannabis before age 15 seems to be linked with increased risk of subsequent psychosis.[w13]

Two small neuroimaging studies found that young adults who had misused or been dependent on alcohol in adolescence had smaller prefrontal cortices and hippocampi than healthy controls.[w14][10] However, it is unclear whether these findings reflect alcohol neurotoxicity or pre-existing developmental vulnerabilities, or both, but animal studies support alcohol neurotoxicity.

BOX 3 CONFIDENTIALITY

"Adolescents are more likely to provide truthful information if they believe that their information, at least detailed information, will not be shared. Before the adolescent interview, the clinician should review exactly what information the clinician is obliged to share and with whom. . . Typically, a clinician should inform the adolescent that a threat of danger to self or others will force the clinician to inform a responsible adult, usually the parents. The clinician should . . . encourage and support the adolescent's revealing the extent of substance use and other problems to parents. In other cases, the clinician should discuss what information that the adolescent will allow the clinician to reveal such as a general recommendation for treatment or impressions rather than a detailed report of specific deviant and substance use behaviors."
Taken from Bukstein et al[13]

BOX 4 CRAFFT QUESTIONNAIRE—BRIEF SCREENING TEST FOR SUBSTANCE MISUSE IN ADOLESCENTS*[14]

C—Have you ever ridden in a Car driven by someone (including yourself) who was "high" or who had been using alcohol or drugs?
R—Do you ever use alcohol or drugs to Relax, feel better about yourself, or fit in?
A—Do you ever use alcohol or drugs while you are Alone?
F—Do you ever Forget things you did while using alcohol or drugs?
F—Do your family or Friends ever tell you that you should cut down on your drinking or drug use?
T—Have you been in Trouble while using drugs or alcohol?
Answering "yes" to two or more questions suggests an important problem

---

BOX 5 TOXICOLOGY TESTING

"Toxicological tests of bodily fluids, usually urine but also blood, and hair samples to detect the presence of specific substances should be part of the formal evaluation and the ongoing assessment of substance use. The optimal use of urine screening requires proper collection techniques including [where possible] visualization of obtaining the sample [to ensure it is genuine], evaluation of positive results, and a specific plan of action should the specimen be positive for the presence of substance(s) . . . Because of the limited time that a drug will remain in the urine and possible adulteration, a negative result of urine testing does not [rule out drug use]."
Taken from Bukstein et al[13]

A small longitudinal study of 113 subjects tracked from infancy showed that frequent users of cannabis in late adolescence had a lower IQ than expected and poorer performance on memory tests than non-users or former users.[11] This effect on memory may be one factor in the poor educational outcomes linked with cannabis use.

How dangerous is substance misuse?

According to UK National Statistics data for 2005,[w3] 8.5% of male and 8.2% of female deaths in the 15-19 year age group were due to misuse of substances; in the male group this is similar to the proportion of deaths due to cancer (8.5%) and far ahead of deaths due to infection, for example. If deaths from self harm (often associated with substance misuse) are added, the proportions rise to 21% and 16.8% of all deaths among this age group. Deaths from accidental overdose tend to occur most often among young adults, leading to substantial "years of potential life lost."[w15] A longitudinal study of 9491 notified teenage opiate addicts indicated that their death rate was 12 times greater than the death rate in the general population of teenagers; the addicts' deaths were mainly due to accidental poisoning.[12]

Management

The capacity for healthcare workers to intervene requires first a preparedness to accept substance misuse as "their business."

Assessing the problem

Assessment searches not only for the time line, dose, type, frequency, and context of substance use, but also for predisposing, maintaining, and protective influences. In straightforward cases, this may be achievable in one interview. Ideally, the history should also enable identification of problems such as school failure, neglect, or physical or sexual abuse. Taking a careful history and explaining confidentiality (box 3) may help to establish good rapport. Consider supplementing a history with screening questionnaires (box 4) and a physical examination looking for signs of physical or sexual abuse, neglect, poor growth, pregnancy, self harm, injury, injection, and infection; also consider toxicology tests (box 5).[13]

Does watchful waiting have a role?

A large prospective study found that rates of substance dependence levelled off at age 18 years, with about 10% of illicit drug users being dependent.[7] Similar trends have been shown in relation to alcohol.[w16] Decreasing 12 month prevalence rates for misuse and dependence in one follow-up study suggested a significant rate of spontaneous recovery.[w10] After assessment, a clinician might conclude that risk is not high and that a role for watchful waiting exists.

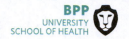

BOX 6 MOTIVATIONAL INTERVIEWING (FRAMES)
Feedback—Give structured and personalised feedback on risk and harm
Responsibility—Emphasise the patient's personal responsibility for change
Advice—Give clear advice to the patient to change his or her drinking habits
Menu—Offer a menu of strategies for making a change in behaviour
Empathic—Deliver these strategies in an empathic and non-judgmental way
Self efficacy—Aim to increase the patients' confidence to change behaviour (self efficacy)[15]

What active interventions can healthcare staff use?

Brief intervention

In a recent randomised controlled trial a brief motivational intervention (box 6) almost halved the frequency of alcohol bingeing at 12 months' follow-up among 13-17 year olds who reported excessive drinking on presentation to an emergency department compared with those who were assessed and given literature.[16] There is recent evidence from an observational trial and a randomised controlled trial that a brief motivational interview versus information alone can substantially reduce the levels of both binge drinking and use of cocaine and ecstasy (3,4 methylenedioxymethamphetamine) among regular teenage users at one year follow-up.[w17 w18] However, reductions of substance use observed in control groups suggest that assessment and information alone may have prompted change.[w17] The following strategies may exert useful effects: a sympathetically conducted history of substance use; thoughtful, knowledgeable interpretation of the findings; and avoidance of lecturing or arguing.

What to advise parents?

A large European survey of 15 year olds found that a confiding parent-child relationship is linked with markedly lower rates of substance use.[17] International survey findings from a range of countries[4] found that parental knowledge of their child's whereabouts was a protective influence against substance use, although greater parental monitoring is likely to be a proxy for a confiding relationship in which the young person informs the parent of their whereabouts. A recent Finnish twin study found that the quality of the parent-adolescent relationship seems to moderate the effects of genetics on smoking tendency.[w19] Whatever other predisposing factors may exist, a strong parent-child relationship could be a powerful barrier to substance misuse.

A nested observation of the intervention limb of a randomised controlled trial examining the effects of multidimensional family therapy for cannabis dependence showed that a good "therapeutic alliance" with the parents as well as with the young person was the best predictor of a good outcome.[w20]

Often troublesome young people do not receive a generous response from education services or the police. Health professionals can support parents to be tenacious in obtaining a more supportive deal from education and other services.

More sustained intervention by healthcare practitioners

Research is limited on the role of healthcare providers in managing adolescent substance misuse. However, it is possible to extrapolate a general approach from relevant if tangential research. For example, a US randomised controlled trial of several interventions for young cannabis misusers reported significant reductions in use after each of these interventions. The authors concluded that the effect was the result of components that were shared between interventions.[18] Interventional studies of adolescent depression and adult alcohol dependence evaluated the effects of seeing a healthcare practitioner as part of a placebo limb compared with specialist psychotherapy for a limited number of meetings over some months. Sympathetic, informed, supportive counselling from a health practitioner approached or equalled the effectiveness of cognitive behavioural therapy for adolescent depression[19] and for adult alcoholism.[w21]

A randomised controlled trial of 90 women with personality disorder (many of the young people receiving help from substance misuse services may be developing serious personality dysfunction) showed that receiving weekly supervised support over a year led to improvement across a range of measures including self harm, depression, anxiety, and anger.[w22] The authors commented that the continuity of care or "relationship focus" buffered the extremes of instability.

Without always consciously doing so, healthcare staff can exert substantial psychological "healing" and stabilisation, which are potentially valuable to troubled young people. The communication skills components of training could potentiate this capacity, particularly with regard to young people. Also, services working with young people need to offer continuity of care as a core feature.

An adolescent oriented service

A randomised controlled trial of 183 substance dependent adolescents showed that compared with clinic based appointments, a form of sustained flexible community outreach was linked with reduced substance use.[20] Services for adolescents could include flexible arrangements to meet, home visits, meetings in cafes, text messages, telephone calls to remind young people of appointments, and help with transport (which is crucial if some adolescents are to be engaged). This effort is required because, among those most vulnerable, lack of external routine and structure (no school, work, family, organised interests), the effects of substances, mental disorder, and perhaps learning disability may be associated with markedly poor self motivation and organisation.[21 22 w23]

Using a range of community systems

Successful intervention often requires channelling a young person away from drug using peers and lifestyle. To achieve this goal, it is often necessary to tackle obstacles such as homelessness, educational exclusion, absence of a carer, continuing mistreatment, or risk of incarceration, all of which require solutions brokered with local services.

A further key strategy is to use other networks that are designed to take the longer term strain. The components of these networks differ across jurisdictions and with age but are likely to include elements from education, social work, criminal justice, non-governmental agencies, health, and mental health. Such a multifaceted system is difficult to test in a conventional trial, but packaged multidimensional or multisystem interventions have shown sustained positive effects.[23 24]

Adjunctive interventions

Contingency management, pharmacotherapy, and motivational enhancement have been studied in healthcare settings. Voucher rewards for "clean" urine specimens and clinical attendance have been shown to be of benefit in managing addicted adults.[15] However, contingency management is

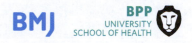

7   Fergusson D, Horwood L, Ridder E. Conduct and attentional problems in childhood and adolescence and later substance use, abuse and dependence: results of a 25 year longitudinal study. *Drug Alcohol Depend*2007;88:S14-26.
8   Crews F, He J, Hodge C. Adolescent cortical development; a critical period of vulnerability for addiction. *Pharmacol Biochem Behav*2007;86:189-9.
9   Hingson R, Heeren T, Winter M. Age at drinking onset and alcohol dependence. *Arch Pediatr Adolesc Med*2006;160:739-46.
10 De Bellis M, Narasimhan A, Thatcher D, Keshavan M, Soloff P, Clark D. Prefrontal cortex, thalamus and cerebellar volumes in adolescents and young adults with adolescent-onset alcohol use disorders and comorbid mental disorders. *Alcoholism: Clinical and Experimental Research*2005;29:1590-600.
11 Fried P, Watkinson B, Gray R. Current and former marijuana use preliminary findings of a longitudinal study of effects on IQ in young adults. *CMAJ*2002;166:887-91.
12 Oyefeso A, Ghodse H, Clancy C, Corkery J, Goldfinch R. Drug-abuse related mortality: a study of teenage addicts over a 20 year period. *Soc Psychiatry Psych Epidemiol*1999;34:437-41.
13 Bukstein OG, Bernet W, Arnold V, Beitchman J, Shaw J, Benson RS, et al. Practice parameter for the assessment and treatment of children and adolescents with substance use disorders. *J Am Acad Child Adolesc Psychiatry*2005;44:609-21.
14 Knight J, Sherritt L, Schrier L, Harris S, Grace C. Validity of the CRAFFT substance abuse screening test among adolescent clinic patients. *Arch Ped Adolesc Med*2002;156:607-14.
15 National Treatment Agency. *Drug misuse and dependence—UK guidelines on clinical management*. 2007. www.nta.nhs.uk/publications/documents/clinical_guidelines_2007.pdf
16 Spirito A, Monti P, Barnett N, Colby S, Sindelar H, Rohsenow D, et al. A randomized clinical trial of a brief motivational intervention for alcohol-positive adolescents treated in an emergency department. *J Pediatr*2004;145:396-402.
17 McArdle P, Wiegersma A, Gilvarry E, Kolte B, McCarthy S, Fitzgerald M, et al. European adolescent substance use: the roles of family structure, function and gender. *Addiction*2002;97:329-36.
18 Dennis M, Godley S, Diamond G, Tims F, Babor T, Donaldson J, et al. The cannabis youth treatment study: main findings from two randomised trials. *J Substance Abuse Treatment*2004;27:197-213.
19 March J, Silva S, Petrycki S, Curry J, Wells K, Fairbank J, et al. Treatment for adolescents with depression study (TADS) randomized controlled trial. *JAMA*2004;292:807-20.
20 Godley M, Godley S, Dennis M, Funk R, Passetti L. The effect of assertive continuing care on continuing care linkage, adherence and abstinence following residential treatment for adolescents with substance use disorders. *Addiction*2007;102:81-3.
21 Craig TK, Hodson S. Homeless youth in London: I. Childhood antecedents and psychiatric disorder. *Psychol Med*1998;28:1379-88.
22 Unger J, Kipke M, Simon T, Montgomery S, Johnson C. Homeless youths and young adults in Los Angeles: prevalence of mental health problems and the relationship between mental health and substance abuse disorders. *Am J Community Psychol*1997;25:371-94.
23 Henggeler S, Halliday-Boykins C, Cunningham P, Randall J, Shapiro S, Chapman J. Juvenile drug court: enhancing outcomes by integrating evidence based treatments. *J Consult Clin Psychol*2006;74:42-54.
24 Liddle HA, Dakof G, Parker K, Diamond G, Barrett K, Tejeda M. Multidimensional family therapy for adolescent drug abuse: results of a randomized clinical trial. *Am J Drug Alcohol Abuse*2001;27:651-88.

expensive, and its effectiveness with younger users has not yet been adequately studied. Combining broader psychosocial and pharmacological interventions to treat adolescent addicts, as has been shown to be effective among adult alcoholics,[w21] has not yet been studied, but this might change with more medical interest in the field.

I thank the *BMJ*'s editors for their help with this article.

Contributors: PMcA is the sole contributor.

Competing interests: The author has received fees for speaking at events sponsored by the pharmaceutical industry and financial support to attend international meetings.

Provenance and peer review: Commissioned; externally peer reviewed.

1   West P, Sweeting H. Fifteen, female and stressed: changing patterns of psychological distress over time. *J Child Psychol Psychiatry Allied Disciplines*2003;44:399-411.
2   National Insitute on Drug Abuse, National Institutes of Health, US Department of Health and Human Services. *Understanding drug abuse and addiction*. 2007. www.nida.nih.gov/Infofacts/understand.html
3   Volkow N, Wang G, Fischman M, Foltin R, Fowler J, Abumrad M, et al. Relationship between subjective effects of cocaine and dopamine transporter occupancy. *Nature*1997;386:827-30.
4   Hibell B, Andersson B, Bjarnasson T, Ahlstrom S, Balakireva O, Kokkevi A, et al. The ESPAD Report 2003. www.sedqa.gov.mt/pdf/information/reports_intl_espad2003.pdf
5   Home Office. *Smoking, drinking and drug use among young people in England 2006: headline figures*. 2007. www.ic.nhs.uk/webfiles/publications/smokedrinkdrug06/file.pdf
6   Wittchen HU, Frohlich C, Behrendt S, Gunther A, Rehm J, Zimmermann P, et al. Cannabis use and cannabis use disorders and their relationship to mental disorders: a 10-year prospective-longitudinal community study in adolescents. *Drug Alcohol Depend*2007;88:S60-70.

More titles in
The BMJ Clinical
Review Series

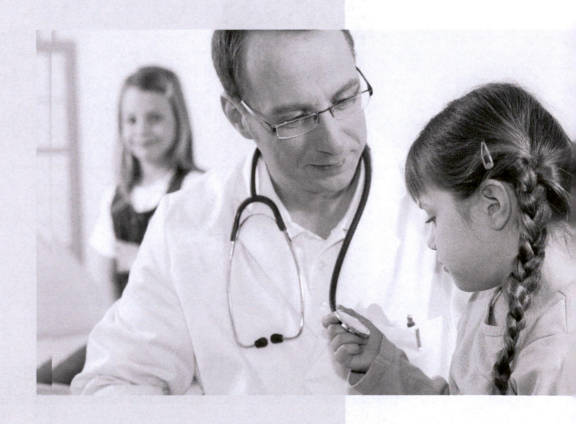

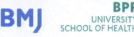
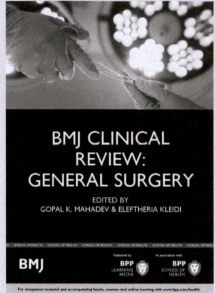
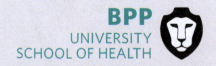

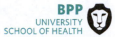

More titles in
The BMJ Clinical Review Career Series

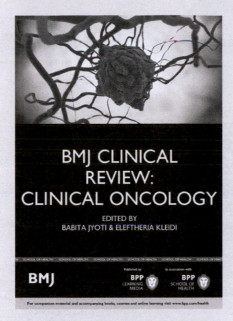

BMJ CLINICAL REVIEW: CLINICAL ONCOLOGY

EDITED BY
BABITA JYOTI & ELEFTHERIA KLEIDI

This volume covers a range topics in the management and treatment of cancer.

Subjects dealt with include:
- The changing epidemiology of lung cancer with a focus on screening using low dose computed tomography
- Identifying brain tumours in children and young adults
- Prostate cancer
- Screening and the management of clinically localized disease
- The management of women at high risk of breast cancer
- Head and neck cancer with reference to epidemiology, presentation, prevention, treatment and prognostic factors
- Malignant and premalignant lesions of the penis
- Melanoma and advances in radiotherapy.
- Melanoma and advances in radiotherapy.

£29.99

August 2015

Paperback

978-1-472739-32-2

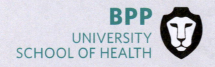

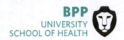

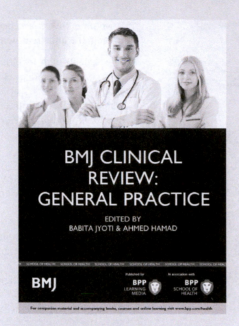
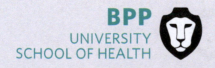

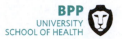

More titles in
The BMJ Clinical Review Series

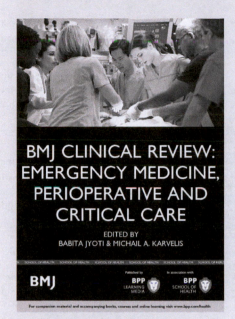

BMJ CLINICAL REVIEW: EMERGENCY MEDICINE, PERIOPERATIVE AND CRITICAL CARE

EDITED BY
BABITA JYOTI & MICHAIL A. KARVELIS

This book discusses a diverse range of traumas which can be presented in emergency medicine and the appropriate treatments to manage them.

Subjects discussed include:
- Emergency and early management of burns and scalds
- Management of the effects of exposure to tear gas
- Pain management
- Sedation for children in the emergency department
- The role of interventional radiology in trauma
- Pre-hospital management of severe traumatic brain injury
- Cardiopulmonary resuscitation
- Managing anaemia in critically ill adults.

£29.99
August 2015
Paperback
978-1-472739-29-2

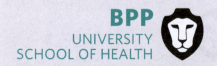

BPP
UNIVERSITY
SCHOOL OF HEALTH

www.bpp.com/medical-series

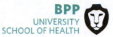
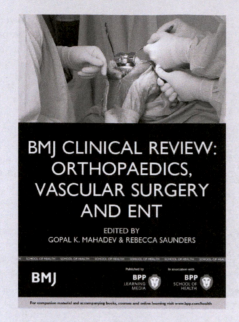
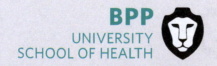

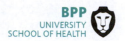
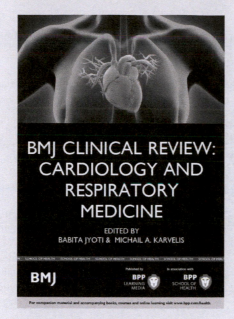
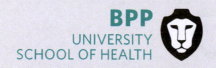

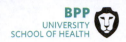
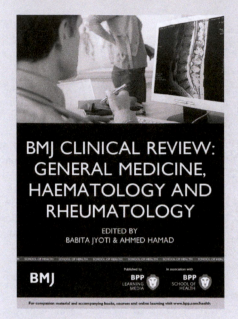
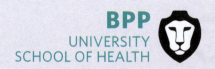

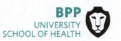

More titles in The Progressing your Medical Career Series

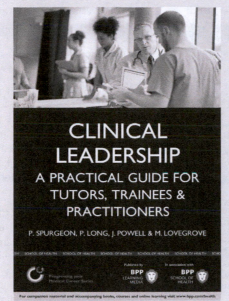

CLINICAL LEADERSHIP

A PRACTICAL GUIDE FOR TUTORS, TRAINEES & PRACTITIONERS

P. SPURGEON, P. LONG, J. POWELL & M. LOVEGROVE

£24.99

June 2015

Paperback

978-1-472727-83-1

Are you a healthcare professional or student who wishes to acquire and develop your leadership and management skills? Do you recognise the role and influence of strong leadership and management in modern healthcare?

Clinical leadership is something in which all healthcare professionals can participate in, in terms of driving forward high quality care for their patients. In this up-to-date guide, the authors take you through the latest leadership and management thinking, and how this links in with the Clinical Leadership Competency Framework. As well as influencing undergraduate curricula this framework forms the basis of the leadership component of the curricula for all healthcare specialties, so a practical knowledge of it is essential for all healthcare professionals in training.

Using case studies and practical exercises to provide a strong work-based emphasis, this practical guide will enable you to build on your existing experiences to develop your leadership and management skills, and to develop strategies and approaches to improving care for your patients.

This book addresses:

- Why strong leadership and management are crucial to delivering high quality care;
- The theory and evidence behind the Clinical Leadership Competency Framework;
- The practical aspects of leadership learning in a wide range of clinical environments
- How clinical professionals and trainers can best facilitate leadership learning for their trainees and students within the clinical work-place.

Whether you are a student just starting out on your career, or an established healthcare professional wishing to develop yourself as a clinical leader, this practical, easy-to-use guide will give you the techniques and knowledge you require to excel.

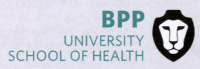

BPP
UNIVERSITY
SCHOOL OF HEALTH

www.bpp.com/medical-series

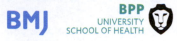

More titles in The Progressing your Medical Career Series

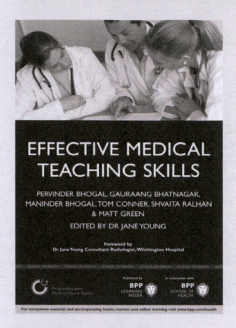

£19.99

September 2011

Paperback

978-1-445379-56-2

We can all remember a teacher that inspired us, encouraged us and helped us to excel. But what is it that makes a good teacher and are these skills that can be learned and improved?

As doctors and healthcare professionals we are all expected to teach, to a greater or lesser degree, and this carries a great deal of responsibility. We are helping to develop the next generation and it is essential to pass on the knowledge that we have gained during our experience to date.

This book aims to cover the fundamentals of medical education. It has been designed to be a guide for the budding teacher with practical advice, hints, tips and essential points of reflection designed to encourage the reader to think about what they are doing at each step.

By taking the time to read through this book and completing the exercises contained within it you should:

- Understand the needs of the learner

- Understand the skills required to be an effective teacher

- Understanding the various different teaching scenarios, from lectures to problem based teaching, and how to use them effectively

- Understand the importance and sources of feedback

- Be aware of assessment techniques, appraisal and revalidation

This book aims to provide you with a foundation in medical education upon which you can build the skills and attributes to become a competent and skilled teacher.

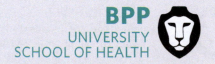

BPP
UNIVERSITY
SCHOOL OF HEALTH

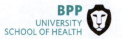

More titles in The Progressing your Medical Career Series

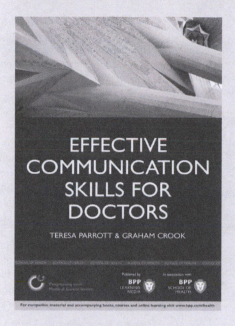

£19.99

September 2011

Paperback

978-1-445379-56-2

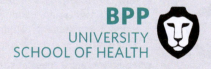

Would you like to know how to improve your communication skills? Are you looking for a clearly written book which explores all aspects of effective medical communication?

There is an urgent need to improve doctors' communication skills. Research has shown that poor communication can contribute to patient dissatisfaction, lack of compliance and increased medico-legal problems. Improved communication skills will impact positively on all of these areas.

The last fifteen years have seen unprecedented changes in medicine and the role of doctors. Effective communication skills are vital to these new roles. But communication is not just related to personality. Skills can be learned which can make your communication more effective, and help you to improve your relationships with patients, their families and fellow doctors.

This book shows how to learn those skills and outlines why we all need to communicate more effectively. Healthcare is increasingly a partnership. Change is happening at all levels, from government directives to patient expectations. Communication is a bridge between the wisdom of the past and the vision of the future.

Readers of this book can also gain free access to an online module which upon successful completion can download a certificate for their portfolio of learning/Revalidation/CPD records.

This easy-to-read guide will help medical students and doctors at all stages of their careers improve their communication within a hospital environment.

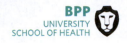

More titles in The Progressing your Medical Career Series

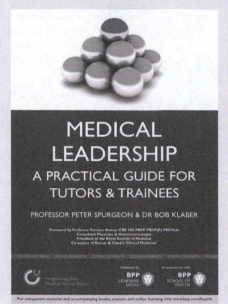

MEDICAL LEADERSHIP

A PRACTICAL GUIDE FOR TUTORS & TRAINEES

PROFESSOR PETER SPURGEON & DR BOB KLABER

£19.99

November 2011

Paperback

978-1-445379-57-9

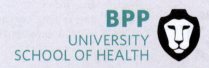

BPP
UNIVERSITY
SCHOOL OF HEALTH

Are you a doctor or medical student who wishes to acquire and develop your leadership and management skills? Do you recognise the role and influence of strong leadership and management in modern medicine?

Clinical leadership is something in which all doctors should have an important role in terms of driving forward high quality care for their patients. In this up-to-date guide Peter Spurgeon and Robert Klaber take you through the latest leadership and management thinking, and how this links in with the Medical Leadership Competency Framework. As well as influencing undergraduate curricula and some of the concepts underpinning revalidation, this framework forms the basis of the leadership component of the curricula for all medical specialties, so a practical knowledge of it is essential for all doctors in training.

Using case studies and practical exercises to provide a strong work-based emphasis, this practical guide will enable you to build on your existing experiences to develop your leadership and management skills, and to develop strategies and approaches to improving care for your patients.

This book addresses:

- Why strong leadership and management are crucial to delivering high quality care

- The theory and evidence behind the Medical Leadership Competency Framework

- The practical aspects of leadership learning in a wide range of clinical environments (eg handover, EM, ward etc)

- How Consultants and trainers can best facilitate leadership learning for their trainees and students within the clinical work-place

Whether you are a medical student just starting out on your career, or an established doctor wishing to develop yourself as a clinical leader, this practical, easy-to-use guide will give you the techniques and knowledge you require to excel.

www.bpp.com/medical-series

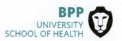

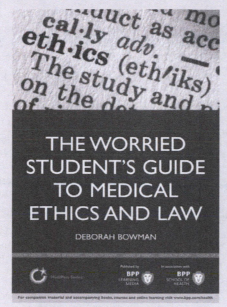
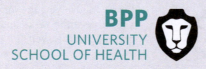

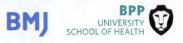

More Titles in The Progressing Your Medical Career Series

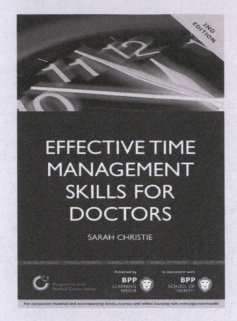

2ND EDITION

EFFECTIVE TIME
MANAGEMENT
SKILLS FOR
DOCTORS

SARAH CHRISTIE

£19.99

October 2011

Paperback

978-1-906839-08-6

Do you find it difficult to achieve a work-life balance? Would you like to know how you can become more effective with the time you have?

With the introduction of the European Working Time Directive, which will severely limit the hours in the working week, it is more important than ever that doctors improve their personal effectiveness and time management skills. This interactive book will enable you to focus on what activities are needlessly taking up your time and what steps you can take to manage your time better.

By taking the time to read through, complete the exercises and follow the advice contained within this book you will begin to:

- Understand where your time is being needlessly wasted

- Discover how to be more assertive and learn how to say 'No'

- Set yourself priorities and stick to them

- Learn how to complete tasks more efficiently

- Plan better so you can spend more time doing the things you enjoy

In recent years, with the introduction of the NHS Plan and Lord Darzi's commitment to improve the quality of healthcare provision, there is a need for doctors to become more effective within their working environment. This book will offer you the chance to regain some clarity on how you actually spend your time and give you the impetus to ensure you achieve the tasks and goals which are important to you.

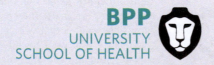

BPP
UNIVERSITY
SCHOOL OF HEALTH

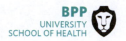
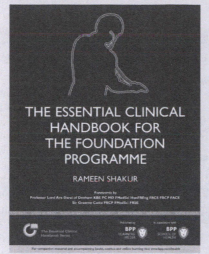
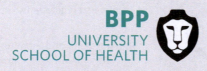

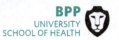

More titles in The Essential Clinical Handbook Series

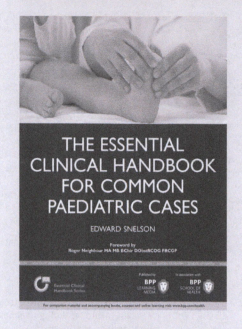

THE ESSENTIAL CLINICAL HANDBOOK FOR COMMON PAEDIATRIC CASES

EDWARD SNELSON

Foreword by
Roger Neighbour MA MB BChir DObstRCOG FRCGP

September 2011

Paperback

978-1-445379-60-9

Not sure what to do when faced with a crying baby and demanding parent on the ward? Would you like a definitive guide on how to manage commonly encountered paediatric cases?

This clear and concise clinical handbook has been written to help healthcare professionals approach the initial assessment and management of paediatric cases commonly encountered by Junior Doctors, GPs, GP Specialty Trainee's and allied healthcare professionals. The children who make paediatrics so fun, can also make it more than a little daunting for even the most confident person. This insightful guide has been written based on the author's extensive experience within both a General Practice and hospital setting.

Intended as a practical guide to common paediatric problems it will increase confidence and satisfaction in managing these conditions. Each chapter provides a clear structure for investigating potential paediatric illnesses including clinical and non-clinical advice covering: background, how to assess, pitfalls to avoid, FAQs and what to tell parents. This helpful guide provides :

- A problem/symptom based approach to common paediatric conditions

- As essential guide for any doctor assessing children on the front line

- Provides easy-to-follow and step-by-step guidance on how to approach different paediatric conditions

- Useful both as a textbook and a quick reference guide when needed on the ward

This engaging and easy to use guide will provide you with the knowledge, skills and confidence required to effectively diagnose and manage commonly encountered paediatric cases both within a primary and secondary care setting.

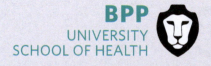

BPP
UNIVERSITY
SCHOOL OF HEALTH

www.bpp.com/medical-series